Our Bodies Belong to God

The publisher gratefully acknowledges the generous support of the General Endowment Fund of the University of California Press Foundation.

Our Bodies Belong to God

Organ Transplants, Islam, and the Struggle for Human Dignity in Egypt

SHERINE HAMDY

University of California Press

BERKELEY   LOS ANGELES   LONDON

University of California Press, one of the most distinguished university presses in the United States, enriches lives around the world by advancing scholarship in the humanities, social sciences, and natural sciences. Its activities are supported by the UC Press Foundation and by philanthropic contributions from individuals and institutions. For more information, visit www.ucpress.edu.

University of California Press
Berkeley and Los Angeles, California

University of California Press, Ltd.
London, England

Library of Congress Cataloging-in-Publication Data

Hamdy, Sherine, 1975–
    Our bodies belong to God : organ transplants, Islam, and the struggle for human dignity in Egypt / Sherine Hamdy.
        p.   cm.
    Includes bibliographical references.
    ISBN 978–0–520–27175–3 (cloth : alk. paper)
    ISBN 978–0–520–27176–0 (pbk. : alk. paper)
    1. Transplantation of organs, tissues, etc.—Egypt.   2. Transplantation of organs, tissues, etc.—Religious aspects—Islam.   I. Title.
    RD120.7.H355   2012
    617.954'—dc23

                                                    2011033137

21   20   19   18   17   16   15   14   13   12
10   9   8   7   6   5   4   3   2   1

This book is dedicated to my parents, Farouk and Mona Hamdy, who had the courage to leave Egypt with dreams of a better life.

And it is dedicated to the courageous revolutionaries of January 25, 2011, who dreamed that Egypt could become a better place.

Contents

List of Illustrations   ix

Note on Confidentiality and Photography   xi

Note on Transliteration   xiii

Acknowledgments   xv

Preface   xxi

INTRODUCTION: BIOETHICS REBOUND   1

1. EGYPT'S CRISES OF AUTHORITY   21

2. DEFINING DEATH: WHEN THE EXPERTS DISAGREE   47

3. FROM SECRET TO SCANDAL: CORNEAS, DEAD DONORS,
   AND EGYPT'S BLIND   83

4. SHAYKH OF THE PEOPLE: GENEALOGY OF
   AN UTTERANCE   115

5. TRANSPLANTING GOD'S PROPERTY: THE ETHICS
   OF SCALE   141

6. ONLY ONE KIDNEY TO GIVE: ETHICS AND RISK   173

7. PRINCIPLES WE CAN'T AFFORD? ETHICS AND
   PRAGMATISM IN KIDNEY SALES   209

CONCLUSIONS: WHERE CYBORGS MEET GOD   239

EPILOGUE: THE ONGOING STRUGGLE FOR
HUMAN DIGNITY   253

viii / Contents

Notes   257

Glossary of Frequently Used Arabic Terms   297

References   301

Index   319

Illustrations

1. Author (left) interviewing cornea opacity patient,
   May 2004   xx

2. Medical outreach program sponsored by Al Noor Society,
   May 2004   xxvi

3. Ragia and her husband   20

4. Elderly woman has her blood pressure checked during
   a public outreach campaign for eye health, May 2004   31

5. An early morning class on Islamic jurisprudence
   at al-Azhar Mosque   41

6. Agricultural highway between Cairo and Tanta   46

7. The grand mufti of Egypt, Shaykh ʿAli Gumaʿa, May 2004   74

8. Patient and family member in a Tanta eye hospital   82

9. Popular 1996 book of Shaykh Shaʿrawi's fatwas   114

10. Nephrologist assesses X-ray of dialysis patient in acute
    renal failure   140

11. Patients in a Tanta dialysis ward   172

12. Cement factory on agricultural land, in violation of the law,
    June 2004   183

13. Nurse bonds with her young patient who is on dialysis 190

14. Khalid, kidney recipient and later father of a twin boy and girl 193

15. Movie poster of popular film *Ilhaquna!* (Save Us!) 208

16. Ola and her husband, Mahmud, who refuses to accept her kidney 238

17. Interior of the Mansoura Kidney Center 240

18. Exterior of the Mansoura Kidney Center 242

19. Interior of the mosque at the Mansoura Kidney Center 248

Note on Confidentiality and Photography

The many people who informed this work were patients, their family members, surgeons, physicians, nurses, hospital workers, religious scholars, medical students, journalists, and lawyers, as well as other Egyptians who do not readily fall into any of these categories. To the extent possible, I have attempted to fulfill their wishes in regard to whether they want their stories to remain anonymous (in which case I have used pseudonyms and unidentifiable markers) or whether they want their stories to be present in a historical record. The public figures involved (e.g., religious scholars, transplant surgeons, journalists) are identified with their real names.

As for the photography, many patients expressly told me that they did not want to be photographed while they were ill and in treatment centers, that they did not like to be reminded of what they looked like when so vulnerable. Others readily asked that I take their photographs and include their names in my research. All the included photographs of patients are of those who expressly asked to be photographed and to be documented in my work.

Often those being photographed shaped their images as much as I did. After several months of knowing me, ʿAbdallah, the man whose image is on the cover of this book, asked me if I would photograph him. Just as I lifted my camera, he gingerly lifted his arms upward in prayer.

Note on Transliteration

In the main text, I follow a simplified version of the standard system for transliteration of Arabic followed by the *International Journal of Middle East Studies*. However, for the purpose of readability, I have omitted diacritics, except in the case of ' for the hamza (a glottal stop) and ' for the 'ayn sound. I also use anglicized plurals (e.g., fatwas, not fatawa), except for when both the singular and plural forms of a word have become anglicized, such as *fellah* and its plural, *fellahin*.

In the Egyptian dialect, particularly in Cairo and other Nile Delta cities, the "j" sound is pronounced as a hard "g." When I quote a person speaking, I use the "g" in the transcription to reflect this (as in *sadaqa gariyya*), but when I translate from an official fatwa, I use the "j" to reflect the standard Arabic *(sadaqa jariyya)*. I also use the hard "g" for personal names as the people themselves pronounce it, such as the muftis Guma'a and Gad al-Haqq.

For the names of Egyptian places, I use the common spelling: for example, Cairo (for al-Qahira), Zamalek (for al-Zamalek) and Mansoura (for al-Mansura). However, for less common names of cities, I use the standard transliteration system (such as Daqahliyya, rather than Dakahliya or El Dakahliya), because in references to them I am generally translating from Arabic texts.

We live in a world in which people who principally speak some language other than English increasingly represent themselves with anglicized spelling, in their e-mail addresses, in instant messaging, or on social network sites. In Egypt, the medical realm in particular relies heavily on English and on non-standardized transliteration of Arabic names. Thus, I use the common Anglicized spelling of Cairo's famous hospitals and medical centers, such as Ain Shaims and Kasr el Aini, rather than 'Ayn Shams or Qasr 'al-'Ayni. In instances in which my informants have published in English,

I use their own spelling (e.g., Safwat Lotfy, not Safwat Lutfi, Dr. Kotb, not Dr. Qutb, and Mohamed Ghoneim, not Muhammad Ghunaym). But for those who have not published in English, I use the standard transliteration as for Mufti ʿAli Gumaʿa, whose name in English also appears as Ali Gomaa. In places where I translate from the Arabic spelling (such as the television reporter ʿAmr al-Laythi and his show *Wahid min al-nas*), I also include in parentheses the name as I have found it spelled on English-language Web sites (Amr el-Lithy, *Wahed Men El-Nas*).

When discussing dialysis, I use the term *ghasil kalawy* or *ghasil al-dam* to mark its entry into Egyptian written Arabic (in newspapers), although a closer transliteration of its colloquial pronunciation would be *ghasil id-dam*. If I use *il* as the article rather than *al* (such as in *il-ghalaba*), it is to mark the term as having strict colloquial usage.

Finally, in my reliance on Egyptian newspapers, I used the standard transliteration system for *Al-Misri al-Yawm* when I am drawing from the Arabic texts, even though their Web site and English editions spell the paper as *Al-Masry al-Youm*. All translations from Arabic into English are my own unless otherwise noted.

Acknowledgments

This project has been long in the making and I have acquired many debts, far too many to mention. I would like to first thank my wonderful dissertation committee: Lila Abu-Lughod, Faye Ginsburg, Rayna Rapp, Talal Asad, and Angela Zito, and also Fred Myers for their intellectual engagement with my work and for their unwavering support throughout my graduate studies. From Lila Abu-Lughod, I learned to think of ethnographic writing as an art and to appreciate the aesthetic and affective dimensions of this endeavor. Faye Ginsburg and Rayna Rapp, my "twin mothers" at New York University, taught me that compassionate listening is the key to ethnographic insight. From Talal Asad and Angela Zito, I learned that one can engage with religious traditions intelligently and interrogate secularist assumptions alongside this pursuit. And from Fred Myers I learned that I really could become an anthropologist.

Several institutions have supported my efforts, from graduate training to field research to the writing of my dissertation, on which this book is based. They include the Foreign Language and Area Studies Scholarship (FLAS) from NYU's Hagop Kevorkian Center, the Center for Arabic Studies Abroad (CASA), the National Research Service Award at the National Institutes of Health (NIH), the International Dissertation Research Fellowship of the Social Science Research Council (SSRC), the program in Societal Dimensions of Ethics, Science, and Technology from the National Science Foundation (NSF), the Charlotte Newcombe Dissertation Fellowship from the Woodrow Wilson Foundation, the Cogut Humanities Center at Brown University where I was a Mellon postdoctoral fellow, the Pembroke Seminar at Brown on "Markets and Bodies in Transnational Perspective" where I was a Faculty Fellow, and the SSRC Book Fellowship Program through which I was fortunate to receive feedback from Mary Murrell.

In Egypt, my work has been enriched by an outpouring of support and help: first and foremost from my aunt Hana Hussein, who provided numerous contacts and research citations for me as well as invaluable emotional support that sustained me throughout my research. I would also like to thank ʿAli Ahmad Hamdi, Shaykh ʿAmr al-Wardani, and Shaykh ʿAli Gumaʿa. I am enormously indebted to the services, wisdom, and generosity of Shaykh Ashraf ʿAbdal-Muʿti. For their unwavering help in Tanta, I would like to thank: Dr. Mohamed Atef Salah, Ms. Fatima Hamdi, Dr. Mamdouh Saweris, Dr. Aziz Kafafy, and Dr. Faten El Shafei. In Mansoura, I would especially like to thank Dr. Mohamed Sobh, Dr. Amr el-Husseini, and Dr. Ahmed Bayoumi. At Al Noor Society in Cairo, I am thankful for the gracious assistance of Dr. Gamal Ezz el Arab and Dr. Ahmed Moussa. I am also immensely grateful to the many unnamed physicians, nurses, hospital staff, patients, scholars, and students who opened their hearts to me and shared their experiences and perspectives that deepened my understandings of medicine and ethics in Egypt that drive the core of this book.

None of my work would have been possible without the love and support of my extended family members in Egypt, and I thank all of them, particularly my aunt Hana Hussein, my cousins Amira and Habiba ElGogary, my grandmother Effat ElBindary, who cared for me and worked to make sure that I was always well-fed and had clean clothes, and my nurturing and loving aunt Fatima Hamdi. In Cairo I was grateful for a full twelve months of fellowship (in both senses of the term) at the Center for Arab Studies Abroad, for the wonderful language instruction teachers I had, and for the lifelong friends I made. During my fieldwork, I felt blessed with the friendship of Amira Mittermaier, Amina ElBendary, Kawthar Jaber, Zareena Grewal, Hamada Hamid, Kirk Johnson, and above all, Ian Straughn. Thanks to the Department of Anthropology at the University of Chicago for providing me with an intellectually stimulating home while I wrote the dissertation on which this book is based. While writing and revising early drafts, I have relied on the support and extremely helpful feedback of many cherished friends and interlocutors, especially: Hussein Agrama, Nidal Al-Azraq, Lori Allen, Sareeta Amrute, Amahl Bishara, Vicki Brennan, Debra Budiani, Jessica Cattelino, Julie Chu, Margaret Cruz, Mona El-Ghobashy, Zareena Grewal, Zeynep Gürsel, Hamada Hamid, Toby Jones, Eleana Kim, Amira Mittermaier, Shira Robinson, Justin Stearns, and Jessica Winegar. I was lucky to have Zareena Grewal, Laura Helper-Ferris, Eleana Kim, and Ian Straughn read and comment on various drafts of huge swaths of material. Zareena Grewal and Ian Straughn in particular have been, from the beginning to end of this project, patient and generative sounding boards for my ideas.

I am grateful for wonderful mentors, colleagues, and interlocutors who paved the way for scholarship on bioethics in global perspective. Thanks to Margaret Lock for providing valuable feedback on chapter 2 and, more important, for being an inspiring role model. Ebrahim Moosa enthusiastically asked interesting and probing questions. The Islam and Bioethics group of the Aga Khan University, including Farhat Moazam and Thomas Eich, helped me think through ideas, as did Jonathan Brockopp. Thanks to the New York University Hagop Kevorkian Middle East Research Workshop, in which I presented a draft of chapter 4 and received wonderful feedback, particularly from Nadia Guessous and Chris Dole. I also benefited from participants in Rutgers University's Bodies and Souls workshop, particularly from Indrani Chatterjee and Julie Livingston. At Brown University, I have found a wonderful community of colleagues who have been generous in their support and feedback. I cannot imagine a more welcoming place to have begun my career. I want to thank especially David Kertzer, Anne Fausto-Sterling, Daniel Jordan Smith, Catherine Lutz, Matthew Gutmann, Lina Fruzzetti, Kay Warren, William Simmons, Deborah Cohen, Michael Steinberg, Paja Faudree, Jessaca Leinaweaver, Yukiko Koga, Elliott Colla, Nancy Khalek, R. David Coolidge, Mark Cladis, Katherine Grimaldi, Jennifer Ashley, and Harris Solomon. Catherine Lutz and Dan Smith commented generously on a complete draft of the manuscript. I also benefited from colleagues' responses as I presented work at the Cogut Center for the Humanities and the Pembroke Seminar at Brown, especially Kay Warren, Catherine Bliss, and Bianca Dahl. I also want to thank the students in my courses for stimulating discussions and for their contagious excitement about learning new ways to interpret our world. Thanks especially to Coleman Nye, Mark Caine, Alexander Wamboldt, and Jennifer Ashley for their wonderful company, good humor, and numerous contributions to the organization and completion of the manuscript. Thanks to Naomi Schneider at the University of California Press for her enthusiasm for this book and for finding me three brilliant, generous, and meticulous reviewers to help me with my revisions, whom I would like to thank by name: Lesley Sharp, John Bowen, and Saba Mahmood. I don't know how I got so lucky. Thanks also to Catherine Bliss, again, for helping me endure the final round of revisions.

I am immensely fortunate to have had consistent support from a loving family who stood by me at every step. My late father, Dr. Farouk Hamdy, spent his first months of retirement accompanying me to the field, arguing amicably with the shaykhs whom I interviewed and helping with archival research. My devoted mother, Mona, faithfully forwarded to me clippings from Egyptian newspapers on organ thefts, on renal toxicity, on polluted water, on hepatitis C, and on all of what she proudly and grandiosely considered "problems Sherine is working on." My mother taught me to be strong in the face of adversity and to believe that I could accomplish my goals. My brilliant sisters, Rana and Dina Hamdy, sustained me with their love and their faith in my abilities. Many thanks to my big-hearted brother-in-law Vinay Parekh and to my generous in-laws Gloria, Bill, and Celka Straughn for their interest in and support of my work. Thanks to all of them, as well as to Afaf Hamdi, who selflessly took time off from her own busy life in the spring of 2004 and enabled me to return to Egypt for the final crucial months of fieldwork.

And thanks, finally and above all, to my husband, Ian Straughn, for listening and believing in what I could do, for seeing me through the ups and downs, and for sharing our treasures, Layali and Amina, for whom I am eternally grateful.

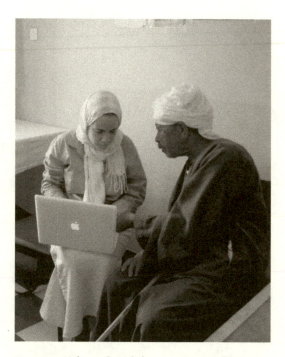

Figure 1. The author (left) interviewing a cornea
opacity patient in the rural outskirts of Fayoum,
May 2004. Courtesy of Al Noor Society.

Preface

I remember clearly the events of one hot day in the spring of 2003, when I was researching life stories of poor rural dialysis patients in a hospital ward in Tanta, a city in the northern Nile Delta. All of the patients there were diagnosed as having end-stage kidney failure and were in critical need of new kidneys. But hardly any of them considered the acquisition of a new kidney to be a viable solution. I was talking to the physician in charge of the ward about this conundrum when I suddenly felt uneasy. I lost my ground and blacked out. The nurses immediately put me on one of the hospital dialysis beds, took my blood pressure, and, when I regained awareness, ordered me to continue lying there. I was soon wheeled to the end of the room and wedged between two of the patients whose life stories I had been recording. I lay on a hospital bed in a cold sweat, intermittently panicking about the fact that many patients had described their first symptoms of renal failure as dizziness. I thought to myself in sad amusement that I had unintentionally slipped into a frightening "native's point of view."[1] Watching the patients' blood move up in their tubes under the flickering fluorescent light, I tried to fight off a feeling of impending doom, the fear that I would be stuck there in that bed, with them, forever. Madame Sabah, a motherly patient in her fifties, insisted that I drink her mango juice to raise my blood sugar. 'Ali, another dialysis patient, pointed at the small fuzzy television screen in the room, showing American troops in Iraq, and prayed aloud for my dizziness to leave me and to fall upon the invaders instead.

There were moments such as these when my fate seemed completely intertwined with the fates of poor patients whose lives were in reality radically different from mine. But while patients were often receptive and grateful for the company and conversation, I grew accustomed to hostility from bureaucrats, officials, and physicians, who would balk at my affiliation with New York University, my "American-style" research project, and would suspiciously ask what I was *really* up to, what I could possibly *really* want from hanging around impoverished medical facilities. Egyptian officials often barred my access to major hospitals in Egypt, suspecting that I had no other purpose than to tarnish the image of Egypt abroad. I grew weary when officials, so accustomed to assuming a defensive posture to cover up the problems of their society, pointed fingers at me accusatorily for wanting to probe into "sensitive" topics like the poor standards of public health facilities and the irresponsible dumping of toxins by local and multinational corporations on agricultural land. The social sciences, more generally, are suspect as a form of inquiry in Egypt, as state bureaucrats, including educators, solely value quantitative indicators as informative. They seemed to regard more "qualitative" questions as both irreverent and irrelevant.[2]

Still, I was taken aback in 2003 when a patient blinded by cornea opacity in a public hospital rebuffed my questions, telling me that he did not want to talk to anyone "from America." He noted sharply, "You are from over there. Why should I help you? Look at how Americans are killing our brothers and sisters in Afghanistan. They blamed us for September 11 and now they say we are all terrorists, and they discriminate against Arabs." Even the patients with whom I had identified so closely at times reminded me of all that stood between us. Facing this patient in a hospital waiting room in Tanta, Egypt, I was surprised at how upset I felt. I threw back, "Yes, and I'm one of those Arabs who gets discriminated against over there! So do you want me to be discriminated against in both places? Is it fair that people should be suspicious of me wherever I go?!"

At one point in the field, my research permissions from the Egyptian Ministry of Higher Education were inexplicably suspended, and I was barred from conducting interviews until further bureaucratic procedures were followed. In frustration, in the spring of 2003, I called my father in the United States to get some advice and counsel from him. Weeks had gone by since I had last spoken with him at length. It was unlike him not to have called regularly, but he had been traveling for a work assignment, and I had been running around Cairo trying to resolve the issue of research permission. When I made the call, his voice sounded strange to me, and whatever he was trying to tell me could not make its way into words. I was suddenly overcome, again, by a feeling of doom. Without thinking it through, I quickly made arrangements to fly home.

Back in the United States, after a series of medical tests, my family received the devastating news that my father was suffering from the most malignant type of brain tumor, for which there was no cure. Questions that had formed the bulk of my research about how people come to difficult bioethical decisions when faced with tremendous pain and the imminence of death were now questions that I was living with. My research on hold, I tended to my father, making sporadic trips back to Egypt after my research permissions were reissued.

Upon my return to the field, the patients for whom I had felt so much sympathy months before now looked at me with sorrowful, concerned eyes. They told me that I had lost too much weight, that I could not let myself be consumed by grief and worry, that I could not torment myself, and that I had to be strong for my family. Their methods of cultivating steadfastness and fortitude in the face of suffering were no longer merely topics I was writing about, but a resource for my own endurance. Together, we meditated on the most difficult of life processes: illness and death.

Months of early fieldwork had turned me off to various practices of organ transplantation. But during the time of my father's illness I would have jumped at the chance to donate a body part, had that been a way to restore him to his healthy self. Now, years after his death, I am sobered by the inevitability of mortality. I wonder about our obsessive quest for the technological triumph over human demise, and how it has left us uninterested in the wisdom that various traditions have elaborated in the preparation for death. I am convinced that decisions about what to do with our failing bodies and those of our loved ones in the face of suffering are deeply contextual.

Organ transplantation is unsettling, in that it disrupts the boundaries between self and other. (Will I be the same "me" with someone else's heart?) Anthropology does this too. As many anthropologists have noted, longstanding fieldwork in a new social-cultural environment renders the familiar strange and the strange familiar. I had set out to study an exceedingly strange practice in a not-so-strange place. The strangeness of illness and death became thoroughly familiar, and the familiarity of my culture, one dominated by illusions of immortality, became strange. I learned about how different people live with their pain as I listened to their stories and tried my best to relate them. I learned more about religious devotion, illness, and ethics as I cared for my father and later helped to bury him.

As this book relates, ethical positions are never static: they both guide our experiences and adapt to them as we inevitably become embroiled in life's messy and complicated social relations. I came to understand this more fully as my ideas continually changed—ideas about the body, death, suffering, and medicine. I knew, analytically, as I set out on this project that understandings of faith, ethics, illness, mortality, and kinship are all subject to social and historical transformation. But in the course of thinking about and writing this book, I was unprepared for how significantly these would all transform for me. As I write and revise these pages, I remain inspired by those who make up its stories.

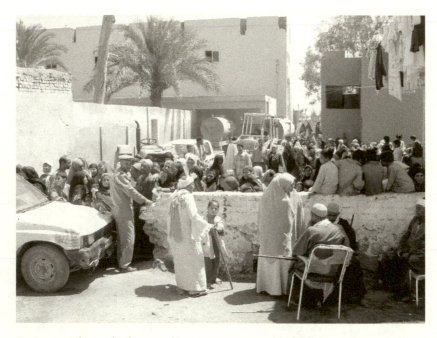

Figure 2.   The medical outreach program sponsored by Al Noor Society, on the outskirts of Fayoum, May 2004. Photograph by the author.

Introduction

Bioethics Rebound

Is it permissible [in Islam] to transfer an organ from one body to another?

The scholars of Islam say: "Human beings do not own their bodies. Buying and selling organs is forbidden, sinful."

Why did the grand mufti declare organ transplantation permissible? Why did Shaykh Sha'rawi object?

We demand a law to permit kidney transplants amid the widespread increase in kidney failure.

This book centers on why transplant medicine surfaced as a topic of much social and ethical debate in Egypt from the 1980s to the early 2010s, amidst dramatic political and economic change. The debate both reflected and shaped the sense of impending crises in medical and religious authority, in the context of mounting dissent toward an unjust and brutal regime, the privatization of health care, advances in science, the growing gap between rich and poor, and the Islamic revival. In the print news, on state television, and in religious sermons, opinions clashed over this life-saving but death-ridden medical practice.[1] As the above headlines indicate, the press often phrases ethical questions in terms of religious authority, and has presented this authority as unclear on the ethics of organ transplants. The media have called for urgent action to be taken, given the desperate fate of patients in organ failure and alarming reports of increases in kidney and liver disease throughout Egypt. Yet there has been no clear consensus on what this action should be.

The debate about transplanting body parts in Egypt presents a number of puzzles:

- All of the official religious scholars in Egypt declared that organ donation is permissible in Islam, yet patients and family members continued to object out of "religious" sentiment, many of them insisting that we cannot donate that which "belongs to God."

1

- Egypt was the "pioneering" Arab Muslim country in the field of transplant medicine and yet has been the most resistant to establishing a national transplant program.

- Egyptian doctors prided themselves on having worked with cornea grafts as early as the 1960s, yet public eye banks were barely operational by the late 1990s.

- Doctors talked about the body belonging to God as a commonsensical basis from which to question the prudence of kidney transplants. Yet they regarded this argument to be a "superstitious" and "backward" impediment to the transplantation of corneas.

- Even more puzzling, people in Egypt have agreed that buying and selling organs is in principle wrong, and yet the majority of transplants have occurred in just this way. The media, medical professionals, and ordinary Egyptians perceive the commodification of organs as a national outrage and at the same time as inevitable and banal.

Making sense of these puzzles requires understanding the social transformations that Egypt has undergone in the past half century and particularly understanding debates surrounding the unfolding of medical authority, political dissent, and the Islamization of public discourse. In the context of political repression and economic instability, the question about how to treat human bodies with dignity in life and in death was bound to be an explosive one. Egyptians face indignities every day, coping with severe overcrowding, housing shortages, unemployment, pollution, police abuse, mass arrests, and rampant corruption. Any sensitive observer would marvel at the strategies that people in Egypt have honed in order to protect their sense of humanity under tremendous political and economic pressures.

But as much as we need to know Egypt to understand its transplant debate, focusing on the transplant debate also reveals new ways to think about and understand Egypt. Anthropologists have shown that studying a contested debate in a given social setting can illuminate deeply held beliefs that are sharply articulated during times of crisis (Turner 1974; Ginsburg 1989; Gusterson 1996; Fassin 2007). In Egypt, debates about organ transplantation have intensified longstanding disputes over social inequalities in basic health care, state welfare, and the place of religious discourse in politics and medicine. Studying extraordinary bodily interventions like organ transplantation helps elucidate the ordinary, everyday ways in which people formulate ethics about caring for their bodies and the bodies of others. A critical analysis of the controversy over organ transplantation thus gives us a privileged perspective onto major axes of social division in one of the fastest growing and changing countries in the Middle East.

WHO OWNS THE BODY?

In the mid-1970s, at a time when organ transplantation was still in experimental phases worldwide, a bold Egyptian surgeon carried out the first kidney transplant, a feat lauded as a national success in the state-run media. After this initial triumph, efforts to initiate a national organ transplant program failed for the next three decades. Legislators continued to disagree about how best to oversee this new medical treatment. The debate among legislators and physicians spilled over into the public domain in the late 1980s, when the mass media began to expose disturbing stories surrounding the exploitation of poor organ sellers and the uncertain outcomes for transplant recipients. Around this same time, all the official religious scholars in Egypt declared organ donation to be permissible in Islam, some even condoning it as worthy of great spiritual rewards. But Shaykh Sha'rawi, a popular television figure, created a stir in 1988 when he stated that you cannot donate a kidney, since it is not yours to give. Sha'rawi was a widely admired figure who was known for his charismatic appearances on his weekly Qur'anic television programs from the 1970s until his death in 1998. Sha'rawi's absolutism heightened the controversy and deepened divisions between opponents and proponents of a national organ donation program.

After a lull, the debate about donating, receiving, and transplanting body parts was waged again following increasing international attention on Cairo's thriving black market in human organs. A report from the World Health Organization placed Cairo among the world's top six "organ trafficking hotspots" (McGrath 2009a). President Mubarak reopened the topic in his November 2008 address to the Parliament, urging legislators to pass a national transplant law so that Egypt could join the ranks of other Arab and Muslim nations that have long-established national transplant programs.[2] In March 2010 a law was finally passed. Yet the new legislation has not resolved the deep-rooted problems in which organ transplantation has become entangled in Egypt.

Until recently, a major sticking point in the debates was the recognition of brain death as legal death. With brain-dead patients hooked to life-support machines, the question about what defines the exact moment of death becomes less clear: Is it the cessation of a beating heart and respiration or the cessation of brain function? Who gets to decide and on what basis?

Given the lack of resolution of these questions in Egypt, organs have not been procured from brain-dead patients on respirators, which has become standard practice elsewhere. The earliest organ transplants in Egypt, beginning in the 1970s, required the extraction of one kidney from a living donor. Two decades later, liver transplantation, a procedure that depends on living donors parting with a lobe of their liver, was introduced. Questions persisted about the ethics of cutting into and extracting vital organs from healthy living donors. What does "informed consent" mean when familial and economic pressures are tremendous, when the risks and benefits of these invasive procedures are so wide-ranging, and when the etiologies of the diseases themselves are unclear? Aside from kidneys and liver lobes, cornea transplants have also occurred in Egypt, beginning as early as the 1960s. These transplants have involved taking corneas from the eyes of corpses in public morgues to transplant into patients blinded by cornea opacity. For over three decades, all these transplants occurred in Egypt's major cities without national or legal oversight.[3]

During the 1980s, private medical clinics began to proliferate well beyond the surveillance capabilities of the Ministry of Health, and it was in these unregulated clinics that the black market in body parts thrived. Rumors spread about children who "disappeared" from an orphanage in Minufiyya, allegedly for the stealing of their body parts (al-Bishri 2001). Kidney theft, the subject of popular films and television serials, became a stand-in for allegations of exploitation and vulnerability. Patients, family members, and physicians in Egypt disagreed about whether it is ethical to take a body part from the dead, whether it is safe or beneficial practice to cut into a healthy living donor, whether organ transplantation actually "saves lives," and about the vulnerability of poor Egyptians to organ theft. With the gap between rich and poor escalating in the context of the demise of the welfare state, the wealthy everywhere seemed to benefit from exploiting the poor, with organ transplantation making this banality ever more visceral.

During the emergence of organ transplantation, Egypt's political regime also generated debate over the relationship between Islam, democracy, and healthcare. Nasser's authoritarian rule (1954–1970) operated under a single-party system, effectively repressing the mobilization of Islam-oriented political groups like the Muslim Brotherhood. In the mid-1970s, however, Sadat began to allow constrained participation by other platforms while still restricting most forms of political expression.[4] While Nasser, like other leaders in the third world in the 1960s, spoke in secular, nationalist, revolutionary language against imperialism and capitalist exploitation, Sadat in the 1970s aligned himself with the capitalist, democratic West and simultaneously attempted to bolster his legitimacy through religious language, encouraging the trend toward religious observance, making a show of his own piety, and rehabilitating the Muslim Brotherhood (R. Mitchell 1993; Wickham 2002). This policy continued under the regime of President Husni Mubarak (1981–2011), and by the mid-1990s, members of the Muslim Brotherhood would wield considerable influence in the Egyptian Medical Syndicate, marking a noticeable change in the orientations of doctors and in their relationship to the state (Wickham 2002).

Nasser tightly controlled and micromanaged the national press, while Sadat's regime-change and opening *(infitah)* to the West included a (still restricted) liberalization of media outlets in which dissenters could voice their criticism of state policies (Hafiz and Rogan 1995; Amin 2002). The economic realignment of the 1970s and 1980s, the increasing privatization of clinics and services and the lack of livable wages for physicians in the public health sector have all contributed to the continued erosion of public health facilities and to the seeming abandonment of socialist ideals (Shukrallah 2012). Since the infitah, biomedical services have proliferated well beyond the surveillance capacities of the Ministry of Health. Stories of physicians' corruption and malpractice persist throughout Egypt. Newspaper columnists and other social critics often focus on untrustworthy physicians in their laments about the current loss of values in Egyptian society. Many see the resurgence of Islam as the solution; others see it as a threat and return to "backwardness." Nasserists wax nostalgic for the days of socialism, during which, it seemed, Egyptian physicians worked out of "love of their country" rather than material greed.[5] With much to differ on, both Nasserists and Islamists nevertheless agree that in an Egypt increasingly directed by corporate capitalism, doctors behave like "butchers and tradesmen" *(gazzarin wa tuggar)*, not caring about integrity or moral conscience, with the suffering bodies of poor patients as the tragic result.

With Islamic revivalism on the rise since the 1970s, educated people in the middle classes and an emergent generation of professionals now teach themselves about Islamic history and scripture, claiming for themselves religious authority that was once dominated by scholars with traditional training (Eickelman 1992; Eickelman and Anderson 2003). Many Egyptians engaging in Islamic reform cast doubt on the authority of religious scholars, or at least on those who hold official positions in the state bureaucracy. At the same time, state-oriented newspapers and television have long portrayed religious figures who operate outside state institutions as dangerous, dubbing them "hard-headed extremists" who grasp at any issue to promote their own agenda. Just as it has been common knowledge that doctors as a whole cannot be trusted, neither, now, can religious figures. They can tout religion for political and social gain or dangerously "play" with religious knowledge without sufficient training. This twin crisis in authority—in the medical and religious realms—has been widely perceived as a serious problem, all the more perilous among a population that official state discourse has long defined as "ignorant masses," unaware of the scientific "truth" of their own bodies and health, and uneducated in their own religion.[6] Many Egyptians express trepidation about untrustworthy physicians who might dangerously manipulate their vulnerable bodies and also about untrustworthy religious figures who might dangerously play with their sacred traditions.

From the 1980s onward, as they have debated the ethics of organ transplantation, neither medical experts nor religious scholars have sought the experiential knowledge of those in need of (new) organs. The experts appear to be uninterested in seeking the perspectives of those who stand most to gain or lose from transplantation. Scientific experts are supposed to know the "truth" of human bodies; medical providers are supposed to restore patients' health; politicians claim to support citizens' rights and bodily integrity; and religious scholars venture to counsel people on choosing right from wrong. Contemporary Egyptian discourse both reflects and solidifies the perception that each of these realms is plagued by a crisis of authority.

Bioethics in Egypt

Amid this predicament, one might think that Egypt would be a fertile ground for the field of bioethics to respond to, or at least explain, the problems surrounding organ transplantation. Within the United States, bioethics emerged during the 1960s and into the mid-1970s as a discrete professional field in tandem with the development of transplant medicine. Bioethicists sought a critical external power check on medical institutions, to advocate for the vulnerable position of patients and subjects of medical experimentation, and to introduce ethical dimensions into what had increasingly become technical clinical practice (Jonsen 1998; Stevens 2000; Martensen 2001). In the early years of transplantation in the United States, ethicists and physicians grappled with the problems of meting out scarce, potentially life-saving treatments, such as long-term kidney dialysis and transplantation for patients in organ failure, and choosing who could serve as suitable organ donors (Fox and Swazey 1974). They also studied the ethical consequences of the redefinition of death that came with organ procurement and the advancement of cardiopulmonary life-support systems (Youngner 1996; Jonsen 1998; Fox and Swazey 2008).[7] Major founding figures in American bioethics insisted on a "common morality" and on universal ethical principles as they worked through the many troubling situations that new medical practices such as organ transplantation instigated (Beauchamp and Childress 2001).

Yet bioethics as a professional field barely exists in contemporary Egypt. Courses on "medical ethics" are taught in Egypt's major medical schools by specialists in forensics. Physicians in public teaching and private hospitals have no external boards of ethicists who oversee difficult patient cases. Where are Egypt's bioethicists? Might a cadre of bioethicists be the perfect prescription to resolve Egypt's organ transplant debate?

Critics of the many Anglo-American manifestations of bioethics have voiced reservations that might signal us to proceed with caution. For many of these critics, bioethical discourse has been overly dominated by neo-Kantian philosophy, without grounding its principles in the realities of political economy, history, anthropology, sociology, or public health (Martensen 2001, Fox and Swazey 2008, Kleinman 1995). The expert voices of the bioethicists—whether as philosophers or as practicing clinicians—have ended up marginalizing those of patients and family members, who have more at stake in their direct experiences of the medical intervention. And as the field of bioethics has become an exportable international commodity, it has remained dominated by the medical concerns of industrialized nations, focusing on individual cases involving high-tech, cutting-edge, and expensive treatments and devoting less time to the ethical problems of routine, everyday care (Kleinman 1995; Fox and Swazey 2008).

By looking at the most extreme and urgent cases, Anglo-American bioethicists have in some senses replicated the *crisis* culture of fast-paced medical dramas and media entertainment in which emotions are tugged about biotechnological capacities to "play God" and choose one life over another (Kleinman 1995). This obscures how we are all already implicated in valuing certain lives over others in our patterns of consuming and distributing resources (Evans, Barer, et al. 1994; Farmer 1999, 2003; Wilkinson and Pickett 2010). In fact, Anglo-American bioethicists and their counterparts in Egypt have had little to say about the great disparities in access and treatment outcome across the world (Daniels, Kennedy, et al. 1999; Martensen 2001; Farmer 2003). Bioethics as a field became institutionalized within biomedicine, serving more to justify than to question biomedical norms and to manage inequalities rather than to address them (Daniels, Kennedy, et al. 1999; Farmer 2003). Medical anthropologists and other scholars have thus repeatedly documented the utter failure of bioethics to address problems that have emerged more globally as biotechnologies are taken up in our increasingly stratified world (Scheper-Hughes 1992, 2000; Kleinman 1995, 1999;

Das 1999; Rapp 1999; Sharp 2000; Inhorn 2003; Moazam 2006; Biehl 2007; Fassin 2007; Fox and Swazey 2008; Petryna 2009; Lock and Nguyen 2010).

Given these limitations, we might question why biomedical practitioners have turned to "ethics," as opposed to analyses of political-economic or social inequalities, to anticipate and resolve the potential social consequences of medical intervention. But rather than move away from the study of ethics, I am committed to expanding it to include questions about broader social and political processes. In the coming chapters, I elaborate on how a widespread agreement on common moral principles such as "do no harm" does not lead to straightforward ethical guidelines, because people with different interests and experiences will necessarily have different ideas about what constitutes harm and how best to avoid it. These ethical arguments are animated not only by the biotechnologies but also by pressing concerns about religious belief and the everyday struggles of life in poverty. Ethics thus remains a crucial site from which to expand the dialogue about social inequalities in health and to seek solutions. Recasting ethics as a necessarily political project is a key aim of this book.

By building on anthropologists' scholarship and critiques of bioethics, this study makes the case for a *bioethics rebound*. I want to argue for bioethics to "bounce back" from its failed relationship with the social sciences in order to engage more productively in these disciplines' intersections with social justice advocacy. Playing on the double meaning of *rebound*, I also suggest that we unbind and "rebind" bioethics, not as a discipline unto its own, but as one fully integrated in social analyses of the political, economic, and cultural terrains that are necessary for bioethicists to effectively promote social justice. From the perspective of many social scientists, bioethics as a field has failed to make important interventions because of its insistence on myopic universalisms (Sharp 2000, Inhorn 2003, Moazam 2006, Hoffmaster 2001, Rapp 1999, Kleinman 1995, Fox and Swazey 2008). And while I agree with this particular limitation, I am less concerned about bioethics being too "culturally specific"; I am more concerned that it is incomplete.[8] In Egypt, one might be tempted to argue that a robust field of bioethics simply does not exist. At least in its imported U.S.-dominated form, the field sees little activity. But given the well-founded criticisms of the narrow limits of the discipline, what counts as a "bioethical" debate when defined more broadly? If we think that only bioethicists or clinicians can adequately address the ethical dilemmas raised by organ transplantation, we will miss the rich discussions and debates that occur among patients and their family members, in the dialysis wards and in outpatient waiting rooms. We might be surprised to find out that much national media attention in Egypt is directed not at clinicians or bioethicists but at the views of Islamic legal scholars, whose answers to ethical questions are circulated and interpreted toward different ends.[9] Theological discussions about God's ownership of bodies, political debates about Egypt's dependence on foreign aid, a toxicology report of a village near a pesticide company, or a family drama about who is most valued—all of these may well be the stuff of bioethics. And conversely, debates that are labeled as "bioethics" in Anglo-American textbooks may bear little resemblance to concerns wrought by biotechnologies elsewhere.

This book thus makes the case for rebinding bioethics' disciplinary boundaries, in order to expand upon and reorient the field to find a better way to meet its original goals of improving health, justice, and medical benefit to the most people. Egypt, which has long conceived of itself as the Muslim Middle East's leader in both medicine and Islamic scholarship, is an ideal site to tap into how people in this region might struggle toward these goals (see Inhorn 1994, 2003). Further, Egypt is undergoing dramatic social, political and economic transformations in which medical and Islamic authority are increasingly challenged. The contestations of authority lay bare the ways in which ethical arguments are always voiced within relations of power. And these power relations are multiple and overlapping, indexing religious authority and medical efficacy as well as kinship and political-economic inequalities. The challenge for rebinding bioethics is to make sense of positions that might appear contradictory, to understand how wider forces are shaping them, and to appreciate how ethical arguments are contingent even when appealing to fixed truths.

WHAT COUNTS AS A BIOETHICAL PROBLEM?

How to recognize a bioethical issue is both a practical and a conceptual question. There is always political and ideological work at play in defining the scope of a problem and making that scale appear commonsensical (Smith 2001; Tsing 2005; Machledt 2007). The standard scale of bioethical analysis—the individual case—can be gripping and morally compelling, because it enables identification with the patient's immediate suffering and ethical dilemma. But focus on the individual pays little attention to how patients are embedded within intricate sets of social relations and within larger political and economic systems of constraints and possibilities (Hoffmaster 2001; Moazam 2006; Fox and Swazey 2008). In Egypt, where kidney-failure patients are completely dependent on living donors, social relations and resources are especially important, as is the degree of pollutants in the physical environment that can predispose the person to organ failure to begin with. In this case, where do bioethical concerns begin and end? Patients might be in need of a kidney from a family member, yet the whole family may live in an area exposed to the mismanagement of toxic waste. Susceptibility to kidney disease can be shaped by particular sociopolitical arrangements and a lack of legal enforcement, which conspire to allow for the dangerous contamination of public water supplies and agricultural land (Sowers 2007, Sowers et al. 2010). The individual scale and the insistence on abstract principles, such as beneficence, justice, and autonomy, often miss what should be the targets of analysis by failing to capture the messiness of bioethical problems.[10]

By contrast, this study examines the layers of social networks that have shaped and been shaped by Egypt's organ transplant debate, interrogating the relationships between social assemblages and ethical formulations, as people's roles shift from being anxiety-ridden medical students to pioneering surgeons, from ordinary people to afflicted patients, from distraught family members to desperate organ buyers, from self-possessed religious scholars to frustrated public figures. Based on twenty-one months of fieldwork between 2001 and 2004 in the three Egyptian cities of Cairo, Mansoura, and Tanta (and brief follow-up visits from 2007 to 2011), I conducted in-depth open-ended interviews with physicians, patients, hospital workers, practicing Islamic scholars, and journalists. This work was complemented by participant observation at medical and religious conferences, hospitals, and dialysis units. I conducted formal interviews with fifty-five patients in renal failure and with twenty physicians involved in kidney transplantations (nephrologists, urologists, vascular surgeons, internists)[11]. I quickly discovered that studying the people who did not pursue transplantation was just as important as studying those who did.[12]

Over the course of my fieldwork, I commuted to Tanta, a city that is an hour's train ride north of Cairo, where I frequented five dialysis clinics. During that time, Tanta's medical landscape was somewhat removed from the scandals of Cairo's black marketing in kidneys and the stark contrasts between sellers in Cairo's slums and treatment for the wealthy at its private five-star hospitals. While the extreme situations in Cairo were spotlighted by the media, the dialysis patients in Tanta were more representative of the overwhelming and growing number of Egyptians in need of a kidney.[13] Patients with kidney failure throughout Egypt who want to pursue transplantation generally seek treatment in private or teaching facilities in Cairo or Alexandria or in the public teaching facility in Mansoura. Because there was no functioning transplant program in Tanta, doctors there did not have a live-organ trade problem to contend with; physicians and patients there were able to reflect on the organ transplant debate and on the high emotional impact that it had in Cairo with some critical distance from these issues. It was in Tanta that I chose one dialysis center as a longitudinal ethnographic setting, and I came to know the kidney-failure patients (twenty-six in total) and the medical staff who cared for them over the period of one year.[14]

In my study of cornea transplantation, I formally interviewed twenty ophthalmologists and twenty patients blinded by corneal opacity, in both Tanta and Cairo, and supplemented these interviews with participant observation in eye hospitals, ophthalmology clinics, and public outreach programs for eye health. I also interviewed many of the most prominent Islamic legal scholars in Egypt (sixteen in total), including muftis, who are entrusted with the task of responding to questions about religion from lay Muslims in the form of fatwas, or nonbinding responses to legal-ethical questions. I also incorporated Islamic legal research studies on organ transplantation into my analysis in order to understand the wider discursive field from which the muftis formulated their positions. Throughout Islamic history, political rulers have attempted to gain religious authority by influencing muftis, yet muftis' authority has often rested on their distance from politics. In Egypt, the modern state most directly sought control over muftis' authority by establishing a state bureaucratic office for fatwa giving, known as Dar al-Ifta' in 1895, at which time the "grand mufti" or the "mufti of the republic" became a government employee appointed by the president of the republic.[15] I analyzed the fatwas of the Dar al-Ifta' archives, as well as those delivered orally in the more informal space of the fatwa committee at al-Azhar University.[16] I also attended classes at al-Azhar University in Islamic jurisprudence *(usul al-fiqh)* in order to understand the formulation of Islamic legal-ethical knowledge. During the time that I spent in Egypt, I did not meet a single Islamic scholar who was not well acquainted with the issue of organ transplantation.

I engaged transplant surgeons and physicians in discussions as they worked in clinical and academic settings, often flanked by residents and medical students. All the high-ranking Islamic scholars and all the transplant surgeons whom I interviewed were men, although I also sought out the opinions of women scholars of Islamic jurisprudence, and many female physicians, medical students, and hospital staff were included in my study. In the overlapping worlds of medical and religious authority, the "expert" voices on ethics are often male, thus contributing to a gender gap in addition to the deep class disparities between experts and patients. The expert-patient interactions that I witnessed were often heavily structured by class difference, and I do not delve into the ways in which gender difference also informed expert opinions. I do, however, analyze the gendered discrepancies in how transplantation from living donors has been experienced by patients and family members.

Given the prominent role that the media play in producing, staging, convening, and at times escalating bioethical debates, I also needed to ask why different media venues have taken up particular bioethical questions and toward what ends. I have incorporated into my analysis the ways in which organ transplantation has been discussed in Egypt's major newspapers for the past three decades.[17] In Egypt, the national media have created a social imaginary beyond the personal experiences of a relatively small number of patients, staging the question of organ transplantation as a national debate that has elicited strong opinions among ordinary people. The media have not only depicted these debates but have shaped them as well, providing the dominant discursive terms by which the public has come to question the ethics of transplant regimes intervening in ailing bodies. Ethical questions about removing a body part from one individual to insert it into another have been debated on various television programs, and both doctors and Islamic scholars have used the state-controlled television and newspapers as a platform to advocate for (and less often, against) organ donation. These figures see themselves as crucial to the education of the Egyptian public, working toward its need to "catch up" to the rest of the modern world and take its place on the global stage. In contrast, in the opposition-party press and on satellite television news exposés, depictions of kidney failure and lack of access to transplants have been framed in nationalist terms as grievances against an irresponsible state—a state that has wasted and mishandled its resources through corruption, exploitation of the poor, neglect of its citizens, and failure to provide adequate health services.[18]

Moving Targets

Part of my challenge in describing ethical formulations around organ transplantation is that people based their decisions on factors that are constantly shifting and evolving. I explore how doctors, religious scholars, patients, and their family members came to bioethical decisions through the fluid and overlapping rubrics of Islam, biomedical efficacy, political-economic exigencies, and kinship. The efficacy of the medical procedure; the etiologies of disease; the political and economic context of health care; the state's inability to manage medical clinics and to curb the market in organs; the extent to which people were being exploited or helped; family relations; the cost, side effects, and availability of necessary drugs; the level of trust in the medical profession—all of these factors, all of which were subject to change, informed ethical decisions. Also subject to change were the frameworks through which patients, family members, doctors, and religious scholars weighed these factors against one another in their ethical and pragmatic calculations.

The rapid process of the deregulation and privatization of major industries in Egypt has led to increased exposure to dangerous toxins through pesticides, chemical fertilizers, and industrial waste that have been dumped onto Egyptian farmland and into the water supply. This has led to Egyptians blaming their government, as can be readily discerned in the daily newspapers, not only for passive negligence in not protecting their bodily integrity, but also for actively harming them through greed and corruption.[19] The disquieting concern with toxicity and disease finds its way into both the official state newspapers and those of opposition parties, as well as into television reports, particularly those on satellite dish channels, into the sermons of Muslim preachers, and into what I call the "political etiologies" of everyday discussions among doctors and patients—that is, the ways in which they link their understandings of the cause of disease to political-economic structures that determine resource distribution (Hamdy 2008). Patients are keenly aware that biomedical outcomes cannot be convincingly attributed to bad genetic luck or their own individual behavior.[20] Their access to health care may be limited to medical services that they have reason to mistrust deeply, having experienced medical mismanagement, from disrespectful treatment to botched operations. This all takes place within the broader context of Egypt's dismantling of public health care and the lack of oversight in public water and waste management, under both external and internal pressures of rapid privatization (Sowers 2007).

Returning to the question of bioethics, these tensions show us that it is futile to seek a unified Egyptian voice of reason. It seems illogical to seek out *the* ultimate Islamic position on complex social issues, especially when people have different experiences, perceptions, and stakes in them. It is especially illogical to imagine that a politically corrupt state can claim the authority to determine what counts as *the* set of Islamic principles. Nevertheless, there has been a pressing desire to determine the Islamic position on organ transplantation in Egypt. And beyond Egypt, Muslims have asked if a distinct field of inquiry exists that could be labeled as "Islamic bioethics" (Daar and Khitamy 2001; Aramesh 2007; Atighetchi 2007; Sachedina 2009). Various parties have sought to address this question, from UNESCO, through transnational Islamic legal coalitions, to hospital administrators in non-Muslim countries flummoxed about how to manage their Muslim patients. But on what basis would one establish *the* Egyptian or Muslim position on organ transplantation, or on any other bioethical problem for that matter?

In trying to find out how a particular culture approaches a bioethical topic, we risk overstating the homogeneity of opinion and further silencing the voices of the marginalized.[21] And here let me note that, in talking about the impossibility of representing *the* Egyptian position, this book focuses on Muslim Egyptians and does not include a study of Coptic Christians, the major minority religious group.[22] My aim is not to find the most legitimate or authentic Egyptian or Muslim position; I am more interested in analyzing the bases from which various groups lay claims to cultural, medical, and religious authority; how they ground their claims in particular arguments and evidence; and which arguments resonate in the public sphere and why.

Aside from the issue of representation, we cannot assume that cultural and ethical norms or attitudes will translate directly into decision-making processes. All the players in this debate—including transplant surgeons, who themselves question the ethics and medical integrity of organ transplantation—are firmly entrenched in the principles and categories of contemporary biomedicine. Similarly, all the informants in my study agreed on a single source of ethics.[23] The Muslim physicians, religious scholars, patients, family members, lawyers, and journalists who inform this book all appealed to Islam as their most authoritative ethical guide, and all have been shaped by Muslim Egyptian culture. Yet this commonality still did not lead to the same decisions or practices about organ transplantation, which is itself a fast-evolving practice.[24]

Further, as Paul Farmer (1999, 2003) has pointed out, "cultural difference" is woefully inadequate in explaining away structural inequality. We cannot talk about the differences in experiences of organ transplantation as "cultural" in a situation in which surgical efficacy rates and access to the transplants are the products of so many other powerful political and economic forces. In the case of medicine, historians have described the paradox of "the unresolved disequilibrium between, on the one hand, the remarkable capacities of an increasingly powerful science-based biomedical tradition and, on the other, the wider and unfulfilled health requirements of economically impoverished, colonially vanquished and politically mismanaged societies" (Porter 1998: 12). Many renal failure patients in this study, connected to the dialysis tubes keeping them alive, weighed risks against benefits as they watched the results of fellow patients who left the ward for the promises that a transplant might bring. Some of these transplant recipients, after their families scraped together all their savings to afford an organ, ended up with "failed" operations in which their bodies rejected the graft. Others never came back, either because they were now better and "free" from the dialysis machines or because they were dead. The historical reality of organ transplantation worldwide reveals a rocky beginning that is both obscured and denied by the popular U.S. rhetoric of the "gift of life." In Egypt, as elsewhere, many of the early recipients of kidneys died shortly after their transplant operations. In the province of Shbin al-Kom, the first three liver lobe transplants in the 1990s resulted in both the recipients and the healthy living donors dying before a moratorium on the procedure was called into effect.[25]

Results, experiences, and perceptions of organ transplantation are as uneven as Egypt's social landscape. Sick patients in organ failure in otherwise socially and economically comfortable families have had much to gain from organ replacement; the poor have had much to fear. Throughout this book we clearly see that no cultural behaviors or religious dispositions are static and that it does not make sense to talk about "the Muslim" or "the Egyptian" view without consideration of shifting political and economic factors, access to resources, and people's different experiences of risk and benefit. Thus, rather than simply asking why "Egyptian culture" or "Islam" operates as a constraint on potential biotechnological solutions, I ask instead why these technologies in fact do not appear to provide solutions to many in Egypt under their present circumstances.[26] While many within and outside of Egypt look to biotechnologies to fix large-scale problems like organ failure, I demonstrate that biotechnologies themselves are products of the same social landscape that they are often meant to "fix" (Winner 1980; Jasanoff 2005; Cowan 2008). Rapidly developing biotechnologies are effectively changing the ways that we experience our bodies and understand suffering and the boundary between life and death. This book is concerned with how people make sense of these changes while remaining committed to timeless theological truths about the created body, the purpose of suffering, and the very meaning of mortal life.

ETHICS EMBODIED: BEYOND ABSTRACT PRINCIPLES

Critical interrogation of ethical problems requires destabilizing units, scales, and categories of analysis. The scale of the individual is often too small for meaningful intervention; we need to expand this unit of inquiry beyond the boundary of the individual's skin to include the larger social and historical forces that have shaped the individual's life. From another perspective, the scale of the individual can be too big, given that biomedical intervention increasingly fragments the body. We need also to shift the scale of the individual *inward* to uncover meanings enshrined in different body parts. Which body part one is intervening in, for what reasons, and how, all make a difference.

The conglomeration of diseases that can be treated with organ transplantation, together with people's understandings of their etiologies, provide another important context for the debates that have ensued in Egypt. Each of the three types of transplants that have been available in the absence of a cadaveric procurement program—the cornea since the 1960s, the kidney since the 1970s, and the liver lobe since the early years of the 2000s—represents a major disease that has come to be identified with Egypt. Cornea opacity has been linked with trachoma, an endemic disease once known as "Egyptian ophthalmia" to travelers of the fourteenth to the nineteenth century, causing blindness to a significant portion of the population in either one or both eyes.[27] Trachoma, a bacterial infection that when left untreated can lead to the loss of sight, has been associated with ignorance and lack of hygiene, particularly after the nineteenth-century European expansion into Egypt (Hamdy 2005).

Diseases of the kidney and liver were generally attributed to bilharzias, or schistosomiasis, an endemic snail-borne parasite of the Nile, also associated with rural poverty. In recent decades, however, epidemiologists have noted a sharp increase of kidney and liver diseases of a different type and of apparently different causes. Doctors and patients alike have linked renal and liver disease to the toxicity of polluted air and contaminated water, the extensive use of dangerous pesticides, and unsafe food storage. Widespread understandings of the cause of organ failure, as the result of the general weakening of the body in a contaminated, corrupt environment, have played a major role in determining patients' decisions to refuse organ offers from relatives. I often heard them argue that they were loath to leave their loved ones "incomplete"—without an organ—in the same environment that made their own "complete" bodies ill. Moreover, in the 1960s and 1970s, a government-backed mass health campaign to treat schistosomiasis involved medical injections with reused needles, which were boiled for sterilization between patient injections. This inadvertently infected a significant percentage of the population with hepatitis C, a heat-resistant virus that survived the attempted sterilization via boiling (Frank et al 2000). Egypt currently ranks as having the highest prevalence of this deadly liver virus in the world, and the devastating repercussions of infection are now presenting themselves clinically, with international reports suggesting an imminent "viral time bomb" (McGrath 2009b). Somewhere between 10 and 30 percent of the entire Egyptian population is said to be infected with hepatitis C, with liver diseases dominating national health concerns. Different parts of the body thus carry with them different social histories, symbolic meanings, and medical outcomes in transplantation, which influence the ethical understandings and consequences of the transplant.

The scale of the individual needs to be expanded temporally as well. We should abandon the assumption, for example, that one can "become an organ donor" by checking a box on a driver's license, as though one is becoming a subspecies or category of person.[28] When I think back to the day that I myself checked the box for "organ donor" as a teenager obtaining my first U.S. driver's license, it no longer makes sense to think that I was "choosing" a timeless identity that would reveal my own interior and personal truths. As a young, healthy person I was fortunate then to have not yet experienced acute or chronic illness and to have never seen mangled bodies or corpses. I had not yet witnessed a brain-dead patient, nor had I experienced the sudden death of anyone close to me. Years later, where is the continuity in this same "me"? Life experiences over the course of thirty or forty years are likely to inform different ethical positions.

And was I really an autonomous and individual agent, of the type often presented in bioethics cases, exerting my will on the basis of my own interior and private code of ethics? Beyond our individual life experiences, various forces shape our ideas and decisions, such as the Department of Motor Vehicles, the U.S. news media's glorification of the "medical miracle" that "saves lives," and high-drama American television programs. These very forces produce and sustain the illusion that the same coherent self who checks a box on a form at the DMV constitutes the "authentic voice" that can authorize life-or-death decisions, no matter what is to come, no matter when, and no matter what the circumstances. Have we rightly assumed that individual choices are static, reflecting a coherent self, whether immersed in news media or ignorant of them, whether inside or outside the threat of immediate danger, whether writhing in pain or enjoying perfect health, whether alienated from kin and other social relations or deeply entwined with them?

When we make any decision about a medical intervention such as organ transplantation, our ideas are informed by what we know scientifically about the procedure and its efficacy. We are also shaped by our moral frameworks, which in the Egyptian context are usually religious. Throughout my analysis, I have drawn on insights from the social studies of science to shed light on the social production of medical and religious truths. In this theoretical framework, science does not constitute the simple outcome of observing and rationally categorizing nature. Rather, science is but one of many social practices that contingently formulate knowledge, whose validity is judged by a variegated social world through preexisting conceptual categories. Science, in this view, is not a locatable fixed entity that resides outside the social sphere; nor is it restricted to certain places (such as laboratories) or confined to particular institutions and peoples (such as scientists). Science and technology are everywhere, materially intersecting with our lives, confirming and revising our conceptual categories through which we judge things to be true.

Understanding religious ethics, too, as a social practice allows me to push the bounds of these two theoretical frameworks by reading one against the other. Scholars of science studies have struggled with how to incorporate the multiple contingencies and possibilities of social interpretations of science with the "givens" of the natural environment that science sets out to describe and manipulate. This is similar to the ways in which scholars of Islam have struggled with how to render the multiple possibilities of religious interpretation and the myriad ways to be a Muslim with the "givens" of the core tenets and texts of Islam. It is important to point to the openness and possibilities of scientific and religious interpretation; just as there is no one way to categorize and interpret the natural material world around us, so is there no single way to interpret and live the canonical texts of Islam. Fatwas of religious scholars cannot accurately represent *the* Islamic position on organ transplantation, much as descriptions in medical transplant journals cannot serve as *the* true or only representation of the human body.

By looking at the ways in which various positions on transplantation are constructed, informed, argued, received, and resignified, this study traces the processes by which medical knowledge and religious knowledge are produced and the different conditions under which knowledge is authorized or contested. In order to comprehend how—and whether—authoritative religious opinions are made meaningful to ordinary people, I had to ask how and why particular arguments resonate with the "common sense" of others. By asking, and not assuming, how particular religious arguments become available, comprehensible, adopted, refuted, or resignified, we can see that Muslim ethics are necessarily shaped by social and historical contingencies, as is the case with scientific and medical theories of the body.

At the same time, we cannot lose sight of the reason that science, including medicine, is powerful precisely because it is able to capture and manipulate the material world effectively (Haraway 1988; Latour 1988). And in a similar vein, religious actors have to make a convincing case for the legitimacy of an "Islamic" argument on the basis of its ability to connect persuasively to the authorizing canonical texts (MacIntyre 1984; Asad 1986; Mahmood 2005; Hirschkind 2006). In exploring, for example, the narratives of patients in renal failure, I have demonstrated that no single, universal experience of kidney pathology exists, but this does not mean that I consider infinite possibilities of bodily experience arbitrarily linked to physiological processes. Similarly, in demonstrating the multiple ways in which people interpret the expression "the body belongs to God," I do not mean to suggest its infinite possibilities of meaning. If it can mean everything, it becomes, in a sense, an empty signifier. In its richness, it offers multiple meanings, but to be recognizable as authoritatively "Islamic," it must ultimately connect in some way to tenets of Islam that Muslims categorize as legitimate. Debate and revision are necessary and integral aspects of both scientific paradigms and religious traditions. Thus, this book does not ask why medicine and religious ethics are not more universal, objective, or stable. Nor does it fault medicine as being "less true" or religious ethics as being "less genuine" because they are dynamic social practices that are context dependent. Instead, the following chapters analyze what is at stake in insisting that science, ethics, and religion should be bound and fixed bodies of knowledge, despite our everyday experiences that tell us that they are not. When we better understand this, we can begin the project of a bioethics rebound.

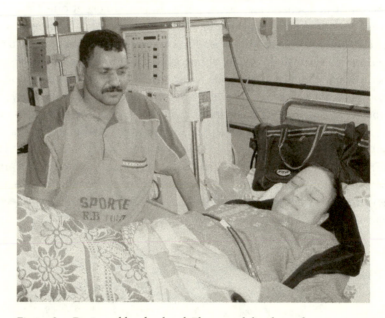

Figure 3. Ragia and her husband. Photograph by the author.

1   Egypt's Crises of Authority

When Egyptian doctors first experimented with kidney transplantation in the 1970s, the wider public had no idea that the number of patients in kidney failure was ominously rising or that this life-restoring surgery would soon become the object of a contentious debate. By the 1990s, investigative reporters for newspapers and local television channels fully exposed the gory and often scandalous details about the transplantation of kidneys, eyes, and other body parts. Doctors, legislators, journalists, and religious figures all argued and debated vehemently about the ethics of procuring and transplanting parts of the human body, with seemingly no resolution. During this span of decades, Egypt's social landscape was dramatically transformed. Significant social changes included the sharp rise in first-generation literates, the massive rural to urban migration, the nation's huge population growth, the diversification of media outlets that exceeded the mandates of the government, the dismantling of the welfare state, the explosion in number of Egyptian migrants seeking work in the newly petro-rich Gulf region, and the Islamic revival across the Arab world that resulted in the increased dominance of religious discourse in daily life.[1] These changes led, among other things, to less perceived social distance between physician and patient and between religious scholar and lay Muslim. In contrast with earlier generations, poor disenfranchised patients actively contested medical practice, and informally educated lay Muslims engaged in religious interpretation themselves. Subsequent crises of authority in both the medical and religious realms resulted in a continuing unresolved debate over organ transplantation, a practice which provoked the reassessment of ideas of personhood, the meanings of death, and questions about the proper treatment of the human body.

This chapter introduces pioneering surgeons, terminally ill kidney-failure patients, patients blinded by cornea opacity, their ambivalent doctors,

21

and religious scholars. Within each of these groups, ideas and arguments are in constant flux. Amid an increasing gap between minimal public services and high-cost, high-tech private clinics, Egypt's medical professionals disagree on how best to practice medicine. Egyptian physicians see medical knowledge as universal, yet also struggle to adapt it to local circumstances. Egypt's religious world is increasingly fractious, marked by state-appointed religious scholars and their critics, who challenge both medical authority and the state's aims, often through newly decentralized media outlets. Ideas about the dead body, human suffering, and divine will are embedded in longstanding theological debates. Meanwhile, since the 1970s, Egypt's political economy has been undergoing the demise of social welfare and the rise of neoliberal policies that have exacerbated the gap between rich and poor (Mitchell 2002). All of these changes have occurred amid a newly articulated Islamic ethic that calls for social justice, yet one that operates within the context of a political regime that has long presented itself as Western-aligned and democratic while practicing brutal intolerance toward dissenters (Ibrahim 1996; Kienle 2001; Wickham 2002; Mahmood 2005; Hirschkind 2006; Rutherford 2008; EIPR 2009).

In this shifting social reality, biotechnologies and new global markets impinge on notions of bodily integrity. And in the fractious realms of religious and medical ethics, patients, religious scholars, and doctors have found themselves faced with questions about life and death with no firm ground to stand upon. Meanwhile, the biotechnology of organ transplantation itself is quickly evolving. The introduction of new surgical techniques, newer generations of pharmaceutical immunosuppressive drugs, and growing clinical experience all contribute to changing rates of efficacy and survival. In this chapter I explore the ways in which various people have engaged with these slippery, moving targets.

BEGINNINGS

In the late 1960s, when the first two dialysis machines were brought to Mansoura, a provincial city on the eastern branch of the Nile Delta, Dr. Mohamed Ghoneim, a young urological surgeon, insisted that they be located in the department of urology rather than the department of internal medicine.[2] His colleagues at the hospital were both baffled and annoyed.[3] Ghoneim did not see the primitive dialysis machines as stations for the life-support of terminally ill end-stage kidney disease patients. Rather, he foresaw them as providing intermittent treatment for patients whom he would eventually treat surgically with kidney transplantation. He planned to carry out this procedure in what he envisioned would be Egypt's first center for treating kidney disease in Mansoura.[4]

Mansoura? The town was so provincial that scarcely a generation earlier any medical practitioner with even a modicum of ambition would have left it to train and practice in Cairo. And even Cairo did not yet have the capabilities for kidney transplantation, a procedure that was still at an experimental stage worldwide. In the United States, where the first experiments were carried out, the failure and death rates of these operations were exceedingly high.[5]

None of this was to stop Ghoneim. With a streak of anti-elitism that marked him as one of Egypt's most beloved medical heroes, Ghoneim famously sneered, "Where *else* would we do it? In Zamalek?"[6] Zamalek is one of Cairo's most exclusive neighborhoods—an island in the middle of the Nile and home to the old-guard elite, five-star hotels, and foreigners. Referring to the high incidence of parasitic schistosomiasis infections among the poor rural inhabitants of the Nile Delta provinces, and hence their susceptibility to kidney and urological diseases, Ghoneim's pronouncement about Mansoura was swift: "Mansoura is the center of the battlefield!"[7]

And, indeed, in 1976, when a mother in Mansoura donated one of her kidneys to her daughter, Dr. Ghoneim carried out the first kidney transplant operation in Egypt. Ghoneim was not interested in merely bringing Egypt up to pace with this biotechnological accomplishment. He envisioned bringing its benefits to Egypt's rural impoverished patients. Ghoneim began with a limited capacity of two dialysis machines and one hospital bed for transplantation at Mansoura University Hospital; in time, he and his colleagues established an internationally renowned national and public institution for the treatment of kidney and urological diseases in Mansoura. The building was erected on the grounds of a famous botanical garden with the help of funds from the Netherlands under then-president Sadat. Thereafter, the beautifully landscaped and curated institution was sustained by government support and local donations. The Mansoura Kidney Center, formally established in 1983, today provides tertiary health care for a population base of seven million.[8] Kidney-failure patients with family members who are willing and medically eligible to donate a kidney can access a transplant, a life-long regimen of immunosuppressants, and follow-up medical care at no cost. Under Ghoneim's strict protocols and his watchful eye, the physicians at Mansoura painstakingly raised the level of nursing and clinical care and carefully screened donors and recipients to ensure the highest success rates. At this center, transplants have all depended on living donors, and after thirty years of experience, the patient and kidney graft survival rates rival those in the best centers in countries with far greater resources, including equipment, staff, and newer immunosuppressants. The center's capacity for transplantation has grown over the years, and since 2008, it has carried out approximately eighty kidney transplants annually.[9]

Cairo's hospitals and private clinics began to carry out transplantation shortly after Mansoura's early experiments. Various medical facilities in Cairo soon dwarfed Mansoura's capacity, carrying out (often unrecorded) operations that were impossible to quantify accurately.[10] During this second decade of transplantation, stories of the black market and theft of kidneys in Cairo began to circulate in Egypt. By the mid-1980s disturbing reports about a thriving market in human kidneys in Cairo hospitals continually appeared in Egyptian newspapers, both the state-owned dailies and, in more provocative tones, in the opposition-party news. Evidence of blatant medical misconduct, including graphic images of people with large, protruding surgical scars, and allegations of organ theft fueled popular resentment against government corruption and the mismanagement of state medical institutions. Criticism immediately spilled into religious and moral discourse about what can rightly be done to the human body as God's creation.

In this period, critics of state institutions increasingly framed their moral discontent with the government in what they considered to be "Islamic" terms. Professionals, including medical physicians, many of whom were members of the Muslim Brotherhood that came to dominate the Egyptian Medical Syndicate in the 1980s, called for a return to religious ideals.[11] While it might have been clear to Dr. Ghoneim of Mansoura in the mid-1970s that the primary battle to be fought was against disease, particularly that which is wrought by endemic parasitic infection among the rural poor, rural disease was much less the priority of elite physicians a decade later and is still less of a priority today. In the first decade and a half of transplant medicine, many Egyptian doctors began to identify other battles to be waged: against the privatization of health care, the commodification of bodies, rampant corruption, government irresponsibility, and godlessness. Who can patients trust, given the ample restrictions on political freedoms, the strained relations between religious and state authorities, and the fact that there has been no tradition of patients' rights and no elaborate system of consent procurement?

ON DIALYSIS, IN THE WASH

Ragia lay on a narrow bed tethered to her dialysis machine. She was now completely blind as a result of her diabetes, which had also devastated her kidneys. Anticipating meeting her again, I walked hesitantly down the hall of the public hospital in the Nile Delta city of Tanta and then fidgeted nervously at the entryway of the dimly lit hospital room. The overhead fluorescent lights flickered arhythmically, and the smell of disinfectant mixed with the human blood moving between the dialysis machines and the patients, was overpowering. The sounds of periodic beeps and swishes of the dialysis machines rarely, if ever, synchronized with the patients' restless movements. The patients lay in rows, each hooked up to a machine.

The Egyptian colloquial word for dialysis is *ghasil-kalawy* (kidney washing) or *ghasil al-damm* (washing blood).[12] *Ghasil*, in everyday parlance, means "laundry."[13] Patients referring to their dialysis sessions said that they came to "wash" or that the doctors "washed" them.[14] When I first met Salih, a forty-year old army retiree whose wife accompanied him on the two-hour trip from their rural village to the dialysis unit, his wife, unaccustomed to hearing the city dialect, asked me to repeat everything I said a number of times. Salih affectionately nudged his wife and joked, "It's true that *I* need to do washing [i.e., dialysis, *ghasil*], but I think *she* needs ear washing *[ghasil al-widan]*!" A younger patient, Ahmad, told me, amusedly, that his children at home learned that their father did "washing" at the hospital and that their mother did the washing at home. As the patients were well aware, the dialysis sessions did not treat their kidney disease or restore their kidney function. Dialysis, a life-sustaining treatment, keeps the diagnosis of end-stage kidney failure from being a death sentence by filtering the toxins in blood that malfunctioning kidneys fail to remove.

As many patients conceived of it, "Food makes blood, and then kidneys clean the blood." Now that their kidneys had failed, machines washed their blood instead. Their toxin levels, they believed, were high not only because of their failed kidneys but also because of their toxic environment. No matter how much washing occurred, their vitality could never be fully restored, because, as they pointed out, the food and water that remade their blood were polluted, just as the blood transfusions they needed might be contaminated.[15] Further, many patients realized that the more time they spent on dialysis, the sicker they were getting, and the less they would benefit from a kidney transplant. As one patient put it, "You wash and wash [undergo dialysis], and just like when you wash your *galabiyya* and it gets frayed and threadbare, the same with the body, it gets worn out from so much washing."

Conscious that they were reliant on dialysis machines for their very survival, patients were also cognizant of their vulnerability to the machines' shortcomings. The dialysis sessions required humans—underpaid and often unreliable—to check, carry, transport, clean, and operate the machines. And dialysis machines relied on hospital and state infrastructure for electric power. In the Egyptian delta provinces of Gharbiyya and elsewhere, patients were vulnerable to the state's irregular power supply and to regular blackouts. Even more frustrating were the more frequent brownouts, periods when the voltage dropped low, threatening the operation of the machines' microprocessing units. The dialysis machines would often let out sharp beeps in response to the drops in voltage. The patients would lift their heavy heads in alarm; the fuzzy picture on a black-and-white television set, which at times emanated melodious Qur'anic recitation and at other times depicted images of war in Iraq, would switch to static. The nurses would run to the dialysis machines and punch buttons until the beeping stopped.

Trying to brace myself for what I might find inside, I had come to the habit of beginning my work in the dialysis unit by counting whose shoes were lying outside the door, trying to anticipate who might be missing by yet another death. Catching sight of Ragia's shoes, then Ragia, I walked in and took my place by her side. I opened my notebook, and she began to speak.

Ragia told me with tears streaming down her face that more painful than the dialysis was the fact that, after years of living in blindness, she had forgotten the face of her seven-year-old daughter. Her husband, at her side, consoled her, saying that he would give her his kidney, and even his eyes, to see her not suffer.[16] They did not have the same blood type, though, foreclosing the possibility of a transplant. Ragia said that in any case she could not bear to see him undergo a major operation for her and that they needed to save all of their resources to focus on their only daughter, who was recently diagnosed with the same diabetes afflicting her mother.

Unlike Ragia, most patients in the public hospital dialysis ward in Tanta did not have family members readily offering them pieces of their bodies. Most of Egypt's poor could not afford to consider transplantation as a possibility. In any case, many patients were not convinced that a transplant would result in more benefit than harm—considering the financial costs, the sacrifice of the kidney donor, and how their lives might or might not turn out posttransplant. They continued to endure difficult and, at times, unreliable treatment and to manage the symptoms of chronic kidney failure and the side effects of medications and hemodialysis, including dietary

restrictions and unpredictable episodes of sharp pain, dizzine
nausea, muscle cramps, and fatigue.[17]

Another young woman, Muna, also fidgeted restlessly in h
too, had a young daughter to care for. Her husband, tiring of t
of dialysis treatment and Muna's inability to conceive and giv ...... to a
son, had left her, a fate not uncommon to women on dialysis. And she had
tried—against her doctor's warnings—to bear another child, but the strain
of the pregnancy resulted in a miscarriage, worsening her kidney function
and precipitating the dissolution of her marriage. In a tired and hoarse
whisper, she explained to me that there was no one who would gift her a
kidney. "Anyway," she sighed, "one cannot give a part of the body away,
since the whole body belongs to God." Then she straightened and forced a
smile, telling me that advances in science happened every day. "Soon doctors may be able to clone a kidney from [my own] cells." Pointing to the
tubes connecting her frail arms to the bright blue dialysis machine, she said,
"I'll be honest with you. It is this hope that keeps me going. It is this hope
that brings me here each day."

At their simplest, accounts of scientific progress assert that the advance of
science and technology necessarily improves the lives of people around the
globe. Even poor rural patients like Muna, in an understaffed and resource-
poor public hospital, live on the hope that advances in scientific knowledge
will directly improve their quality of life.[18] Yet anthropologists and postcolonial scholars have demonstrated that the increased sophistication and circulation of science and technology have generally continued to privilege those
already most advantaged (Mitchell 2002; Harding 2006). Skills, techniques,
expertise, and pharmaceuticals generally tend to follow the flows of global
capital. In the visceral case of organ transplantation, the actual kidneys and
other body parts, too, tend to move "from poor to rich, from black and brown
to white, and from female to male" (Scheper-Hughes 2000: 193).

The majority of dialysis patients with whom I spoke told me that they
refused the premise of organ transplantation, the idea that one could "give"
a piece of one's body, that they could "take" such a thing from someone
they loved or, even from someone they paid to part with an organ.[19] "The
body belongs to God," they would say. This sentiment is generally unre-
markable and obvious in the context of the lives of believing Muslims who
in illness turn to God more fervently. Yet it has been a sentiment that
people constantly evoke and iterate in discussions of organ transplantation
in Egypt. Shaykh Sha'rawi (d. 1998), a popular religious figure, first asserted
this statement as a challenge to the biomedical treatment of body parts as
interchangeable commodities. With each utterance, patients, doctors, and

religious scholars with whom I spoke imparted new meanings to the idea that the body is divine property *(inna al-jasad milk allah)*.

Something deeply disturbing about the prospects of organ transplantation precluded Ragia, Muna, and other patients from considering it as a viable treatment. Muna's hope focused on stem cells and the future possibility of a technique in bodily regeneration. This position challenges doctors' assumptions that their patients' refusals of organ transplantation are due to "fatalism," a fear of human intervention in a divine plan, or anxieties about technological intervention in "natural processes." At the time of my fieldwork, a certain irony unfolded: In the United States, stem cell research, the very hope that Muna said kept her going each day, had provoked major ethical and political discussion, while organ donation in dominant North American discourse continued to be depicted as an act of altruism, that well-known "gift of life." In contrast, most of the Egyptian patients with whom I spoke felt uneasy about organ transplantation, but they had no such qualms about ideas of "therapeutically cloning" kidneys or about "artificial kidneys" in the form of the dialysis machines that were sustaining them.[20] The positions of these Egyptians may initially seem strange, considering their avowals that "the body belongs to God." Why did organ procurement *from another human* trouble the premise of the body as divine property, whereas the therapeutic cloning of kidneys, or their replacement via a dialysis machine, did not? I soon learned that transplantation did not appear beneficial as a medical "solution," because patients often resisted the idea of turning to a family member as a potential kidney donor. Most patients did not experience their illnesses as isolated in their kidneys. Neither did they conceive of their body parts as interchangeable with those of others. Many patients did not accept what medical expertise has defined as a "tolerable risk," that is, the opening up of a healthy human donor and extracting a vital organ. They expressed their frustration at being vulnerable to the stresses of daily life, to the mismanagement of toxic waste, to the dumping of pesticides on agricultural land, and to a generally polluted environment. The polluted cities and farmland and their mismanagement through corruption and exploitation profoundly influenced patients' ethical dispositions toward their treatment options. They saw themselves as the most damaged cases in a place where everyone was vulnerable to organ failure, including would-be donors.

Dialysis units began proliferating across the country in the 1990s, expanding into smaller cities in the provinces, often in the form of private clinics.[21] For most of the patients I interviewed, the mushrooming of dialysis units, each one teeming with people diagnosed with end-stage kidney failure, was not read simply as progress in medical treatment or as improvement in medical access. Both patients and experts interpreted the rise in diagnoses of kidney failure as an indication of increased vulnerability to toxicity and exploitation. Many editorials in the state-owned newspapers *(Al-Ahram* and *Al-Akhbar)* as well as in opposition newspapers consistently asserted the links between pollution and kidney disease. Investigative reporters on popular television shows linked laboratory results of unclean water in particular urban quarters, slums, and villages with high rates of kidney and liver disease.[22] Witnessing the affliction of entire villages with kidney disease, their agricultural lands poisoned by toxic waste, chemical fertilizers, and bungled sewage draining, they argued that the Egyptian state not only did not care for its citizens but also negligently left them exposed to toxins and vulnerable to substandard medical practice.

Indeed, despite a mandate for universal health coverage, general government expenditure on health under President Mubarak amounted to 2 percent of total GDP (Fouad 2005; WHO 2007). Under Mubarak's regime, the Egyptian government contributed only 38 percent of the country's total health expenditure; the rest came from private sources, including out-of-pocket expenses paid by the poor (Fouad 2005; WHO 2007). The percentage of cost borne by patients out of pocket has only increased in recent years, with most Egyptians scraping together what little they have to pay for outpatient care at private clinics. As opposition party leaders complain, government resources are spent paying off foreign debts and interest on the financing of imports, upon which the Egyptian economy has been made to depend.

As I will detail more extensively in chapter 3, in the 1950s patients in public teaching hospitals served as the unwitting experimental subjects of Egyptian ophthalmologists' cornea transplants. In contrast, at the time of my fieldwork, beginning in the 2000s, patients at public facilities were vigilant about medical mistreatment; they were informed by national television and other media about religious debates in medical practices. Many were acquainted with the criticism expressed in opposition-party platforms regarding the shortcomings of the Mubarak regime. Patients were particularly suspicious of eye and kidney specialists because of allegations of "eye theft" from the morgue and reports of the vibrant market in human kidneys. It was well known that Egyptian doctors participated in these practices, and, as noted by the opposition-party newspapers, they were rarely held accountable for transgressions.

The dialysis patients whom I interviewed, even those who needed to embark on painful and onerous travel from the countryside to reach a clinic, learned to tolerate the burdensome regime of dialysis treatments in order to survive without recourse to a new kidney. Many were aware of the reported scandals in medical malpractice and of their particular vulnerability in terms of their dependence on surgery, dialysis, blood transfusion, and pharmaceuticals. Understanding that organ failure is a terminal illness that can be offset by procuring a "new" organ, some patients turned to their family members as resources. There was a lucky minority of patients with family members willing and medically eligible to donate kidneys to them, and with the resources to go through with the operation and follow-up treatment. Others felt the need to protect family members, particularly those most vulnerable. Many patients described themselves as undergoing a trial from God, during which they would remain steadfast in faith. They struggled with whatever resources were available and worked to cultivate dispositions of acceptance of God's will for the suffering that they could not end. In this context, patients extolled the virtues of cultivating steadfastness *(al-sabr)* during God's trials *(al-ibtila')*. Reliance on God and acceptance of divine will *(al-tawakkul)* are far from a passive or fatalistic attitude. Patients did not irrationally refuse positive change; instead, they conscientiously and rigorously trained themselves to accept God's will in regard to that which they could not change without unacceptable costs.

In some cases, people eventually turned to an eager supply of organ sellers in Cairo who were ready to part with their kidneys for fast cash. Young patients often passively accepted the decisions of their parents, who sacrificed significant resources and exerted tremendous effort to procure "new kidneys" for them. In desperation, parents resorted to what they themselves called "the unsavory option" of buying a kidney from a desperate seller in Cairo in order to see their sick sons and daughters live, grow, marry, and have children of their own.

JUST A LITTLE BIT OF SIGHT

"Come here, my daughter. What is this you are saying? I cannot see you, but God has blessed me with the sound of your voice."

At the time of my fieldwork, cornea transplant operations were hard to come by. Yet unlike kidney transplants, they were highly sought after by the patients who needed them. At the public eye hospital in Tanta, the phrase I heard most often among poor rural in-patients in the Eye Ward was: "I just want a little bit of vision—just enough to see and work throughout the day so that I am not a burden to others." Patients called for a health care system that would make corneas available to all those who were blinded by cornea

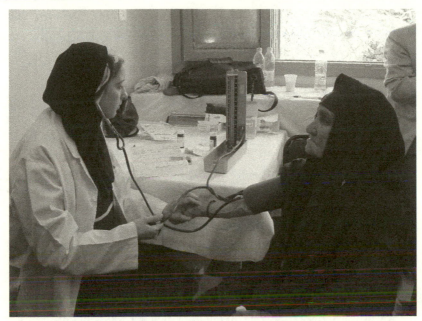

Figure 4. An elderly woman has her blood pressure checked during a public out-reach campaign for eye health, May 2004. Photograph by the author.

opacity. Even though cornea transplantation was looked upon favorably, here too patients and doctors blamed a corrupt government and dysfunctional political system for preventing their access to good treatment.

The elderly rural patients whom I saw consistently thanked God for what little they had left of their vision. They told me that they sought medical treatment not for a cure, not to restore their vision, and not because they felt ungrateful for what they had; what brought them in was their need to "see a tiny bit more" so that they could be of use to their family members. One older woman pressed her creased thumb and index finger together tightly to illustrate to me the small amount of vision with which she would be fully content.[23] I observed several adamant older patients refuse to undergo surgery, out of a refusal to spend scarce family resources on themselves.[24] A full restoration of vision seemed to lie beyond the imagination of many elderly patients I saw, and, in any case, they wagered that it would not be worth the cost or the potential risks.

In contrast, cornea opacity patients who described themselves as young (*shabab*), often meaning that they had yet to be married and start their own families, expressed frustration at their conditions and had higher expectations of their access to basic medical provisions. For example, ʿAziz, a young lawyer and cornea opacity patient, stressed that people with eye diseases in Egypt are in a particularly critical state: "Eye disease is very important to study, because there are a *lot* of Egyptians who suffer from it. And it's not like the kidney that a dad can give to his son, because God gave us two kidneys. With vision, you can't live without it. It is the whole life and soul. The kidney—it would be bearable to be sick in that, but vision, light, eyes . . . The eyes are the windows of the soul [*al-ʿayn nafizat al-ruh*]."

I met Muhammad, a young man of twenty-five, who was also "searching" for a cornea at Cairo's Maghraby Eye Hospital, a large private eye care center that has an outreach and charitable wing for the poor.[25] He was one of six siblings, five of whom suffered from the same genetic cornea opacity condition, which he attributed to the close genetic relationship of his parents as first cousins. He and his four sisters had spent the last decade trying to find the means to undergo cornea operations to improve their plight. As Muhammad narrated to me:

> When I was born I could see well. This happened to me in middle school. It became a real problem, and my vision got worse and worse. By the time I was thirteen, I had to drop out of school because I could no longer see. All my classmates now are pharmacists and doctors [highly esteemed professionals], and I swear they were not that smart, not as good in school as I was. But because of this cornea condition, I couldn't see, and so I couldn't continue with my studies. This gets me emotionally upset to think about, because I was very intelligent in school, and I could have been anything. But I had to drop out [when I lost my vision]. . . .
>
> This has been very upsetting emotionally to be young and to have to go through all of this. . . . I have gone to about ten doctors, trying to look for a cornea. Each time the exam is about 100 £E, and they keep saying that it will be thousands of pounds for the [cornea transplant] operation. . . .
>
> This could break someone, being young and not finding a way to live. I became one of the old and destitute; I worked sweeping the streets. But I should have had my whole life in front of me.

Muhammad appealed to the ideals of state welfare and the idea that just as citizens sought to be productive, so should the state care for them. Social mobility through education, however difficult in Egypt, was never even a possibility for him. And with corneas available only in private clinics at high costs, Muhammad's lack of access to what he saw as a basic health provision infuriated him. Hoping that my record of his narrative might raise awareness to his plight, Muhammad continued:

I want you to write all of this. And I am happy that my name is on it. I am not ashamed.[26] People should know that we are young and we had everything in front of us. We want to be productive like everyone else; I want to get married and have children. I want to be able to make my [future] children something good, educate them, so that they can be engineers or doctors. Imagine someone who is disabled and can no longer do anything. No productivity. The eye is the most important thing in the body. If your eye all of a sudden went out, you wouldn't be able to function at all.

When the doctor saw my eyes, he started to cry. I swear to God, he felt so bad because I am so young, and I had my whole life in front of me. But what can we do? You go to the public hospital, and they say there are no corneas. They say wait for years until the bank opens, until your turn comes, for years. I can't wait for this. This happens daily; you should see all the young people there, all the children and women. It is unconscionable [*haram*] to leave us like this.

Look at us; we are six in the family. Where am I going to get all this money [for private operations] for my sisters? How can I myself afford to live, let alone support others in these difficult times? I was in my youth, at the time when I am most supposed to be enjoying life. But I was so depressed, so upset, all the time. So irritable. Mentally I couldn't take it; if anyone talked to me I just wanted to scream. Anytime I tried to move or walk I would bump into everything, and I felt horrible.

As for me and my siblings, the longer we wait, the worse our eyes will get. So we have to come [to the clinics to keep trying to find a cornea graft]; we can't afford to wait until the day that we are old and completely blind.

As if conjuring an image of a surviving family member reluctant to turn over the corneas of their dead, Muhammad offered matter-of-factly: "That person already died; he won't use [his cornea] anymore. The worm is going to eat it. But if he donates it, he can help someone to see. God would forgive him for all his sins in life because he helped another person."

Out of the twenty Egyptian ophthalmologists and thirty cornea opacity patients that I interviewed, all unanimously agreed on the clear benefits of cornea grafting. They all argued that the rights of the living should supersede the rights of the dead. They differed on the best means of procuring the grafts, but they all agreed in principle that cornea donation is a necessary and commendable act. Cornea opacity patients and ophthalmologists alike were infuriated that public discussions about transplantation (*naql al-'ada'*) had conflated such widely different issues: the procurement of an outer tissue after death, they argued, is completely different from the extraction of a vital organ from the living, with all its attending problems involving exploitation, immune suppression, and black markets.

Dr. Mustafa, for instance, an ophthalmologist at a private eye hospital, complained to me that the only reason why people had suddenly become so excited and upset about cornea grafting in the 1990s is that they had confused it with the issue of kidney transplantation. Like other ophthalmologists, Dr. Mustafa argued that the cornea is so materially slight that no one should or can claim emotional attachment to it, especially when there are desperate people whose lives would be radically improved with a cornea graft. Shaking his head, he told me:

> It is just nonsense that people have confused this with the issue of kidneys and markets. People are afraid of organ theft, and they are right. Terrible things really are happening in that respect!
>
> But the cornea—this is totally different. It is not an organ. It is nothing, completely immaterial, it will disintegrate in a matter of days. It is only taken after death, the operation is simple, low cost, and the patient's life is saved. It is only taken after death, so there is no market for people selling their corneas.
>
> It is not like the kidney recipient, who will have to spend the rest of his life on immunosuppressive drugs. The patient will be fine and will be able to see right after the operation. We have had great success rates with this. Unfortunately, people don't understand this. It evolved into a discussion of what is *haram*. But it is not like a kidney for sale or something.

Given the material insignificance of the cornea, Dr. Mustafa viewed discussions about donors' consent and patients' rights to be inapplicable and impractical to cornea grafting. Poor patients like Muhammad only suffered, he suggested, while policy makers, religious scholars, and legislators took the luxury of debating abstract questions about the ethics of removing body parts from the dead or living, which has nothing to do with the practical matters of cornea grafting.

Notably, all of Dr. Mustafa's arguments *for* cornea transplantation implicitly argue *against* the transplantation of solid internal organs. He resented the debates around kidney transplantation and the black market and its attendant corruption for having instigated a national debate about cornea transfer and eye banking. Thus, while the idea that "the body belongs to God" came to stand in as a challenge to the transplantation of body parts, the statement is not as clear-cut as it seems.

The key issues and nuances that have shaped whether and how transplantation is accessed have been missed in legislative, jurisprudential, and bioethical debates that have ignored the direct experiences of patients when addressing the transfer of tissues and organs from one body to another. Patients' experiences tell us that the malfunction of different body parts can have different cultural associations and consequences. Different parts of the body necessitate different methods of procurement, and the surgery and follow-up treatment of transplantation can involve varying degrees of complication. While all patients agreed that their bodies were not their own property, *how* exactly the body belongs to God is subject to continual reinterpretation and resignification with each bodily intervention.

complex

TRANSPLANTING WITH TREPIDATION

Medical experts have differing opinions about whether a market in body parts is an inevitable outcome of organ transplantation and whether such marketing can be effectively stopped. As with patients, they anxiously wonder: is the risk of surgery and extraction of a vital organ (a kidney) from a living, healthy donor acceptable and justifiable? What counts as true "consent" for kidney donation, given the pressures of familial relations, discourses about altruism and sacrifice, and economic desperation and promises of "fast cash"?

Dr. Walid, a young nephrologist who had carried out kidney transplants in Cairo for thirteen years, told me that morally, legally, and ethically he was quite confused on this issue and that he was not sure if his reservations were of a religious nature. He told me, "Of the specialists who should have convinced me [about organ transplantation]—whether scientific or religious—no one has convinced me either way. I feel hesitant about this point. Maybe it is *haram*. Maybe not. If I felt for sure that it was *haram*, I would leave it at once."

Dr. Walid's ambivalence rested on his inability to assess whether organ transplantation brought more benefit than harm to Egyptian society. Many physicians and patients with whom I spoke reasoned that because there is harm to the donor and no clear or guaranteed benefit to the recipient, then this practice must be *haram*. But the questions then became: how is "benefit" to be assessed, by what criteria, and by whom? Dr. Walid went on to tell me: "I am not a religious scholar, but I think . . . I think the One who creates [bodies] is the One who owns [them]." He began with this well-known religious precept but then asserted that he was not convinced that particular medical practices such as kidney transplantation should be avoided simply because God owns our bodies.

Dr. Farida, a nephropathologist at a public facility, was a member of the pioneering medical teams that carried out the first kidney transplants in the 1970s. She had since worked on thousands of kidney failure cases in which patients received grafts from family members or unrelated donors. In our interview, she told me with certitude that she herself would never consider undergoing a transplant. "Why would I be afraid?" she asked. "If I were dying of kidney failure, I would return my body to God, who created it in the first place." Upon my further questioning, she conceded that she would certainly consider donating a kidney to one of her children if they were ever in need. But she would never think of receiving one.

For some physicians with whom I spoke, such as Dr. Ghoneim of Mansoura, biomedicine's ethical imperative to "save lives" was universal and applicable to all situations. For others, the issue was less clear. Their ambivalence toward organ transplantation in particular marked a departure from the role that the Egyptian doctors had generally taken in accommodating biomedical practice to Egyptian life. Physicians have historically played a major part in maintaining biomedicine's social and cultural authority in Egypt as a "universal science." In other societies that are heirs to complex textual traditions, such as those in China and India, postcolonial nationalists borrowed from modern institutions to systematize "alternative" medical traditions. In Maoist China, traditional Chinese medicine developed along these lines as a sign of national culture (Farquhar 1994; Zhan 2001; Scheid 2002), as did what became known as Ayurvedic medicine in postcolonial India (Burgel 1976; Leslie 1976; Gran 1979; Langford 2002). Throughout the Arab world there has been no such modernization of indigenous healing practices, even if other medical and healing traditions continue to exist (el-Aswad 1987; Watson 1992; Early 1993; Morsy 1993; Inhorn 2003; Sholkamy and Ghannam 2004). Muslim reformers from the late nineteenth century to the present have argued that modern science, including biomedicine, is "universal," stressing its continuity with the knowledge produced by medieval Muslim scientists. In the case of Egypt, biomedicine is perceived as *the* national medicine, and in official nationalist discourse it is the only true and appropriate means by which one can act responsibly toward one's own body.[27] In Egypt the major issues in biomedical debates are not about the legitimacy of biomedicine itself but rather about the ethics of its application.

It became evident, in the course of my fieldwork, that an ideal type of trustworthy Egyptian physician, the "doctor of confidence," has been largely responsible for maintaining this biomedical authority. The doctor of confidence is entrusted to adapt what is held to be a "universal science" to the Egyptian context.[28] This figure, often described as someone who is "close to God" (*'arif rabbina*), is one who upholds "Egyptian" and religious values and, through his or her high ethical and scientific standards, decides which medical practices are to be accepted and which are to be filtered out.[29] Dr. Mohamed Ghoneim, the surgeon who performed the first kidney transplant in Mansoura in 1976, is perhaps one of the best examples of the doctor of confidence and is often described by fellow Egyptians as such. He is known throughout Egypt as an exemplary medical physician. Dr. Ghoneim successfully accommodated biomedical treatment to the needs of his local rural population rather than merely reproducing the medical practice of Western countries, where he had undergone specialized training. Ghoneim proved his status in the international realm of urology and urological surgery through numerous publications in medical journals in the United States and Europe. As the national narrative goes, Ghoneim was never seduced by the potentials of power and fame abroad; his goals were to improve medicine in "his country."[30] His "homeland" (*balad*) refers not only to Egypt but also to his provincial home city of Mansoura. Ghoneim gained tremendous moral capital throughout Egypt both for having reached a high stature in medical science and for not forgetting the rural poor. Throughout the eastern delta provinces, inhabitants thank God that his heart and his surgical skills remained in Mansoura. As we will see in chapter 2, the idea of a "Muslim doctor of confidence" (*al-tabib al-muslim dhul-thiqa*), someone who would practice medicine within a specifically Islamic ethical framework, is offered in contemporary fatwas as the final authority in bioethical conundrums.

At the same time, mistrust in biomedicine is pervasive; corruption and greed in public and private medical institutions are rampant; and medical malpractice and exploitation of vulnerable patients remain largely unaccounted for.[31] Though several other well-respected doctors, motivated by Dr. Ghoneim's wider goal to serve poor rural patients, also led Egypt to excel in kidney transplants, still others profited in private practice by turning a blind eye to the obvious buying and selling of the organs that they were transplanting, yielding uneven surgical results. This has led many of their colleagues and the general public to decry organ transplantation as *haram* and to question the authority of biomedical practitioners.

Caught between a dominant religious discourse that now pervades the medical profession and the sobering realities of exploitation and an informal market in organs that has become common in Cairo's public and private hospitals, the next generation of physicians, those who went into medicine under the influence of inspiring, yet intimidating, figures like Ghoneim, have grown *unconfident*. Most doctors that I interviewed nervously eyed my pen and notebook in response to my questions and claimed that they did not want to "talk politics." These physicians have avoided sensitive political issues, like organ transplantation. The debate around organ transplantation has further split medical professionals who were already divided. Those doctors who have argued that organ transplantation is wrong "because the body belongs to God" could be dismissed as "extremists" and suspected of affiliations with political Islamist organizations that are critical of the government. On the other hand, those who have been involved with transplantation could be suspected of participating in irresponsible and corrupt practices such as the black market in organs. [32]

While trust in biomedical practices still hinges on the doctor of confidence, since the 1990s in particular, people everywhere feel that current conditions have made it nearly impossible for doctors to "do good" for their countries. Medical education is a case in point. Though medicine has remained one of the most prestigious specialties in Egypt, medical education has come under fire as a broken and corrupt system that leads to a broken and corrupt health-care industry. [33] Although the doors to higher education were theoretically open to the poor under Nasser's regime, [34] by the 1990s sustaining a discourse of equal opportunity was much harder. At one time, a nationalist ideal held that doctors could come out of poor classes and, in turn, do good to help the poor. With the concomitant privatization of medical education and medical services, it has been harder to maintain the notion that doctors are those who want to serve the poor and benefit their country. Coveted medical positions and clinics have even become inherited, passed from father to son or daughter. [35] An agitated opposition party press often fans the flames of these discussions by providing detailed accounts of cases in which doctors' primary goal appears to benefit financially, and often at the expense of the poor.

It is true that the medical faculty's official salaries are so low that to survive they depend on the fees that they accrue in their private clinics, and, in some cases, by offering private medical-school lessons. Some of these professors offer underground anatomy lessons in their homes, teaching on cadavers illegally obtained, because there are so few corpses per student in Kasr el Aini's main lecture hall. [36] Others in the medical faculty have been so overburdened by other commitments that they do not show up to teach the students, and they have no financial incentive to treat the patients in the public teaching hospitals. The official income of medical faculty comes from the Ministry of Education rather than the Ministry of Health, and thus their low salaries are fixed by the lectures they give in the medical school; the number of patients they attend to (or not) in the adjacent teaching hospitals do not bring any increase in their pay. Some residents have accused their senior physicians of refusing to teach them certain new procedures in the public facilities so as to maintain a monopoly on the procedures in their own private clinics. As a result, many of the extremely poor patients I met raised money to afford a visit with a physician at a private outpatient clinic rather than risk mistreatment in public facilities (see also Kamal 2004). Ironically, in many of these cases, the physicians who had the private outpatient clinics were the same physicians who worked in the public facilities.[37]

Diminishing confidence in physicians, wrought by these structural factors in public and private medical institutions, has extended to outright charges of corruption. The public dispute around organ transplantation that has polarized its potential benefits and harms seems to have exacerbated the polarized potentials of biomedicine itself. Scandals about a black market in human organs and, even worse, about physicians in league with middle men convicted of organ *theft* from unwitting patients have occupied the press and sullied the claims that organ transplantation is simply a life-saving procedure. Take, for instance, the 1998 book written by the journalist 'Abd al-Hamid al-'Irqsusi, titled *Anqadhuna . . . fishash wa kalawi al-Misriyin lil-biy*'*!* (Rescue Us . . . Livers and Kidneys of Egyptians for Sale!) (al-'Irqsusi 1998). A young doctor wrote the preface to this piece, which extolled six ideal virtues of the physician: compassion, love, trust, confidence, self-sacrifice, and ethics. He asked rhetorically whether these virtues are still relevant to doctors in Egypt today, implying that doctors' participation in a black market in human body parts has forever tarnished the medical profession, which was once seen as the very moral fabric of the nation.

The virtues of the doctor of confidence in resolving irreconcilabilities between biomedical science and "Egyptian values" can no longer be counted on in assessing the appropriateness of organ transplantation. Physicians have been deeply ambivalent about the ethics of transplantation, because they have negotiated their multiple subject positions as experts, as family members, as potential patients themselves vulnerable to illness, and as religious devotees. This has led to a widening of the debate among religious scholars, who also are wondering: is organ transplantation suitable to Egyptian needs, or does it carry more potential harm than benefit?

FROM AN ISLAMIC FRAMEWORK?

Shaykh 'Amr, a young religious scholar whom I first met and observed at al-Azhar University, was a figure who struggled daily with contestations over Islamic authority. He was part of a small elite dedicated to reviving the "traditional Islamic curriculum" *(al-manhaj al-Islami)*. He was usually at the Azhar mosque in Old Cairo by sunrise, where he began his workday by sitting cross-legged on the carpeted floor surrounded by young students, male and female, whom he would ask to read aloud from classical texts of jurisprudence, classical Arabic grammar, or Sufi philosophy of worship, intermittently adding his explication and interpretation. The students explained to me that these are the classical texts that require a *shaykh fattah*, a scholar who can "open" the meaning of the texts in a small face-to-face setting, something that cannot be achieved through the "modern" curriculum established in the secularized and nationalized lecture halls of al-Azhar University.[38]

Shaykh ʿAmr was able to articulate the dominant views of the traditionalist Azhar scholars and present them in a way that was accessible to those foreign to that education. For this reason, I attended several of his classes during the course of my fieldwork and listened attentively while he captured his audience by stressing the value of regaining a sense of the inner beauty and wisdom of the Muslim scholarly traditions. Occasionally street beggars would wander into the lesson and interrupt with an outburst, and Shaykh ʿAmr would calm them with a litany of blessings and direct them to one of the mosque caretakers responsible for charitable cases. He would severely chastise any student who exhibited annoyance at the interruptions of the beggars, reminding them of their duties of acting out of compassion and patience toward those less fortunate.

Always at least a half a dozen students vied for Shaykh ʿAmr's attention after the lesson. After several days of unsuccessfully attempting to make my way through them, Shaykh ʿAmr saw that I was trying to approach him. He brushed the more assertive students aside and beckoned me so that I might come forth and ask my question.

"Organ transplantation?" Upon hearing me utter these two words, he nodded seriously. This was a question that had become one of those "contemporary issues" *(qadaya muʿasara)* about which all the students and scholars at al-Azhar were well-versed and opinionated. I was curious about how Shaykh ʿAmr would respond, for he constantly cautioned against those "hard-headed" elements of Muslim society who feel as if they have the right to spout religious opinions without proper training or scholarship. He had harsh words for those who think of Islam as rigid and inflexible. He lectured constantly about the genius of the Islamic jurisprudential tradition, which looks at every case from several angles to assess the utmost spiritual benefit for the community. He pointed out that one of the bases of Islamic

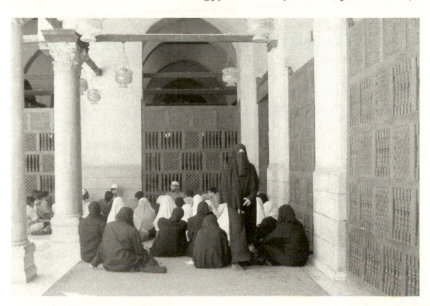

Figure 5. An early morning class in Islamic jurisprudence at al-Azhar Mosque, Old Cairo. Photograph by the author.

jurisprudence is that any act is assumed to be *halal* (permissible) unless proven otherwise by revealed texts or legal reasoning, and he lamented that "ignorant extremists" operate from the reverse premise: assuming that all is *haram* unless they can find evidence of permission in the Qur'an, in the traditions of the Prophet, or in those of the early Muslim community.

Out of modesty, Shaykh 'Amr would never look directly at me, and yet I still felt his piercing gaze somehow, holding me to high expectations: "You will present this research abroad. But you will have to study it carefully first, gathering all the different perspectives. I will not prejudice you now with *my* opinion. I want you to read all the texts, to hear from everyone." He then jotted down a list of citations for me to pursue.

I followed Shaykh 'Amr's suggestions and read many of the scholarly texts, during which time I continued to research this issue in medical clinics among patients and doctors in the Nile Delta cities of Tanta and Mansoura. I also intermittently attended some of Shaykh 'Amr's classes on the days that I was in Cairo. More than a year after this initial conversation with him, I approached him and again posed my question. I was still curious to know what he thought and whether he would tell me. He paused in contemplation. Then he said, "Your topic necessarily proposes a philosophical question about the ontology of the body and its relationship to its Creator. . . .

So you must begin your work with a discussion of basic philosophical questions.[39] When you see this, you will have the right framework to understand everything."

Taking out a pen and pad from the upper pocket of his *galabiyya* (an ankle-length dress shirt), he drew a circle with a dot in the center: "This dot and the circle represent the relationship of the human being with his Creator. This is the relationship of 'abudiyya [slavery/worship/utter submission]. Everything a human does is within the bounds of this relationship."[40]

By then I had attended enough of his lessons and had researched this topic long enough to understand what Shaykh 'Amr meant. The specifics of organ transplantation in and of themselves were hardly relevant to Shaykh 'Amr; more pressing for him was what this medical practice represented more broadly and how it interfaced with a larger "Islamic worldview" *(manzur islami)*. Shaykh 'Amr was implicitly complicating the logic of proponents of organ transplantation, who have argued that it is permissible in Islam to donate or receive a human body part because it "saves lives" and therefore fulfills criteria for *maslaha*—the attainment of overall social benefit, or welfare. *Maslaha* is a tool of Islamic jurisprudence that has served as a cornerstone for modernist scholars who seek to bring various modern practices into accord with Islamic thought, arguing that anything that serves the greater social community is therefore permissible in Islam (Krawietz 1997; Skovgaard-Petersen 1997; Dallal 2000; Johnston 2004). Yet for Muslims, Shaykh 'Amr stressed, the premise and end of *maslaha* is not the human being. It is the human-Creator relationship.[41] Thus, he argued that we should not ask if something serves our interests without also asking if it serves our relationship with God.

Shaykh 'Amr explained that the main challenge is to ascertain which aspects of modern knowledge are useful and coincide with "the Islamic framework" *(al-itar al-islami)*. He asked whether organ transplantation *necessarily* portends a different ontological understanding of the human body, one that lies outside an Islamic framework. Does the act of donating or receiving a body part necessitate a particular attitude toward one's relationship with God? Does organ transplantation, for example, necessitate an understanding of the body as a mere mass of parts? Or can organ transplantation be used merely as a technique that can be reworked and resignified, given different meanings depending on its various applications and contexts?

Shaykh 'Amr's well-reasoned questions seem worlds away from the predicaments of end-stage kidney-failure patients in the Tanta dialysis wards. He believed that if we were all certain about our place within God's plans of

Creation and servitude, then none of these "contemporary" questions would be ethically vexing. Yet, among the Egyptian public, doctors, and patients, and especially among interlocutors in the Egyptian media, questions about organ transplantation *have been* quite troubling. Religious discourse in Egypt is marked by schisms in understanding issues of moral responsibility, the acceptance of God's will, and, as detailed in the next chapter, the role of the dead body. But scholars like Shaykh 'Amr are in consensus that one must, in any case, assess to what extent any given procedure is beneficial when considering its ethics. For this assessment they have turned to the doctors. But the doctors too have been in disagreement among themselves.

CONCLUSIONS

Biomedical authority remains *the* national medicine of Egypt; no other medical traditions are given credence in dominant state discourses related to health.[42] Similarly, religion is *the* code of ethics that Egyptians say they turn to when in doubt about a particular practice.[43] But this agreement on the source of knowledge about bodies and ethics has not led to uniform positions on the human body or to a singular form of moral reasoning. Religious scholars, medical practitioners, politicians, the media, and patients in Egypt are in disagreement over the efficacy, safety, religious permissibility, and legality of organ transplantation.

Debate continues over which field of expertise should be given the most weight and, even more fundamentally, over who qualifies as an expert. There is much discomfort with the increased (com)modification of bodies and the privatization of medicine, as well as the significant demographic change that the medical profession has undergone, now representing the interests of a wider array of social classes, religious dispositions, and geographic origins.[44] Discourses surrounding cornea transplantation in the 1950s did not refer to Islamic reasoning or fatwas, whereas those in the 1980s with kidney transplantation did so as a matter of course. Public religious discourse in the contemporary Middle East should not be taken as a fixed measure of religious sentiment writ large (Bouzid 1998). It ebbs and flows according to the strategies and exigencies of political players, namely, the state and its critics.

In describing patients, physicians, and religious scholars who launch criticism of the state, medical authority, and the pronouncements of religious officiates, I am discussing a much broader swath of Egyptian society than Cairo's "counterpublic" (Hirschkind 2006). With this term, anthropologist

Charles Hirschkind refers to people in Egypt associated with social movements galvanized by preachers who are outside state official positions and who promote greater religiosity in everyday life through the circulation of decentralized media, such as cassette sermons. Those devoted to listening to these sermons as a practice in moral edification work to cultivate dispositions that they imagine to be essentially "Islamic," contra the pressures of modernity, nationalism, and secularization (Hirschkind 2006). Many of those whose stories inform my work were also wary of falling into godlessness, but at the same time they were fully indoctrinated in the ideas of "modern progress" and felt the need for Egypt to "catch up to the West." Many questioned the relevance of Islamic authorities' pronouncements about medical science and at the same time sought confirmation that their medical decisions were in line with Muslim ethics. These are people who straddled the line between state-oriented discourses and new forms of religious revivalism; many held multiple and seemingly contradictory positions, depending on which of their many roles—as workers or patients, as family members or religious devotees—they were foregrounding at any given time.

At one point in my fieldwork I attended a public outreach campaign relating to eyesight at which a medical assistant harshly scolded the rural peasants for their "ignorant" beliefs about the "body belonging to God," arguing that in a matter of days bodily tissues would be eaten by worms and that it was their duty to donate the eyes of their dead for cornea transplantation. Upon my private questioning of him later, he told me that as someone who came from a humble rural background, he was completely opposed to transplantation in all forms and believed that the body, as God's creation, was not something to exchange, cut up, and meddle with. In his position in the public health campaign, however, he could engage with only one vocabulary, which I suspect he may have also partly believed.

Throughout my study, I also encountered religious scholars who might have been appointed by the state and yet who were critical of it, transplant surgeons who worried about the ethics of their practice, and patients who both trusted and mistrusted medical authority. Some people turned to the market in organs while articulating their disgust with it. Doctors poked fun at patients' fears that they might need all their body parts in the afterlife and simultaneously felt uncomfortable with the idea of parting with their own organs. Deep ambivalences seem to be intrinsic to organ transplantation wherever it is practiced, putting its medical practitioners and patients in contradictory positions (Fox and Swazey 1974; Joralemon 1995; Sharp 1995, 2006; Scheper-Hughes 1996, 2000; Lock 2002a, 2002b; Crowley-Matoka and Lock 2006). Biomedicine, as powerful and as pervasive as it

has become, is never fully totalizing of our ideas about bodies, em'
life, and death.

And at this historical moment in Egypt, a shifting social landscape ⸻
rendered medical authority even less certain. Broad changes in economic
and social policies, in rural and urban demography, and in the dramatic
escalation of public religious discourse have yielded rapidly shifting social
norms. Patients I spoke with often simultaneously articulated their hopes
for biomedical intervention and criticism of its false promises. As forthcoming chapters detail, this plurality of patients' experiences, opinions,
and perspectives is too often ignored, in part because of the assumption
that there should be a singular truth in matters of religion and science.
The cacophony of expert opinion also ignores the perpetuation of social
inequalities through biomedical intervention. In the next chapter I explore
how the impetus to locate a single moment of death and to codify a single
"truth" about the human body comes up against the necessarily multiple
and messy realities of bodily demise and the end of human life.

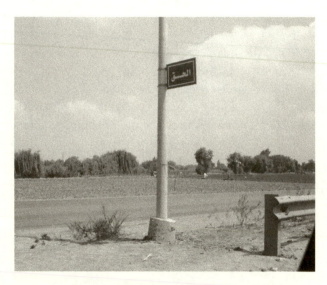

Figure 6. Agricultural Highway between Cairo and Tanta.
Many patients diagnosed as brain-dead are victims of auto-
mobile accidents. Ninety-nine signposts are located along
this highway in Egypt, each one spelling out one of the
ninety-nine *asma' allah al husna* (the divine attributes),
also known as "the beautiful names of Allah." This one
reads "Al-Haqq" (The Truth). Photograph by the author.

2. Defining Death

When the Experts Disagree

Shortly after Egypt's first kidney transplant, doctors sought legislation to initiate a national program for organ transplantation, like those established in other countries, to regulate the procurement of organs from both living and dead donors. But opponents to the proposed legislation insisted that the "cadaveric sources" for organ transplants were in fact dying patients, not yet cadavers. This claim formed a major obstacle to the passage of a bill. The already thorny question about the rights and ownership of deceased bodies was now further complicated as doctors and others began to ask who counted as "really" dead.

This chapter details the arguments among religious scholars and doctors over the status of brain-dead patients. By unpacking the intricacies of their arguments, I examine why the debate about brain death has remained unresolved for so long, as the various voices involved have continued to misunderstand their points of disagreement. Legislators, in taking up these questions, have depended on a religious "stamp of approval" for organ procurement from the official state muftis, and yet the muftis have been influenced by disagreements among doctors about the definition of death. Without resolution on whether organs can be legitimately harvested from cadaveric sources, patients in organ failure have continued to face the predicament of whether or not to seek a living donor.

When it comes to medicine-related fatwas in contemporary Egypt, religious scholars generally defer to the doctors, even when, ironically, it is the doctors who solicit the fatwas. And the fatwas issued are often based upon information that the physicians give to the religious scholars. This circular production of knowledge between the religious and medical realms generally works to resolve bioethical questions through the "doctors of confidence," as discussed in the last chapter. By the 1990s, physicians and the official religious scholars of Egypt reached consensus on the ethics of most of the questions raised by organ transplantation. They decided that a family member *can* ethically donate a kidney but that it is wrong to buy or sell one. And they agreed that a person *can* voluntarily bequeath organs upon death.

In the case of brain death, however, fatwas and medical opinions have swirled in *circuits of doubt*. The mechanism for issuing a medical fatwa for the entire nation within the confines of the Egyptian state bureaucracy necessitates a singularist vision that does not account for differences of opinion among the medical scientists or practicing physicians. The assumption underlying the state-institutionalized practice of fatwa giving is that the experts will speak in a unified voice. Yet, to date, no such voice has come forth.

The story of Egypt's brain-death problem begins with Shaykh Gad al-Haqq, who was the grand mufti of the republic when doctors first began to organize a proposed transplant program in the 1970s. When directly asked about the problem, he stated that the brain is but one of many parts of the body; its cessation does not necessarily indicate the death of the entire person. A group of physicians, led by a certain Dr. Safwat Lotfy, further cast doubt on the soundness of the category "brain death," arguing in terms of medical science that life persists after the cessation of brain function. In the 1990s, frustrated proponents for an organ transplant law sought a new fatwa and turned to Shaykh Muhammad Sayyid Tantawi, the rector of al-Azhar and the former mufti of the republic, in the hopes that his ruling would be more sympathetic to their aims. Tantawi, upon being asked whether it is permissible in Islamic law to procure organs from heartbeating, brain-dead patients, stated simply that this question is "medical, and not religious."[1] Physicians had full authority over this issue, he claimed, and Islamic legal scholars had no business getting involved. But Lotfy and his group betrayed disagreements within the medical profession, causing some religious scholars who had earlier permitted cadaveric organ procurement to revise their positions. The doctors' medical arguments also prompted another important religious voice, that of Shaykh ʿAli Gumaʿa, the current grand mufti, to question the legitimacy of brain death criteria for determining complete death.

Laying out these arguments requires disentangling them from the ways in which they have been framed in legislative debates and in the media hype surrounding the debates. The chapter concludes by juxtaposing the reluctance to accept brain death criteria in Egypt alongside muted reservations about cadaveric procurement in Euro-American countries. In this juxtaposition, I expose the inadequacies of culturalist analyses that deepen the imagined divide between the Muslim world and the West.

ENCOUNTERING THE BRAIN DEAD

Brain-dead patients are generally the victims of accidents in which major injury to the brain has occurred, leaving respiration and heartbeat to continue only with the support of medical technologies, including the artificial ventilator (Lock 2002a, 2002b: 1).[2] The idea that brain death should be equated with the death of the person was explicated in the United States in 1968 in a report by the Ad Hoc Committee of the Harvard Medical School to Examine the Definition of Death. In proposing a new definition of death, the committee responded to two new developments in medicine: the use of the ventilator to mechanically maintain the heartbeat and respiration of a brain-dead patient for an indefinite period of time, and the growing recognition of the need to transplant organs that would no longer be useful once "conventional" cardiopulmonary death had set in (Lock 2002a, 2002b; Crowley-Matoka and Lock 2006; Sharp 2006). This redefinition inspired discussion among medical experts and bioethicists and shaped legislation in the United States over the course of the next decade. As organ transplantation developed globally, the redefinition of death led to controversy in other countries as well, perhaps most notably in Japan, where the brain-death problem was discussed exhaustively in the national media, comprising Japan's most contentious ethical debate of the last thirty years (Lock 2002b:3).

Brain-dead patients are, as Margaret Lock has put it, "betwixt and between"—warm to the touch, yet unable to breathe spontaneously (Lock 2002a, 2002b). They appear to hover eerily between life and death, dependent on an assembly of machines, which also, in the case of the heart monitor, attest to their continuous heartbeat. Despite the urgency to pass a national organ transplant law in Egypt, the more that clinicians have studied and experienced the strange status of brain-dead patients, the more divided they have become over what precisely to do with them.

Dr. Ahmad, the chief resident in anesthesiology and intensive care at a public hospital in Tanta, is an example of someone confounded by brain-dead patients. According to Dr. Faten, who is his mother and also his medical colleague, his confusion over how to treat them is the reason for his disquiet and moodiness. Dr. Faten, who is a clinical pathologist, told me:

> He was not always like this!
> He only got this bad temper after his work in the ICU . . . it is terrible there. They have the patients on the machines, and the families in the hallways crying and wailing and wanting to take them home. And they have to tell them that they can't take their relatives home, because once they take them off the machine, they will die.

And the family is upset, and the attending physicians are always yelling. . . . Once, about five patients in the ICU died around the same time, and the attending physicians were screaming at the residents, and the families were screaming at the residents, and they didn't know what to do. Since that day my son [who was one of the residents] has developed a very bad temper.

With furrowed brow, Dr. Ahmad himself told me about his training in the ICU with patients on life support. He described the different attending physicians as battling out their moral positions, often to the confusion of the residents and to the detriment of the patients. "You see it a lot of times," Dr. Ahmad told me.

A patient is brain-dead, on life support, and all of a sudden his heart stops. And the attending physician says, "Fast! Start CPR!"

And you are about to, and then another attending physician says, "*Haram 'alayk!* [Shame on you!] Can't you see that he wants to die? Be merciful and let him die!"

And the other one says, "*Haram 'alayk!* Don't just leave him there to die!" And you are left not knowing what to do.

Placing his shaking head between his hands, Dr. Ahmad said, "Even now, I still don't know the right thing to do."

As medical students, they had no problem accepting what they were taught in lectures, namely, that brain death is the total death of the individual and that this is a "technical, scientific matter." But upon clinical experience in the intensive care unit, several medical residents with whom I spoke, like Dr. Ahmad, felt ill-equipped to confront and settle ambiguous cases of patients who teeter on the border of life and death.

Dr. Nuha, a resident in internal medicine in Tanta, told me about a case involving a twenty-three-year-old woman on a ventilator in the ICU, who had been on life support for five months:

Of course during these five months, other patients have needed the ventilator. But to take her off? I don't know. This is an issue that I myself don't know. The decision is so hard, even though she is brain-dead. . . . Her family started to understand that she is living because of the machine, that if she is taken off, she will die. But just by her being there, they feel better emotionally. She is only twenty-three. Her lungs spontaneously collapsed and caused her respiration to fail. We resuscitated her, and she came back, but on a ventilator.

When I asked her if she thought the patient should have been on the respirator all this time, Dr. Nuha answered:

This is a really hard question; I can't reach an answer. I don't know. It's like making a decision about whether a patient should die. It is very difficult, and I think no one can make it except her family. If that decision could be made by us, I think she would have been disconnected a long time ago. But the family didn't ask for her disconnection. They know that she'll never wake up, that's been told to them, but they are okay with the situation. They have never asked for disconnection. . . . I think it's hard for them to understand brain death. . . . I think they think she is in a deep coma or something and might wake up.

When relating details about the family's hopes despite the young patient's grim prognosis, Dr. Nuha was in tears. She had a difficult time reconciling the family's seeming acceptance of their daughter's status and their hopes for a miracle. She told me that Islam should provide the answer to all of these ethical questions, but at the same time she did not always know what the right balance is when considering the lives of her patients. "But religion and medicine should always go together," she said. "The knowledge of one leads to more knowledge of the other."

Both Dr. Ahmad and Dr. Nuha encountered brain-dead patients in the Tanta hospital only as *living patients* and never as potential sources for organs. Their respective specialties, as an anesthesiologist and an internist in Tanta, did not place them as squarely in the debate about the passage of a law permitting organ harvesting. When I asked them if they thought these patients could ethically be sources for organs, neither was able to answer.

In contrast, many of the physicians who did have a working relationship with transplantation—nephrologists, urologists, liver surgeons, vascular surgeons, and ophthalmologists—did not have much clinical experience with patients categorized as brain-dead. I spoke with several Egyptian physicians who had witnessed for the first time the procurement of organs from brain-dead patients during their fellowships abroad in Europe or in North America. These physicians had mixed reactions to what they had seen. They returned to Egypt as "native ethnographers" in a sense, trying to explain what specifically about Egyptian society precludes what has become routine abroad.[3] One nephrologist-urologist working in Tanta University Hospital explained to me, in outrage, the way that brain-dead patients were treated in an American hospital where he had trained under a fellowship:[4] "Their hearts are still beating; they are still breathing. They don't turn off the machine. And they split him open and take from him what they want. They crack open the rib cage and pull out the heart while it is beating! *I seek refuge in God!* What do they think this is? A lamb to be slaughtered?! We treat our animals better than that!"

Another physician, a heart surgeon who worked for many years in Germany, told me that he too had been greatly disturbed when he observed the surgical procurement of the heart while it was still beating. He looked at me intently and told me that he was willing to swear before God that the soul of the person was still present in the brain-dead body. While working in the German hospital, he explained to his senior attending physicians that his religion prohibited him from participating in such operations. He was both surprised and relieved to find that his German colleagues respected his request to abstain from organ procurement.[5]

Dr. Mustafa, an ophthalmologist, described what he witnessed while working abroad in a French hospital: "After they took all the organs and the machine was turned off, then they would also take the corneas. The first things they would take were the lungs, kidney, and the heart, *all before they turned off the machine.*"

When I asked him what he thought about this, he replied, "I think this is *haram*, because they should be really dead. In our religion we can't allow this, because the soul is still there. He is still breathing, and his heart is still beating. We can't say, "Let's take him off now." This issue is different for Egypt from what it is in Europe and the United States. For us, he has to be *really* dead."

For Dr. Mustafa, a different ontological understanding of the soul and death characterizes practice in Euro-American countries. But this was not the only difference; he also noted that the higher standard of care and cleaner environment in those countries have enabled brain-dead patients to survive long enough for it to be thinkable that their organs should be taken and used elsewhere:

> In Europe, they can leave him like that for up to six months. There the patients won't get bedsores or anything, because the nursing is so good. The standard of care is so high that they have the ability to keep them for that long. . . . They are very clever abroad in the ICU, so people who are brain-dead or in vegetative states can survive for a long time. . . .
>
> Here there is a lot of [environmental] stress, and the patient gets infections and dies quickly. We have a very, very, very small number of cases where the patients can live for months and up to one year in a coma. Because of the bad care and high rate of infection, the patients die. Abroad they can get people to live much longer, so they can use their organs for transplant.

Dr. Mustafa thus contrasted the relative wealth, resources, and sterile environment of European hospitals with the harsher conditions and "environmental stress" in Egyptian biomedical clinics, noting that this discrepancy bears important ethical implications for understanding the issue of brain death.

Indeed, ethnographic research has shown that North American intensive care specialists do worry about their brain-dead patients potentially existing for a prolonged period "on machines," in limbo, between life and death (Lock 2002a, 2002b). Those involved with organ procurement in North America have stated that being definitively killed through organ procurement would be better than remaining technologically trapped for an indefinite period of time (Lock 2002a, 2002b).[6] The fear of lingering near death and "on machines" is much less common in Egypt, in part because most people still die outside the hospital and because death is not as technologically or clinically managed (Kaufman and Morgan 2005). For Dr. Mustafa, a scarcity of resources spares Egyptians from developing what he considers to be unethical practices toward end-of-life patients, because they are less likely to survive long enough for their organs to be harvested before complete (cardiopulmonary) death.

REDEFINING DEATH

As my conversations with Dr. Ahmad and Dr. Nuha illustrate, even short of the question of organ procurement, a great deal of uncertainty and clinical inconsistency already exists in treating brain-dead patients in Egypt. Doctors have no clear consensus on whether they should remove patients from life support, whether they should initiate CPR when patients' mechanically assisted hearts stop beating, and whether CPR is a show of heroic persistence or an exercise in medical futility. Is it ultimately callous or more merciful to allow them to die? The possibility of using these patients as sources for organs has only exacerbated these dilemmas.

The first public attempts to clarify whether brain-dead patients can ethically be used as sources of organs in Egypt took place in 1979, when legislators sought to organize a national transplant program. It occurred to a young legal scholar that physicians, in pushing for organ transplantation, were redefining what can and cannot be done to the body and where the boundary between life and death is. The young legal scholar sent in a lengthy, eight-part question to the grand mufti of the republic, asking for Islamic legal perspectives on the permissibility of organ extraction, from living, dead, and brain-dead patients.[7] By bypassing medical debate and addressing the mufti directly, he seemed unaware of the ways in which physicians, too, were concerned about what Islamic legal ethics had to say about new medical practices.

As I discussed in the Introduction, the late 1970s and early 1980s in Egypt saw a period of rapid transformation in the role of Islamic discourses in the public and political spheres. Under Sadat, in 1971, Constitutional Amendment 1(2) stipulated, "Islam is the religion of the state; Arabic is the official language; and the principles of Islamic shari'a are a principal source of legislation." In 1980, this was changed to "*the* principal source." Sadat's regime initiated a delicate balance in claiming to operate under modern secular law while also claiming that Islam guided this law.[8]

On the one hand, the new regime catered to increased popular concerns about ruling in "Islamically ethical ways." But on the other hand, the state was unable to convince the public fully that it had legitimately co-opted Islamic authority. Many political "Islamic-oriented" groups *(al-tiyar al-islami)*, such as the Muslim Brotherhood, held little appreciation for state-appointed religious scholars and even, more broadly, for elite Islamic scholarship and formal religious training. With little or no formal religious education, members of these groups felt that they could teach themselves what they needed to know about Islam (Eickelman 1992, 2000; Skovgaard-Petersen 1997; Eickelman and Anderson 2003).[9]

The grand mufti, a position appointed by the president, has stood in an uneasy position as both state employee and representative of Islamic scholarship and rulings within the state bureaucracy. Particularly since the 1970s, with the semiliberalization of opposition parties, their newspapers, and the increased circulation of media that were outside the direct control of the state, the grand mufti has become an easy target of attacks and suspicions that he is merely a "government functionary" who will give anything an "Islamic veneer" to legitimize state aims (Skovgaard-Petersen 1997). As social historian Skovgaard-Petersen argues:

> The Islamist movement presents a threat to *'ulama* [religious scholars'] authority in religious matters, and the man who is increasingly [since the 1970s] targeted is the State Mufti.
> Since he has to pronounce the position of Islam on all new inventions and ideas, hardly any initiative or idea of Islamization is introduced before someone asks the Mufti about the matter. And in many cases there is no middle way; either he must confirm the Islamists' claim that the old order is un-Islamic [and thus legitimate their aims at Islamization], or he must come up with some impressive fatwa that supports the government. (Skovgaard-Petersen 1997: 226)

Notably, not all people interested in *the* Islamic stance on a particular question hold such cynical views toward the mufti. Many appeal to the mufti for religious guidance and with the hope that he would bring state laws closer to Islamic principles of justice.[10] The young legal scholar who initiated the request for an official fatwa on organ donation in 1979 expressed concerns about the proposals submitted by Egyptian physicians to initiate an organ donation program similar to those established in Western countries. He stated in his request for a fatwa that he "wanted to facilitate their humanitarian goals [in helping dying patients] but feared that there may be some contravention to religious principles or improper treatment of the human body." He assumed that Egyptian physicians had relied on Euro-American ethics in their justifications of a new definition of death, the treatment of patients on life support, the cutting into bodies after death, and the possibilities of allowing the donors of kidneys to receive compensation for their "sacrifice." The legal questioner wondered if Islamic jurisprudence might have something different to say.

The grand mufti at the time was Shaykh Gad al-Haqq 'Ali Gad al-Haqq (d. 1996), who had been appointed by Sadat in the previous year.[11] He issued a complex response to the eight-part question, which became an influential ruling on organ donation for subsequent fatwas of other Muslim Arab countries.[12] Shaykh Gad al-Haqq argued that because the preservation of life is an overwhelming principle in Islam, dire necessity, in the case of a dying patient, overrides what is otherwise forbidden—that is, cutting into and extracting a body part of another person, living or dead. Trustworthy medical authorities—the doctors of confidence—would have to guarantee that the would-be recipient was in a dire medical situation and that the donor had consented before his death. Like earlier-issued fatwas allowing for autopsy, the mufti's official 1979 fatwa indicated that extracting organs from the dead may be permissible in the case of overwhelming need and benefit. Also, the mufti stipulated that the donor *could not be financially compensated*, because the human body is outside the purview of market transactions.[13]

Despite these fatwas, the argument that it is *necessarily* sinful to cut into the dead held much sway with the public.[14] At this time, in the late 1970s, the only organ transplant operations publicly known in Egypt involved the kidney, which had proceeded from *living* donors. The fatwa stating that organs can be legitimately taken from the dead thus facilitated the development of various transplant initiatives and was regarded as permissive, exonerating the plans of the physicians. The doctors of confidence had to establish that, in the case of a living donor, he would not be harmed by the operation or by the extraction of his body part.

But what about the fatwa's stance on brain death?[15] The mufti specified that no body part can be taken from a dead person until his death. In the text of the fatwa, Gad al-Haqq wrote, clearly in response to the medical profession's insistence that it can define death by measuring brain activity:

> There is nothing to forbid the use of medical equipment to establish the death of the nervous system, but this is not the only indication of death; rather, the end of all life signs [is what confirms death].
>
> The continuation of breathing and heart beating and heart function is an indication of life. If medical equipment confirms the loss of nervous system function specifically, this is just one system of the body, and a human being is not considered dead when *one part* of his body loses life . . . for death is the loss of *all* signs of life [emphasis added].

Life, in this view, is animated by the soul, which is *not* discretely located in the brain. The brain is just one part of the body, Gad al-Haqq argued, as are other parts that can also cease to function while the person is still alive. Much of Islamic philosophy has, indeed, drawn on the concept of the heart *(al-qalb)* as the metaphysical seat of the soul, mind, and body. And much of Arabic poetry extols the liver *(al-kabad)* as the center of vitality and strength. On this basis, reconciling a beating, functioning heart—and other vital organs—with the death of the person and the departure of the soul is counter-intuitive.

At the time (in 1979), this fatwa did not cause much legal or medical controversy. Its major practical effect was to declare permissible the available forms of organ transplantation. It established that body parts can ethically be taken from living donors (in the case of kidneys) and from corpses (in the case of eyes) for the purpose of transplantation. Yet after kidney and liver lobe transplantation from living donors had taken off in Egypt's major hospitals, and the black market in organs in Egypt's major cities was growing intransigent, proponents of organ transplantation, including doctors, lawyers, and journalists, reinstigated the debate about brain death in the national press. They were furious that the dispute over brain death—which they at times characterized as a "trivial detail" and at other times as an abstract philosophical question—stood in the way of life-saving operations for patients in organ failure. Proponents of organ transplantation vociferously argued that the fatwa's "obsolete" definition of death as the "loss of all signs of life," taken from earlier sources of Islamic jurisprudence, was hindering the establishment of a national organ transplant program.[16]

In the late 1980s, the next grand mufti, Shaykh Muhammad Sayyid Tantawi, issued his own fatwa about organ transplantation.[17] The official press repeatedly printed his arguments that organ transplantation is permissible and that the definition of death is for medical experts to determine. He stressed that Islamic scholars (including himself) should not interfere in medical issues. Other fatwas issued in the 1990s from international Islamic legal conferences (Majmaʿ al-Fiqh al-Islami), as well as from the Islamic Research Academy (Majmaʿ al-Buhuth al-Islamiyya) in Egypt confirmed Tantawi's position (see Moosa 1999; Krawietz 2003).

However, Shaykh Tantawi faced continued opposition from unofficial religious scholars and commentators in the press who voiced suspicions about organ transplants and brain death criteria. They maintained that Tantawi was nothing more than a state official, using religion to pave the way for government interests to establish more elaborate medical centers that would cater to the elite. Shaykh Gad al-Haqq, in his position as shaykh al-Azhar, did not change his ruling on brain death, and Shaykh Tantawi alone as grand mufti did not have enough authority to make a difference on the floor of the Parliament, where members were themselves polarized over the question.

CONVINCING THE MUFTIS, CONVINCING THE DOCTORS

As the practice of organ transplantation proliferated in Egypt, it became clear to both doctors and the newspaper-reading public that the vast majority of operations had transpired through the local sale of live-donor kidneys. Various investigative reports revealed the abundance of Egyptian "donors" willing to sell their kidneys, the sufficiently desperate renal-failure patients ready to buy them, and the numerous doctors eager to play a role in, and profit from, this new medical practice. Physicians pushing for the initiation of a national cadaveric transplant program argued that those who opposed the procurement from "cadavers" were in a sense responsible for the proliferation of a black market in live-donor organs. The unmet demand for kidneys, established as fact, had to be met by another supply.[18]

And now with two conflicting Islamic scholarly opinions on cadaveric procurement there was even greater debate about organ transplantation. Under the assumption that religious stringency had become the chief obstacle to Egypt's national organ transplant program, proponents of organ transplantation worked hard to convince muftis and other Islamic scholars of the legitimacy of cadaveric procurement. A parallel effort was made in other Muslim Arab countries to "educate" muftis about the medical and scientific realities of brain death. One such effort was initiated by a physician who worked in an organ transplantation center in Kuwait. This physician Dr. Al-Mousawi sent a questionnaire to fifty senior religious scholars in Kuwait, Saudi Arabia, Iran, Egypt, Lebanon, and Oman to gauge their views

mis-information

on the permissibility of organ donation during life and after death, the removal of life support from brain-dead patients, and the buying and selling of organs. Twenty-nine (91 percent) of the thirty-two who replied initially rejected the concept of brain death. Al-Mousawi then met personally with nine scholars to explain brain death to them. Seven out of nine changed their views after this medical explanation.[19] Al-Mousawi concluded on an optimistic note: his little experiment was evidence that proponents of transplant legislation could overcome the "religious obstacle" by merely "educating" religious scholars on the "true" medical meaning and clinical definition of brain death (Al-Mousawi and Al-Matouk 1997).

Ironically, one of the major forces pushing against the medical community's efforts toward Egypt's transplant legislation was not its religious authorities but rather another small group of doctors. Dr. Safwat Lotfy, a senior anesthesiologist and intensive care specialist from Cairo University Faculty of Medicine, had initiated a campaign to convince doctors and religious scholars about the "dangers" of accepting "brain-death" as medical fact. In a personal interview, Lotfy explained to me how he became animated around this issue: he had been appalled upon learning about the practice from reading European and North American medical journals.[20] But his real shock came closer to home after reading that, in 1992, Egyptian surgeons had performed transplant operations using organs from executed prisoners. Presumably, the harvesting had to be done before what Lotfy considered to be "total death." Lotfy eventually formed a group that he called the Egyptian National Medical Ethics Committee (*al-Jama'iyya al-Misriyya li-l Akhlaq-iyyat al-Tibiyya*) with the intention of halting what he considered an inhumane, barbaric, and unethical practice.[21] His use of the term *al-akhlaqiyyat al-tibiyya* was a direct translation of the English term *medical ethics*. Yet rather than establish a scholarly field to study the ethical dimensions of different practices, what Lotfy established was a lobbyist group agitating against the practice of organ transplantation. And whereas formal ethical debates in Egypt were often conducted in terms of religious scholarship—for Muslims, in the field of Islamic jurisprudence *(fiqh)*—Lotfy circumvented the scholars by circumscribing his own "medical ethical" domain.

Like Mousawi, Lotfy described the muftis and other religious scholars as having been "misled." However, Lotfy worked in the opposite direction— he thought the culprits creating confusion among the religious elite were self-interested physicians (like Mousawi) who used deceptive language to argue for the legitimacy of brain-death criteria. He thus spent much of his time "reeducating" the public and his medical colleagues about the category of brain death and influencing the major Egyptian newspapers. Dr. Lotfy and his group generated a large number of reading materials on the issue, much of them from British medical journals, where debates over brain-death criteria are particularly pronounced within anesthesia, Lotfy's profession. He circulated pamphlets and flyers among his medical colleagues, the press, politicians, and Islamic scholars. He wrote his own publications about why the practice was *haram*, and picking up on the popular fervor of Shaykh Sha'rawi's statement (discussed in chapter 4), he premised his arguments on the notion that God alone owns our bodies.

Although he started with this seemingly religious premise, he relied on medicine to argue that insurmountable problems were associated with organ transplantation. For example, he pointed to the lack of any clear established way to prevent recipients from rejecting organs as foreign tissue without pharmaceutically "knocking out" the immune system; Lotfy described this practice as doctors "giving the patients a form of 'artificial AIDS.'" He also argued, from a public health perspective, that the cost of such expensive, highly technological interventions could be better channeled into preventative health measures, like cleaning up the water and land that had predisposed Egyptians to renal and liver failure in the first place. He argued vehemently for why organ transplantation leads to overall harm in society. His more reasonable public health concerns—about access, immunosuppression, and the lack of focus on prevention—got lost in his more hyperbolic statements. Each time a parliamentary committee was scheduled to discuss the question of organ transplantation, Lotfy would submit materials to be reviewed, bearing titles such as "Essential Information about the Most *Dangerous* Issue to Appear before Egyptian Legislation!!!"

One such pamphlet written by Safwat Lotfy in 1996, addressed to "My fellow doctor and Muslim brother," urged doctors to reconsider the ethical implications of organ procurement. Focusing on brain-dead patients, the pamphlet ominously reminded the doctors that they would soon stand before God on the Day of Judgment and be held to account. While the original pamphlet offers a hodgepodge of fifteen scary questions for doctors to consider, I have re-sorted his points here into four major categories of argument, for analytical clarity. The first argument Lotfy makes is that the concept of brain death is an "invention" to facilitate organ transplantation and that the patients are not truly dead. In his words:

> Can we consider a "concept" to be the same as a "fact"? How can the concept of brain death be considered the same as the fact and certitude of death, which is defined by God? The certitude of death is what humans have known for centuries, whereas the concept of brain death is a recent invention by doctors less than a quarter of a century ago.

Doesn't it seem suspicious that this brain-death concept is defined by different criteria according to different countries and even from state to state within the same country?

For those who think brain-stem death is a true category, I ask: can truths differ according to a person's age? Many countries' protocols warn against applying the brain-stem death category to children under the age of five, as do many medical references . . . because of scientific studies showing that children have an amazing capacity to recover from major brain damage after long-term medical care.

Even if the diagnosis of brain-stem death does mean that the patient is in a state close to death, is this justification for harvesting his organs? The answer, my Muslim brother, is that the concept of brain-stem death was concocted merely as a justification for the procurement of organs.

If patients diagnosed as brain-stem dead are really dead, then why do protocols require the use of anesthesia and muscle relaxants during the procurement of organs? The answer, my Muslim brother and doctor, is clear: brain-stem-dead patients are capable of movement, for example, in their limbs flailing [as though] attempting to defend themselves against their organs being harvested.

They also make attempts to breathe, their blood pressure rising, their heartbeats accelerating, their levels of adrenaline and hormones increasing . . . the same signs that happen if any patient is not given enough anesthesia; this has resulted in organ procurement teams needing psychological care, because they are told that these patients are dead although they clearly express signs of life.

One of the indications of the presence of a soul in life is its body temperature. Many brain-stem-dead patients suffer from infections of their lungs or kidneys, and they develop fevers: how could a dead person develop a fever?!

The soul, a matter solely for God, exalted and sublime, animates the rest of the body and keeps it from decomposition. If a person has died and his soul has left his body we would see that: (1) his body gets cold; (2) all of his bodily functions stop working; (3) his body begins to decompose. The question is: do these three conditions apply to the brain-stem-dead patient? The answer, of course, is no.

Lotfy's argument that death has been redefined by brain criteria to justify the procurement of organs is, in fact, not contested among international bioethicists and historians. This is Lotfy's strongest point and the one that most closely aligns with Shaykh Gad al-Haqq's position that the death of the brain does not necessarily equate with the death of the entire person. In his official fatwa, Gad al-Haqq had clearly stated that the dying patient— even one whose condition is *irreversibly* heading toward death—should simply not be treated as though he were already dead. For Gad al-Haqq, death is a divine sign calling on people to remember the sanctity of life and the ultimate return to the divine. Death in this framework has its own purpose and meaning outside the utilitarian logic of organ shortages and the impetus to "recycle" life (see also Sharp 2006).

Upon careful reading of Lotfy's material, we can see how he capitalizes on the tensions between the religious and the medical treatments of death and sensationalizes the deep-rooted ambivalence around brain death along the lines of a "clash of civilizations." They in the secular godless West, he implies, don't care about the status of the soul. We as Muslims must. These arguments resonate with the above-mentioned narratives and experiences of the physicians who had trained in Europe and North America.

Once Lotfy has reeled his readers in by demonstrating inconsistencies in medical practice toward brain-dead patients, he moves toward less solid arguments. In contending with the fact that his medical colleagues in other countries have already, for years, been procuring organs from brain-dead patients, he goes on to claim that these doctors have been improperly hastening the patient's death in an act akin to murder:

> Can the role of the intensive care unit doctor change from extreme care of the patient and a fight for his survival to hastening his death?
> Should the time of death for the brain-stem patient be decided by God, most exalted and high, or by doctors? My fellow Muslim brother and colleague: I leave this question to your conscience to answer.
> If the brain-stem-dead patient's family members refuse to take him off the artificial respirator for the harvesting of his organs, are you capable, Muslim physician, of taking him off the artificial respirator yourself and issuing a death certificate for his burial?
> When the brain-stem-dead patient's heart finally stops beating, can all the scientists of the earth gather to return life to him? Can they make the organs [that had been working while the brain-dead patient was on a ventilator] return by reconnecting him to the machine? Can they now stop this body from decomposing?

Lotfy states that by prematurely declaring patients dead, doctors usurp the rightful command of God. If doctors cannot make their dead patients alive simply by calling them "alive," they similarly cannot claim to make patients dead by merely calling them "dead."

His third, most provocative, argument is that there may be a small, lingering chance that the patient can "come back":

> If a brain-stem dead patient's heart were to stop beating and we doctors perform CPR, is it not possible that the patient's heart would continue to beat? This has led an established anesthesiologist at Cambridge

University to ask: "How many of the patients used for organ harvesting worldwide might have recovered had CPR been continued?"

Can you with absolute certainty attest that those patients defined as "brain-stem dead" will never return to life? The answer, Muslim doctor, is no! Some cases have returned to life, and some others have reverted to persistent vegetative states.

Lotfy labeled transplant legislation as "dangerous" by suggesting that doctors might prematurely take life that could, however small the chance, potentially continue. Those who were more familiar with transplant medicine dismissed his claims in frustration, because one of the basic definitions of brain death is, indeed, the irreversibility of the condition. For those cases of "brain-dead" patients in other countries who had indeed "come back to life," physicians later admitted to diagnostic error.[22] Lotfy points to the troubling circular logic of brain death, which is defined by its irreversibility, such that if any diagnosed cases do later prove to be reversible, they are retrospectively "explained away" as "misdiagnoses."

Lotfy argues, in the same breath, that it is "murder" to procure organs from the brain dead *and* murder to withdraw artificial life support from them. In his view, all medical efforts should be made to keep the patient alive until his heart and lungs give out, because the "irreversibility" of brain death cannot actually be known. His argument to keep all patients on life support is an extreme position within the Egyptian medical profession and also extremely impractical, given that, in their everyday work, medical practitioners face heart-wrenching decisions about the allocation of scarce and expensive resources. In any case, most Egyptian patients strongly prefer to die "naturally" in the home, away from medical technological intervention.

In his argument that patients might "come back," Lotfy's position is distinct from Shaykh Gad al-Haqq's 1979 fatwa that addressed brain-dead patients on life support. Gad al-Haqq did not question the irreversibility of brain death. Whether or not the patient is definitely dying was not the issue for him. Shaykh Gad al-Haqq saw no problem with withdrawing end-of-life treatment. Withdrawal of mechanistic support, Gad al-Haqq argued, facilitates a process already set in place. In fact, he questioned whether the dying patient, on an irreversible path toward death, should be put on life support in the first place. The fatwa even condemned those who continue to prolong the process of dying through the continuation of artificial life support. As Gad al-Haqq wrote in his fatwa, "It is forbidden to cause or prolong suffering to this dying patient by using medical equipment that will do no good to him, as the body is in a state proceeding to death. For this reason it is not wrong to stop the artificial ventilator if the medical expert knows that the patient is in an irreversible process toward death." For the mufti, then, the goal should be to treat the process of death with humility, respect, and awe, not to question whether it is actually taking place.[23]

Further, Mufti Gad al-Haqq did not hold Lotfy's view that, by diagnosing a patient as on an irreversible path toward death, the doctor "usurps" the command of God. The mufti did not believe that the diagnosis of imminent death was outside the purview of medical expertise. And he also did not hold Lotfy's view that death needed to be overcome at all costs. Mufti Gad al-Haqq refused to accept the idea of "brain death" as universal, because he did not view "defeating death" as a universally worthy goal. He insisted that death was inevitable and, indeed, that preparation for death—that is, recognition of our limited time on this earth—should be a primary focus in the struggle to live a virtuous life.

In contrast, Lotfy argued that there was no justification for giving up hope on patients' lives, no matter how dire the circumstances. Lotfy was a thoroughly modern anesthesiologist with biomedical sensibilities through and through; he was not offering a broader critique of medical hubris in the face of death. He invoked the problem of the "slippery slope," often telling people that giving up hope on the brain dead precludes medical researchers from trying to improve their care and finding treatments for them. Lotfy also pointed to the widening eligibility of "dead" organ donors with the increasing global demand for organs. If we take organs from the brain-dead now, he argued, tomorrow we may decide to take them from the comatose or the disabled.

Lotfy's fourth and final argument took him the furthest afield from both the mufti's position and that of the majority of his medical colleagues. He argued that it is unethical to procure organs, even if the patient is completely dead. In clear opposition to earlier official fatwas that allowed for procurement from the dead under conditions of "dire necessity," Lotfy argued that death should be sanctified. The procurement of organs, he maintained, is a clear desacralization of divine property: "Even for the sake of argument, if we were to agree that these patients are really dead, then do we Muslim doctors have the right to procure and harvest their organs?"

Lotfy scoffed at the idea that only official muftis or those with formal Islamic scholarship can pronounce on religious issues, reflecting a more broadly held view among Egyptians. Lotfy claimed to work in the name of Islam and "Islamic ethics," yet he was at the same time little interested in the reasoning and evidence that scholars of Islamic jurisprudence have drawn upon to come to their conclusions. Indeed, Lotfy's own direct appeals to doctors, the newspapers, and the Parliament bypassed the authority of the muftis. He was a rogue scholar with maverick views as compared with both his medical colleagues and with the established religious scholars. In this sense, he represents what political scientist Carrie Wickham has termed the "counter-elite." This shift became apparent in the mid-1980s, when the "Islamic trend" *(al-tiyar al-islami)* took control over professional associations such as the Medical Syndicate, transforming them from "elite institutions with relatively small, privileged memberships into mass institutions marked by sharp generational and class cleavages" (Wickham 2002: 183). Regarding the permissive official state fatwas on organ transplantation as untrustworthy and therefore irrelevant, Lotfy was personally against organ transplantation in all of its forms. He ends his pamphlet with the following:

> The final question is: If we look at all the lively debates that have ensued in different conferences throughout the Muslim world over the question of brain-stem death, we see the hearts of Muslim doctors filled with doubt over this practice, which comprises the murder—or at least something like murder—of those labeled as brain-stem-dead.
>
> The answer right before our eyes is the saying of the Prophet, may God's blessings be upon him: "What is permissible is clear, and what is forbidden is clear, and between these two lies that which is doubtful. Whoever stays away from these is blameless in his religion, and whoever falls into the doubtful has fallen into that which is forbidden." [24]

Though Lotfy's position against organ transplantation in toto was a marginal one in the wider Egyptian Medical Syndicate, his argument about the ambiguity of brain death as a category and its use to justify organ procurement does, indeed, touch on something troubling in contemporary medical practice. Most Egyptian physicians did not believe that organ transplantation *in all forms* should be condemned, even if many of them held ambivalent positions about its more controversial permutations. Yet even those colleagues who were offended by what they characterized as Lotfy's flamboyant and aggressive manner admitted to me that the questions he brought to the surface are disconcerting and raise many legitimate concerns about the category of brain death. His lobbying efforts had a palpable impact in the media, in the Parliament, and among his medical colleagues and religious scholars, so much so that the head of the Medical Syndicate, Hamdi al-Sayyid accused Lotfy and his group of being extremist doctors seeking to draw attention to themselves for personal gain. He did, indeed, succeed in "reeducating" those who had been previously convinced by medical statements that brain death is a valid scientific category based on robust criteria assessing neurological activity.[25] And in these types of arguments, his credentials and status as an attending physician at Cairo's most prestigious medical school and teaching hospital, Kasr el Aini, served him well. Lotfy, as a "medical expert" who argued against the category of brain death as legitimate, convinced several religious scholars to revise their positions after they had stated that it was permissible to donate organs.[26] Several journalists took up the issue and began publishing a series of columns about the artificial invention of this new "clinical death" *(al-mawt al-kliniki)*. Because of the question of brain death, several important parliamentary members remained adamantly against establishing a national organ transplant program that would include cadaveric procurement.[27] In 2001, ultimately unsuccessful initiatives were on the floor, heavily citing Lotfy's materials, to specifically *criminalize* the recognition of brain-dead patients as dead.[28]

BODIES AND SOULS

Lotfy and his group spread doubt among their medical colleagues, raising concerns about the category "brain death" by demonstrating that signs of biological life continue in brain-dead patients. This evidence was not denied among North American and British proponents of brain death, and indeed most of Lotfy's evidence came from North American and British medical journals. The key difference was the interpretation of these biological signs: whether or not they mean that the *person* is "still there." Lotfy assumed the self-evidence of signs of biological life indicating the presence of the person's soul. He argued that intensive care specialists in North America, where this "new death" was "invented," have disingenuously called living patients "dead" in order to facilitate transplantation. In his view, transplantation, a lucrative medical specialty, can profit from dying people who will otherwise be a drain on resources. He saw North American transplant professionals as utilitarian, godless people who have perpetuated a lie, a lie that "people of Islam" must stand against.

But medical practitioners in these countries are not being deceitful about the patients being "actually" dead, because in their terms patients *are* dead. As comparative ethnography in North America and western Europe shows, medical practitioners have come to see brain-dead patients as dead, not by denying signs of biological life, but by reinterpreting them. In Margaret Lock's study of North American intensive care specialists, all recognized that the brain-dead are in a sense still biologically alive.[29] But they argue that the person is located in the brain, and thus the person, soul, or spirit is no longer present in a brain-dead individual, despite the continuance of biological life. Following what Lock has described as the Cartesian mind/body problem permeating Western biomedicine, they argue that in a sense "two deaths" occur: first the person, then the body (Lock 2002a, 2002b: 248).

Dr. Lotfy and Shaykh Gad al-Haqq, in contrast, negated the possibility of a person existing separately from the functions of his or her anatomical body. The soul, in their conception, is what animates biological life. Thus, any sign of biological life is a sign of the presence, even if lingering, of the soul. The vast majority of Egyptian physicians, patients, and Islamic scholars with whom I spoke shared this understanding of the connections among life, soul, and body. And, indeed, these more ambiguous views about the status of the soul and death have also persisted among lay people in North America. As anthropologist Lesley Sharp reports from her study in the United States, surviving family members of dead donors have defined death as the moment of departure of the soul from the body, which, as in Egypt, is thought to coincide with biological death. Thus, family members in the U.S. also talk of their loved ones "dying" at the moment that their organs are procured by surgeons, and not when their brains have stopped functioning (Sharp 2006).

U.S. and European transplant procurement professionals have long assumed that such a confusing "betwixt and between" state (Lock 2002a, 2002b) will discourage surviving kin from consenting to donation. Consequently, like Dr. Al-Mousawi and other transplantation advocates in the Arab world, they have worked hard to stress that brain-dead patients are in fact dead and only deceptively seem alive. As Sharp's (2006) work shows, however, family members of patients in the United States have not always believed this. Perhaps more surprisingly, they also have not necessarily let the idea that their loved ones are "not quite dead" prevent them from consenting to donation. This is partly explained by a general disinclination toward intensive technological management of death and fears that people will be "trapped indefinitely" in states between life and death through high-technological intervention. In this view organ donation can help bring closure to the patient's suffering or to the family's liminal state between anxiety and grief, or to both, by finalizing an inevitable process toward death.

Shaykh Gad al-Haqq and Lotfy both argued, for different reasons, that brain-death criteria, far from being universally applicable, are based on godless disrespect toward human dignity and human life. Yet in the United States, where this "universal" medical practice was instantiated, it appears that, far from being prompted by a disenchanted secularism, transplantation has been driven by the impetus to *sacralize* the dead, albeit in a different form. As anthropologist Lesley Sharp (2006) writes, the U.S. transplant world is driven by paradoxes and "ideological disjunction." Sharp explains, "Whereas transplant recipients are encouraged by hospital staff to depersonalize their new organs and to speak of them in terms that can sometimes even approximate car repair, procurement staff regularly tell donor kin that transplantation enables the donor's essence to persist in others who are thereby offered a second chance at life" (2006: 14). In the United States, a major motivation of donor families has been to "make meaning" out of "senseless loss" or to "make good" come out of a sudden tragedy (Joralemon 1995; Lock 2002a, 2002b; Sharp 2006). Procurement professionals in the United States have encouraged donor kin to "imagine their lost loved ones as living on in donors, their life essence persisting in the bodies of strangers" (Sharp 2001: 114).[30] Thoughts of "transcendence," more so than ideas of the materialist utility of dead bodies, have formed the overriding impetus for organ donation in the United States (Lock 2002a, 2002b; Sharp 2006). The restoration of meaning is located in the idea that a "freed soul" will, through an act of altruistic sacrifice, offer good to the world after tragic loss.

These notions of transcendence, or "recycling life," are muted in U.S. medical discourse on transplantation, which presents itself as a secular science devoid of religion rather than as a rearticulation of religion in a different form. Notions of transcendence were also virtually unintelligible to the wide range of Egyptian patients, doctors, and religious scholars with whom I spoke. When I attempted to explain to them this motivation among American family members, many looked at me incredulously, telling me that it sounded more like Hinduism and reincarnation.

This does not mean that no Egyptian Muslim would ever agree with the notion of organ procurement from brain-dead patients. Those who argued for cadaveric procurement did so from the logic that the patient *was* truly dead, not that the patient's soul might be freed or recycled in the process. They believed that both body and soul must be dead and that it was the ventilator that was *deceptively* showing signs of biological life, much like many lay people's views and those without intimate connection to organ donation in North America and Europe (Lock 2002a, 2002b; Sharp 2006). In Egypt, people do not speak in terms of "making meaning" out of senseless loss or living on, in spirit, in the life of another. They argue instead that the donor will accrue spiritual rewards during his or her time in the grave between death and the Day of Judgment. Thus, while many physicians and legislators have pushed for a national organ transplant program in Egypt on the model of Western countries, they have offered in some instances parallel and in other instances divergent arguments to legitimate organ procurement from the brain dead (Lock 2002a, 2002b; Sharp 2006).

PROPONENTS OF BRAIN DEATH

Dr. Badr, a nephrologist and transplant surgeon in private practice whom I followed, shook his head cynically: "Oh they've made it into a big drama in the Parliament. Those doctor-lobbyists who like to make noise, they go in and say: 'Stop! If you pass this law, then doctors will be killing patients! A brain-dead patient can come back to life!' And then the legislators gasp, 'Oh! Let's stop this law now! They can really come back to life!'" Dr. Badr let out a chortle, "It's nonsense. It's really nonsense. Transplantation is not their specialty. They are bitter, they want to make a name for themselves somehow. And since they are ICU doctors, they want to make money off the families of brain-dead patients."

Many Western-educated elites like Dr. Badr have been confounded by what they see as the usurping of control, in professional associations and in public and cultural life more broadly, by an embittered middle-class "counterelite" who speak of "Islam as the solution" *(islam huwwa al-hal)* (Wickham 2002). They attribute increased "backwardness and decline" *(al-takhalluf)* to "religious extremism" *(al-tatarruf)*, which has been posited as a major obstacle to the advancement of science, technology, economic progress, and cultural "openness." The only solution, they maintain, is to fend off these "extremist" movements that are evidently making Egypt only "more backward." In this view, religion is a private matter. When it leaks into public forums, Egypt only falls more and more "behind" the rest of the world, by restraining itself from developing out of fear of transgressing God's will.

Layla Marmush, an investigative reporter and former editor-in-chief for a news publication specializing in health issues *(Dar al-Hilal al-Tibbi)*, agrees with Dr. Badr's sentiments. For many years, and especially during the most heated times of the media debate between the late 1980s and early 1990s, Marmush covered stories on organ transplantation throughout Egypt. She reported on the first liver transplant in Shbin al-Qum and had traveled on several occasions to Mansoura to research stories on the Kidney Center.[31] When I met to speak with her, she stated upfront, "I am pro–organ transplantation and pro–brain death as clinical death. What does this question have to do with Islamic law? This is a scientific definition that we must apply. I am against them interfering with science." While I first thought Marmush might be speaking about muftis when she spoke of "them" interfering, I soon realized she too was speaking specifically about a group of doctors whom she regarded as "fundamentalists" in their attempts to bring Islamic principles to bear on medical practice.

Marmush pointed to Saudi Arabia's long history of recognizing brain death and said that this is proof that opposition in Egypt has to do with "fundamentalist" movements, not with "real religion":[32]

> With these fundamentalist movements, these people are moving backward in time. And now this fundamentalism is a movement among the *doctors*. They are only about five doctors whose voice is very loud. And they are the ones stopping everything from moving forward. This is not on a scientific basis, because these people don't think scientifically. It is on a religious level—but a backward understanding of religion, not enlightened religion.
> These people, they are looking for a role to play. Shouldn't they be spending their time saving people's lives? What is better in the eyes of God?[33]

Marmush and her colleagues charged the "fundamentalist doctors" with political selfishness: "They are very conservative; they don't want to progress with contemporary issues or with freedom. And it's not really a question of whether the shari'a says it is *halal* or *haram* or what the definition of brain death is; they are just using it as a political issue for their own conservative agenda." She sneered at Lotfy's arguments, such as that a brain-dead pregnant woman can keep a fetus alive in utero if the woman is hooked up to life-support and that this is evidence that the woman could not be truly dead.

"But this is true," I offered. "There really are cases of brain-dead pregnant women, and the fetus survives."

"Yes," Marmush answered, "But the brain is dead. You are just keeping the organs alive by the machine, and the IV fluids are what is nourishing the fetus. For them to say that there is no such thing as brain death and that all the organs must stop—then there wouldn't be organs [for transplantation] anymore. This is a big waste. If you wait for complete death, only the bone is still useful; all the organs will go to waste."

As someone who is "pro–brain death," Marmush argued that the donor is actually dead. This first argument legitimated a second, more implicit one: that to insist on the older criteria of death is to waste organs and lose lives. Like Marmush, many of the transplant-proponent physicians argued that (1) the brain-dead person is already dead, (2) procuring organs from brain-dead patients would curb the black market in live organs, (3) it would solve the problem of unacceptable harm posed to the living donor, and (4) it would alleviate the recipient's psychological burden and guilt at having received a gift that can never be fully repaid. (See also the "tyranny of the gift," discussed by Fox and Swazey 1974, 1992.)[34]

Further, for these "pro-brain-death" physicians and especially for journalists like Marmush, who consider themselves "progressive," what they see as Egypt's "lack of ethics" and its "inferior science and technology" are implicitly conflated. They link the "scientific and technological advances" in the "developed countries" with the advanced ethics of those countries. It is in the West, Marmush imagined, that doctors concern themselves with patients' rights, with informed consent, with efficacious and beneficial medical procedures. Countries in the West have excelled in medical transplantation and saved lives, so opposition to such advances must be pure backwardness. On separate occasions, Dr. Badr and Layla Marmush had both asked me rhetorically, "If it is unethical to procure organs from the brain dead, then why do all those countries do it? Do these people [Lotfy and his group] think they are the only ones with ethics?"

Importantly, I also spoke with many Islamist-oriented physicians who were active members of the Muslim Brotherhood who also accepted the idea of brain death. Many of these doctors worked abroad in Gulf countries such as Kuwait and Saudi Arabia, where cadaveric transplant programs are in operation. One Mansoura nephrologist who had worked for many years in Saudi Arabia believed that brain-death criteria are based on sound, scientific evidence and that when patients labeled as "brain-dead" in fact recover, these cases result from diagnostic errors by inexperienced physicians. Convinced that organs are procured only *after* the donor's death, this physician, Dr. Karim, remarked that the donor will receive spiritual rewards because even in death he will continue to be "beneficial for people."

Saudi Arabia was able to initiate a program while Egypt has not, he explained, because the Saudi government has taken a "strong political position" in favor of transplantation, encouraging donor families with money, the best hospital treatments, and reduced fares for transportation and insurance:

> Thousands have agreed to donate [in Saudi Arabia], from all different cultures and nationalities, different people. They did this because they see that the government is encouraging them; they see that it is logical. . . . Why should they be afraid? They would already be dead. And what will happen to them anyway after they die? Not only is there no harm to [the dead donor], he will even get [spiritual] rewards after he dies. Also strict rules and regulations are in place. If anyone [e.g., the doctor] goes outside these regulations, he is severely punished.

Yet Dr. Karim also noted that Egypt does not have the infrastructure to support such a program and acknowledged the difference in economic resources in Saudi Arabia and Egypt, especially with respect to government expenditure on health care:

Imagine if someone in Asyut [a city in Upper Egypt] dies, and he could help someone in Mansoura [in the lower Nile Delta]. The government would have to help with the transport; we'd have only a short time and we would need integrated circuits between the centers, a computer system that connects everything, planes between the two places. If I suddenly got a kidney from Asyut, what would I do with it?

There has to be organization at the national level. . . . And for me, I wouldn't just give an available kidney to someone who hasn't had really good training in how to do the surgery and follow-up. Is Asyut like this? Minya like this? No . . . In Saudi Arabia there were teams. We Egyptians were the ones who put the system there for them.

This physician, despite his own doubts as to whether Egypt is "ready" for a cadaveric transplant program, insisted that there is no religious problem with procurement from brain-dead donors. As an active member in the Muslim Brotherhood, Dr. Karim felt comfortable interpreting Islamic ethics and arriving at this position by himself, not through religious scholars. Dr. Karim argued that religious scholars are not specialized in neurology or neurosurgery and so should not speak about the definition of death. As he reasoned:

The shaykh [religious scholar] should not be getting into the details of these issues. This isn't his specialty; it is ours. He should tell the doctors, "Make your best decisions and best efforts so that there are no problems."

Brain death is the irreversible loss of all brain function. There is no hope of reversibility. From the medical point of view, it is death. [The religious scholars] can argue what is *halal* or *haram* on the basis of the principle of lesser harms. But they can't discuss the definition of what constitutes death.

And anyway, it is a team of different people who don't know each other, from different specialties: anesthesia, ICU, general medicine. Each person writes a report, and they don't meet. There should be a strong decision that this is the irreversible loss of brain function and life. The majority of [religious] scholars in Dar al-Ifta' here [in Egypt] and in Saudi Arabia have allowed for donation from both the living and the recently dead [i.e., the brain dead], as long as there is consent from the donor and his family.

Dr. Karim thus took self-contradictory stances, as did many of the Islamist-oriented proponents of brain-death criteria in Egypt: they argued that religious scholars should not interfere in defining death but also that religious scholars should convince the public that Islam allows for this type of organ donation. And while they noted that the lack of necessary infrastructure in Egypt prevented a cadaveric-procurement program, they simultaneously blamed the religious scholars, as though the muftis themselves were responsible for the logistical issues standing in the way of developing such a program.[35]

MUFTI GUMAʿA: WHY DOCTORS ALONE CAN'T RULE ON DEATH

In 2003, a new scholar was appointed as grand mufti of the republic: Shaykh ʿAli Gumaʿa. A young scholar with a secular, untraditional education, Shaykh ʿAli Gumaʿa was known to argue against the "extremists" in Egypt and to insist on the flexibility of the Islamic legal tradition.[36] He was appointed during Tantawi's rectorship at al-Azhar, and, given Tantawi's adamant support for organ donation, proponents of the organ transplant law hoped that Gumaʿa's appointment would swiftly and finally put an end to all debates on the matter.

But this was not to happen. I conducted a private interview with Gumaʿa in the spring of 2004, in the office of the grand mufti of the republic. Gumaʿa, who is himself positioned against what he sees as threats of godlessness and secular utilitarianism, responded to the issue of brain death thus:

> It is the *doctors* who have differed on these issues, not *us* [the religious scholars]. There is a disagreement among them about the definition of death and brain-stem death. When does the human's life cease: when the brain stops functioning, or when the heart stops beating? Here the laws of different countries have differed, between those who say it is when the brain-stem stops functioning and those that say that the brain-dead person is still alive.
>
> Now if someone goes to an intensive care unit and kills a brain-dead patient with a gun, did he commit murder, or did he merely commit the crime of desecrating a dead body? Here in Egypt [with the existing criminal laws] the person would get the death penalty for murder, because he killed the patient with intent.
>
> Now I approach this as a scholar of the shariʿa. So I would say: Why are you [doctors] in disagreement over the definition of death [*taʿrif al-mawt*]? Why do you play with it?
>
> This [problem of brain death] has arisen as an issue only because of organ transplantation. The person who is diagnosed as brain-dead, they

[handwritten margin notes: "seriously", "takes Muslim text", "Muslim family"]

cut him up and take out his heart, his kidney, and his liver, all whole and functioning, for transplantation. Because [if they waited for] the person whose heart has completely stopped beating, his organs would not be good anymore.

In Islam we have a holistic view of the human in Creation: the human is not like any other creature. [He should not be] relegated to the status of a material object, as though he were made of a piece of wool or steel. He is the viceregent of God over Creation [*mukhallaf*]. But he is also a *part* of this Creation; he is not the dominator [*musayyad*] over it.

The scientist can [ethically] research anything he likes: the intricacies of the cell, the genome, the function of organs and tissues. But how will he use this knowledge? Will he use information from the genome for the control of a select group over others?

Will organ transplantation be used for the poor to sell their organs to the rich? for the rich to take over organs? for the world to be further divided between the North, the rich, and the South, the poor? We have finally ended slavery and colonialism, and now will they come back?

To Shaykh Guma‘a, more than just the artifice of redefining death is problematic; also the intention and motivations behind that definition make the concept of brain death unacceptable. Further problematic are the practices in organ transplantation that reify inequalities, such that organs move from poor to rich, from South to North, and from postcolonial nation to past empire. As he argued, "We see that this issue is necessarily tied to economic, political, and social incentives. It is *not* just a technical medical issue. It's also a human and moral issue. Therefore, the doctors *cannot* say it is only for them alone to decide. We *must* get involved. And we have to say, 'Define death as you will, but the issue is not about definitions [*al-ta‘rif*]; the issue is about uncovering the truth about something [*al-ta‘rruf*].' "[37]

He thus rejected Shaykh Tantawi's assertion that this is a "medical, and not a religious," question. Shaykh Guma‘a also rejected the argument among those "pro-brain-death" physicians and journalists that brain death is a sophisticated concept, and that those who opposed it out of religious backwardness or ignorance simply did not understand. He clarified that the mufti must be involved in judging the ethics of a particular medical practice when he finds that it is clearly tied to larger economic, political, and social incentives. As he reasoned:

It is not up to the doctor to say, "Why does the mufti have to get involved with organ transplantation?" I am not telling him how to *do* organ transplantation; I am saying what is permitted and what is not. I don't know the mechanism of how to do it; I don't know the conditions

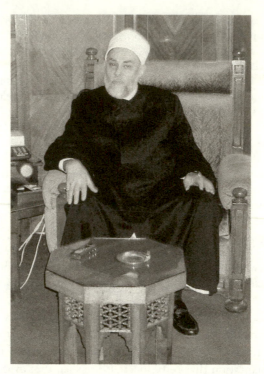

Figure 7.   The grand mufti of Egypt Shaykh
'Ali Guma'a, in May 2004, resolved in his stance
against the death of the brain signifying the
death of the person. Photograph by the author.

that determine which patient can have a transplant and which cannot. I
don't know how to match tissues or what the surgical procedure is.

But I *can* say: Here a human being has been relegated to the status of
a *spare part* that can be bought and sold; a person has been rendered into
something that is cut up, whose parts are distributed. Now we are returning to slavery, after we had already gotten rid of it. It is coming back in a
different form. We got rid of colonialism, and now it is coming back after
we fought against it and developed freedom. Why are they doing this? It
is because of economic interests and the laws of the market.

So we *have* to get involved. And we have to say, "No, this is not
permitted." Because it goes against our understanding of the human's
divine duty of representing God and assuming his sacred responsibilities on this earth. . . .[38]

I could ask [the doctors], If you want organs from someone after he
has died, can you go to the grave and take them [to use for transplanta-
tion]? They will say, "No, we can't do this. Who knows if it would work

Wrah what abt just people changing another @ life

or not?! But the one who still has a heart that's beating, that organ is still good." . . .

Defining death is now suddenly a problem among those who are within the practice and institution of organ transplantation and the circulation and trade of human body parts.

Defining death wasn't a problem throughout history. It doesn't need a sophisticated philosophy. I can show anyone what death is; let us go to the grave, and I can point to it. Let us stop anyone in the street and ask, "Is this person dead?" Death is known and has been known. It doesn't require a new definition.

This question now [of playing with the definition of death] is built on the principle that humans are composed of spare parts. . . . So now we have turned a person into a material thing. The human is *not* [in this framework] the one divinely entrusted to cultivate human society on earth [*al-insan al-mukhallaf fi 'imarat al-ard*].

Shaykh Guma'a here followed a larger trend of state muftis in Egypt who have seen their roles as protecting the integrity and relevance of the shari'a in the face of forces of secularization and godlessness (Skovgaard-Petersen 1997). He saw particular medical practices, like the procurement of organs from brain-dead patients, transsexual surgery, and active euthanasia as interventions in processes of life and death that reduce the theomorphic human into an arbitrary, material object.

Thus, an important distinction occurs between the outlooks of Guma'a and Tantawi, and it does not involve a question of who was more or less "flexible" with Islamic legal interpretation. Tantawi's fatwas, particularly those deferring to "the experts" as authorities, seemed to assume that Muslim ethics already reigns in Egyptian society. Tantawi seemed to imagine that doctors, unless they are criminals who should be stopped through legal means, would proceed according to Muslim ethics. And he viewed organ transplantation as sound medical treatment. Hence, for Tantawi, questions about whether certain medical procedures are *religiously* permissible are inappropriate, because it is up to the doctor to decide. For Guma'a, in contrast, Islamic legal principles and Muslim ethics are marginalized in Egyptian society: social life in Egypt, he maintained, generally proceeds *without* recourse to Islamic law. Unlike Tantawi, Guma'a questioned whether "treatment" is the sole motivation behind organ transplantation. He pointed to economic incentives as well as to a larger social worldview of Euro-American hegemony and the exploitation of the poor by the rich in which transplantation is embedded. Guma'a resented the marginalization of Muslim ethics in Egyptian society and the tendency, nevertheless, in the state-oriented media to blame "Islamic stringency" for any problem.

Significantly, in the disagreement between Shaykh Gumaʿa and Shaykh Tantawi, the point of difference is over the social constitution of organ transplantation, not over the textual interpretation of scripture or religious law. Further, their contrasting fatwas on brain death complicate simplistic assumptions of "liberal" versus "conservative" politics mapping onto Muslim legal interpretation or, for that matter, onto permissiveness regarding medical practice.

A CLASH OF DEATHS?

Contemporary Egyptians are made ever more aware of U.S. militarization and intervention in the Middle East, which has resulted in the bolstering of brutal dictatorships "friendly" to the United States. They witness through their smartphones and satellite receivers the mass civilian casualties in the military attacks on Iraq and Afghanistan, the bolstering of Israeli attacks on Lebanon and Palestine, the erosion of state welfare policies, and, especially, open hostility to Muslims and Islam more generally. The "clash of civilizations" rhetoric between the Muslim world and Euro-America often boils over in the general public, as the Arab mass media portray social injustices caused by their own and other governments like the United States (Said 1979; McAlister 2001; Qureshi and Sells 2003; Khalidi 2004, 2009; Mamdani 2004; Shaheen 2009). The rhetoric takes on a new life with each political conflict, as we saw with the events of September 11, 2001, the Islamic Revolution in Iran in 1979, the U.S. hostage crisis there in 1979–80, and the Arab-Israeli War of 1967.

We should not be surprised, given the entrenchment of this discourse, that it would inform medical and scientific debates as well. When the U.S. medical establishment decided that death occurs when the brain irreversibly stops functioning (Lock 2002a, 2002b; Sharp 2006), religious scholars and physicians in Egypt were primed to interpret this move as yet another sign of the prioritization of material gain over human life, an argument whose logic coincided with analyses of U.S. imperialism in the region. Egyptian doctors who expressed horror at the way organ harvesting occurs in the United States and western Europe were struggling with the discrimination against Arabs and Muslims that is palpable in the public rhetoric of the host countries in which they trained. They continue to grapple with the superiority of Euro-American standards of medical care and their own convictions about the authority of Muslim ethics. Of chief concern is how western European and North American medical institutions have routinized a practice that curtails remaining moments of one patient's life in order to make use of vital organs for another "more productive" life. Critics feel that this utilitarian façade has masked material gain, echoing the logic of U.S. hegemony from which these Muslim doctors and religious scholars have felt politically embattled.

At one point in our interview, Shaykh Guma'a expressed concerns over the ways in which human life, however unproductive to society, can so easily be dismissed in biomedical practice. He stated in frustration, "[This question about brain-dead patients] is like what they [unbelievers] call 'mercy killing.' [Looking at a dying patient,] they say, 'Isn't he dead yet? What use is he to us like this? Let us just kill him and end his/our suffering!'" Guma'a implied that Islam forces into the open what others try to obfuscate, such as the notion of "mercy" masking unwillingness to invest in the terminally ill. He couched his anti-utilitarian criticism in Islamic philosophy and made apparent the postcolonial realities and socioeconomic inequalities in which the category of brain death has emerged.

Unfortunately, Shaykh Guma'a and other Muslim intellectuals who shared his views (e.g., al-Bishri 2001) did not link their own criticisms of materialism and utilitarianism with similar criticisms coming from Western theorists. In Germany, for example, there have been heated debates about organ procurement from brain-dead patients (Hogle 1996). Memories of the abuses of medical authority under National Socialism rendered all too apparent the historical connection between biomedicine and state violence that is elsewhere easily denied (Hogle 1996; Porter 1998). In the early 1990s, many books were published in Germany voicing fears and criticism of organ harvesting from brain-dead patients, one of which reproduces an old German folktale as its frontispiece:

A wolf approaches a herd of sheep.
   "Do you know me?" says the wolf.
   "I know your type," says a sheep.
   The wolf explains that he is not a danger but a friend to sheep because he eats only dead sheep that are left to rot in the field. "I don't eat live sheep. Couldn't I just stay by the herd in case one of you dies?" he asks.
   The sheep forbids him, saying, "An animal that eats dead sheep learns quickly out of hunger to see sick sheep as dead ones and then healthy ones as sick ones."[39]

This fear of a "slippery-slope" echoes the worries of people in Egypt. Yet figures such as Dr. Safwat Lotfy and Shaykh 'Ali Guma'a have placed their criticism in terms of a Muslim defense against Euro-American moral imperialism. By failing to recognize that their criticisms in fact match the voices of many critics in Euro-America, they thus perpetuate a dichotomous conception of the world, divided along a cultural clash between Euro-America and Muslim countries.

In all these various contexts, the push to codify medical practice into laws or firm bioethical principles relies on the modernist and nationalist goal of singularization. This contributes to an anemic notion of both "Islamic" views and what "the West" stands for. In the United States and western Europe, moral doubts (e.g., about changing gender roles or in attitudes about death) are often, in public rhetoric, streamlined in opposition to "cultural" attitudes in "traditional" places, including Muslim societies (Cohen 1998: 37). Similarly, when people in other societies voice antipathy toward medical procedures like organ procurement, they explain their own stance in terms of "culture," such that similar feelings of antipathy from within the U.S. dominant culture are rendered imperceptible.[40]

Despite Euro-American media images of organ transplantation as the manifestation of the "gift of life," ethnographers and social analysts have uncovered fears, anxieties, and criticisms about the utilitarianism of organ procurement in western European and North American societies as well (Fox and Swazey 1992; Joralemon 1995; Fox 1996; Hogle 1996; Youngner, Fox, and O'Connell 1996; Agamben 1998; Lock 2002a, 2002b; Sharp 2006). Lock (2002b) has argued that, in contrast to other countries like Japan, within the U.S., medical arenas hostile to public debate ultimately shaped legislation on brain death. Further, in the 1990s, ethicists in the United States reignited the debate about death after physicians widened the criteria of "dead donors" to include patients whose brains might still be functioning but whose hearts have stopped beating. As anthropologist Lesley Sharp explains:

> An even more unsettling intervention within the realm of organ transfer involves a recent, albeit still limited, shift to obtaining organs from what are referred to as "non-heartbeating donors" (NHBDs), and the procedure itself as "donation after cardiac death" (DCD). This protocol, which has expanded the boundaries of death, concerns specifically those patients who are maintained on ventilators yet who fall outside the criteria for brain death, their failing health instead indicating signs of imminent cardiac arrest. Their potential donor status is dependent on there being a do not resuscitate (DNR) order entered in their medical chart. At the moment the heart stops beating (either on its own or after the patient is disconnected from a ventilator), medical staff make no attempt to restimulate it but, rather, rapidly prepare the patient-turned-donor for the surgical removal of his or her organs. (2006: 21)

The ethical questions raised by widening the criteria for organ donors to include patients with brain function still remain unresolved in the United States, with the President's Council on Bioethics releasing a report on these controversies as recently as 2008 (Thomas 2010).[41] Yet the "clash of civilization" rhetoric, as well as what Mamdani (2004) terms "culture talk," has obscured the similarity in misgivings that people in various cultural contexts have voiced in relation to biotechnological interventions. In this way, we lose sight of the chance to engage in bioethical discussion across places, communities, and interests.[42] And we miss the opportunity for a broader interrogation of the ways in which moral uncertainty about brain-dead patients gives way to the routinization, bureaucratization, and, ultimately, the banality of organ procurement.

CONCLUSIONS

In contrast to North America and other Muslim countries, physicians and legislators in Egypt have been less successful via the media in "reinventing a new death" (Lock 2002a, 2002b). The United States, Canada, Saudi Arabia, Iran, Jordan, and Kuwait have passed laws recognizing brain-dead patients as dead, thus enabling organ procurement from cadaveric sources. But in Egypt, a national transplant program has remained suspended. Legislators, legal theorists, religious scholars, and physicians have argued about whether the death of the brain can legitimately and ethically be equated with the death of the person. To the frustration of many proponents of organ transplantation, this impediment to national legislation has exacerbated the problem of an organ shortage and the related problem of a black market in organs from living donors. The policy implications have been considerable, given that tens of thousands of patients are in desperate need of kidneys, let alone other organs. Yet, this circumstance on its own has not been able to resolve the confusion that doctors experience when faced with the clinical realities of brain death.

The case of the brain-death debate in Egypt demonstrates the failure of the Egyptian state to deal productively with the plurality of voices that have emerged in assessing the status of brain-dead patients. One way to engage productively with this plurality would be to distill the various issues that have come to be attached to this debate—from social inequalities, to the efficacy of transporting and coordinating organs, to the financial costs of these operations, to respect for the dead and the dying. We need also to focus attention to the question of scale. That is to say, "Is this brain-dead person dead?" is a different question from "Can we legitimately weigh the benefits of treating organ failure patients against the costs of precipitating the cardiopulmonary death of patients who are brain-dead?" Because the multitude of views and perspectives have been cast negatively, as a "crisis" or as an indication that the experts have not been able to speak authoritatively on the subject, movement toward a national transplant program has been held in limbo for over three decades. This case serves as an important lesson for conceptualizing bioethics in a way that can use multiple perspectives as a strength—in that each reveals a different aspect of a complicated question—rather than as a failure to find clear answers or firm principles to complicated, messy questions.

Narrating the issue of defining death in terms of "civilizational clash" has further obfuscated the great antipathy that already exists toward medical intervention in death and dead bodies more generally in Egypt. No matter what religious and medical experts decide, it is unlikely that a substantial number of family members in Egypt—given the worsening state of the health care system—would knowingly and willingly allow loved ones in a state of brain death to be cut open, with their hearts still beating, for the removal and allocation of their organs to strangers. Death in Egypt is still not as technologically managed, nor has it been rendered as invisible as it has been in places where brain death has been accepted medically. And death in Egypt is already understood as saturated with religious meaning, such that new meaning need not be assigned to it in order to "make sense of senseless suffering," which is how surviving U.S. family members are apt to explain their impetus to donate the organs of their loved ones (Youngner, Fox, et al. 1996; Sharp 2001, 2006; Lock 2002a, 2002b). Whether or not family members know the intricate details of these debates, concerns linger about medical treatment of the dead and dying in Egypt (see also Hirschkind 2006). The next chapter illustrates the debates and controversies over cornea transplantation, which relies on tissues from those who Egyptians perceive as "really" dead.

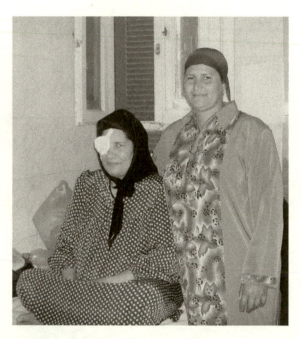

Figure 8.   Patient and family member in a Tanta eye
hospital.

3. From Secret to Scandal

Corneas, Dead Donors, and Egypt's Blind

In February 1996 in a public morgue in Cairo, a son discovered that the eyes of his deceased father were missing. While preparing his father's body for burial, he found that in place of his father's eyes, two pieces of cotton had been stuck into the emptied sockets. His complaint against Ain Shams Teaching Hospital led to a police investigation that found the medical staff guilty of procuring eye globes from the dead *without consent* for use in cornea transplants. The prosecutor general interrogated the director of the eye bank, arrested a laboratory technician, and ordered the eye bank to be shut down.

Or so the story went. The shutdown was, in fact, not the result of any single case or sudden event; rather, it resulted from the accumulation of numerous complaints over the years of eye "theft" from the dead for the purposes of cornea transplantation.[1] Both public eye banks in Cairo—the one in Ain Shams and the older one, at Kasr el Aini Teaching Hospital—were subsequently closed.[2] The highly publicized theft of eyes scandalized a public now weary of stories of kidney theft and the black market in organs, which opposition-party newspapers in particular had been exposing for over a decade. At the time of my fieldwork, cornea grafts were difficult to come by in Egypt. Cadavers at Cairo's public teaching hospital morgues—the only source that had been routinely used—were now strictly off limits.[3] The public prosecutor of the 1996 case accused the eye bank of not having obtained the surviving family members' consent. Physicians protested that this condition was impractical given the short time in which the cornea must be taken—within six hours after death.

I argue in this chapter that the scandal around cornea grafting touches on difficult and long-unresolved religious and cultural debates in Egypt about the proper treatment of dead bodies. The biomedical notion of death as the irreversible cessation of all consciousness is held simultaneously with several other competing understandings of death in Egypt, particularly those emerging from religious teachings.[4] Neither religious nor medical fields speak in one voice on important and even basic questions such as these: What is the relationship between the person's soul and his or her dead body? What are our responsibilities toward the dead? Are the religiocultural rituals for dealing with dead bodies necessary for an easy transition to the afterlife? Or are they more for the spiritual well-being of the loved ones who remain alive, in grief? Would the extraction of tissues or body parts of the dead disrupt their smooth entry into the afterlife? Would it signal the failure of the living to care properly for the dead?

As we saw in the previous chapter, in the debate about brain death, most of the disagreement has had to do with the sociomedical understanding of the brain-dead patients: are they dead or alive? In contrast, the scandal around procuring eye tissues reveals medical *and religious* debates about the proper interpretations of dead bodies—that is, *unquestionably* dead bodies. Egypt's eye bank scandal was entrenched in these and in yet other unresolved issues of Egyptian medical practice, namely, (1) the exploitation of the poor, including the dead; (2) whether and how to obtain informed consent from patients in the context of a strongly paternalistic medical system; (3) the privatization of medicine and the related marketing of body parts, the eroding quality of medical care, and struggles in class inequalities between professionals and poor patients; and (4) longstanding cultural associations of eye disease and blindness with Egyptian "ignorance." Whereas in the debate about brain death, lobbyists mobilized in terms of a "clash of civilizations" rhetoric between supposedly "Western" and "Islamic" values, the debate around cornea transplants revived a longer and more deeply entrenched discourse on the struggle within Egypt between enlightenment and backwardness.

WHY NOW?

With the abrupt shutdown of the national eye banks, Egyptian ophthalmologists were quick to point out that they had been carrying out cornea transplants for over half a century. Why *now*, they asked, would our medical expertise, our surgical and technological advancements, and our life-saving procedures be so suddenly ground to a halt? Ophthalmologists, journalists, and others protested that Egypt's technological progress was being "set back in time." In fury, they asked, How could anyone now claim that procuring eyes for the purposes of transplantation is religiously reprehensible when we have been practicing cornea grafting without any problems for over half a century? Eye doctors offered various explanations; the two most popular were that the "religious extremists" had taken over Egypt and wanted to take things "backward" and that the problems with *kidney* transplants had confused people on the issue of cornea transplantation. Ophthalmologists argued that transplanting corneas is completely different: it should not, they maintained, even be considered of a piece with any of the issues plaguing the transplantation of vital organs, such as the poor selling their body parts, muddled rates of success, procurement from the brain dead, and cutting into and extracting internal parts of dead bodies.

My research into this topic revealed that, contrary to the doctors' rhetoric, no contestation about cornea transplantation had existed before the 1990s simply because the general public did not know about it. It had been a professional medical secret that eyes were taken from the dead in hospital morgues, sporadically starting in the 1950s and routinely since the 1980s. Scant mention of new "eye operations" appeared in the official press and never with an explanation about the transfer of corneas from a dead person to a living patient. The *demystification* of the procurement process is what outraged public opinion, not any change of heart over the procedure. Opposition-party newspapers revealed details of "eye theft," some with gory pictures of bloodied eye sockets, in the midst of coverage about wider problems with organ transplantation.

Further, by the 1990s, a social criticism had emerged around the previous elitism of the medical profession as a consequence of the demographic shift among lawyers and physicians, many of whom were now people with much less social distance from the poor (see Wickham 2002). Indeed, the Cairo prosecutor involved with the investigation into the public eye banks had himself originated from the rural peasantry. In my interviews with him, he related to me that his roots "among the fellahin" motivated him to act on injustices against the rural poor that his senior colleagues neither recognized nor cared about. Before being transferred to Cairo, he had worked in a provincial area, and he told me about a case that had stuck with him ever since. A farmer's water buffalo was killed by the electrical output of a nearby factory. When the farmer wanted to file a suit and reclaim reparations for his lost property, the lawyers in the office laughed at the notion that a poor peasant could file claims against factory officials. The young prosecutor himself took on the case, and in the end the factory was compelled to compensate the farmer: "Because I know, coming from the fellahin myself," he explained, "that the water buffalo was his entire livelihood."

In the 1950s, when cornea transplants were first practiced in Egypt, a poor illiterate peasant was much less likely than today to hold a medical practitioner legally responsible for wrongdoing. By the 1990s, media outlets were more diverse, the literate base was broader, and the public was more engaged in a "hyperessentialized" Islamic discourse that could be mobilized to reign in the misconduct of state institutions (Salvatore 1997). The same young prosecutor, now working in Cairo, was called in to investigate the case of a young rural girl whose untimely death was made even more painful for her family members when they discovered that she had been defaced: her eyes had been emptied from their sockets while she lay dead in the hospital morgue.

As I describe below, Cairo professionals often dismiss excessive attachment to the dead as "ignorant superstition" among what they see as the poor, more tradition-bound segment of society. Hospital staff tend to discourage and sometimes outright prevent patients' families from moving dying or recently dead patients to rush them home. Village practices of caring for the dead are particularly denigrated as excessive in emotion and lamentation, as inappropriate in their religious interpretation, and as "ignorant" and ill-suited to biomedical practice. Further, patients in public hospitals, having received their treatment free of charge, are generally regarded as unentitled to demand better care. Yet against this backdrop, the young prosecutor took the case seriously. He initiated proceedings that ultimately led to the closure of the eye banks.

THE PROBLEM OF CONSENT

From the earliest cornea transplants in the 1950s and 1960s, when preservation techniques were still lacking, few operations took place (fewer than twenty per year in each of the two major public teaching hospitals in Cairo). In the mid-1980s, Egyptian public hospitals in Cairo received a series of donations to set up a system for eye banking.[5] What had been a dream was now finally realized. With the proper equipment, preservation fluid, and refrigeration techniques, corneas could be stored for use, dramatically increasing the number of cornea transplant surgeries. These operations were largely successful, low-cost, and relatively simple, with dramatic effects for the recipients. The donated equipment now allowed for the tissues to be screened for major diseases and preserved in a bank. Corneas could theoretically be obtained from dead patients under unrushed conditions; rather than hurrying to the morgue to find an adequate graft at the time of an operation, the medical staff could presumably turn to a supply that was now preserved in special solutions in a refrigerator. Further, American workers taught the Egyptian medical staff how to extract only the thin cornea tissues from the eyes and replace them with a lens—rather than using the entire eye globe—a process that results in minimal disfiguration of the donor corpse.

After the establishment of the eye bank facilities, the capacity at Ain Shams Teaching Hospital grew to more than a thousand cornea transplants per year. With the institutionalization of the procurement and preservation of corneas, it became less evident that procurement was being done solely in "conditions of dire necessity" *(darura)* or "for overall public benefit" *(maslaha 'ama)*—the two major arguments that had legitimated taking eyes from the dead. With more and more eye tissues being taken from the hospital morgues, some of them could easily slip outside protocols and regulations; that is to say, not all of the eye tissues went into the eye banks of the public hospitals for the poor. Some were shipped abroad to wealthy Arab Gulf states, some were taken to private clinics, and others were used for hospitals elsewhere in Egypt. And not all were extracted by the newly trained staff; unskilled hospital workers who took corneas, often out of expediency, would cut out the entire eye globes and not just the thin outer tissue. It was cases such as these that led to the district attorney's investigations of the bloodied eye sockets and the subsequent shutdown of Cairo's two public eye banks in the late 1990s.

I frequented one public hospital in Tanta, which had failed to establish its own eye bank. It was there that I met Shadi, the worker responsible for traveling to Cairo to obtain eye globes from the morgue. At age fifty-three, Shadi had an elementary school education and had worked as a medical technician and physician's assistant in a Tanta public hospital for the past twenty-four years. Working under a particularly forceful "big" (prestigious and powerful) ophthalmologist, Shadi was for years sent to Kasr el Aini, Cairo's largest public hospital, to procure eyes to be used in the cornea transplant operations in Tanta. He explained that the eyes were taken from corpses in Cairo because the guard of the morgue at Tanta Hospital, where Shadi worked, was vigilant in protecting the dead bodies, because he feared possible retribution from the family members of the deceased. If he was given enough money, however, the morgue guard would offer the eyes of an accident victim whose body was already damaged, in which case the family members were less likely to find out that eyes were missing. But this supply was not guaranteed. Cairo's larger public hospital, Kasr el Aini, was more anonymous, and the "procedure" could be done without anyone noticing.

Shadi said that sometimes they tried to take the eyes from executed prisoners, who would show up at the Tanta morgue in their red prisoner jumpsuits. Some of these people had family members who never claimed them. They would take the eyes from them and bury them in charity graves. Shadi said they tried to get some samples from the regular patients in the morgues in Tanta after they could no longer obtain them from Kasr el Aini, but the Tanta morgue guards were stricter than those in Cairo had been, and eventually everything just shut down. When I asked Shadi if anyone ever tried to ask the family members' permission, he seemed to find this question ludicrous: "No one can ask for permission. Say I have someone [in my family who died] and someone says: 'I'll take your family member's eyes.' I'd slit his neck." He gestured to his neck and laughed. "Isn't this the truth? Isn't this the natural response? Isn't it? That's the natural response of a family member."

When I talked to Shadi, he insisted that it was natural to believe eye procurement was *haram* and some unconvincing fabrication on the doctors' part to think otherwise. I told him, "Well, maybe you would agree to this [procurement] because you might think you could help someone else." He had clearly heard this argument before and did not think much of it:

> I say this is *haram*. A lot of people tell me this is *haram*. It is *haram* to take from the dead, I would say this to [the famous doctor he worked for]. How many times I went into his office and said, "I *don't* want to do this; this is *haram*!"
>
> And he [the doctor] would say: "My son, [think of] all of these people who work in a factory and who can't see and they say, 'If you can't see, you lose your job.' This person is in need, without this he can't see, without seeing he can't work, and without working he and his family can't live. But the dead person is dead. The worms are going to eat it. He won't get use out of it."
>
> And the pediatricians would even take whole, entire children from the morgue so that they could study from [the dead bodies]. The obstetricians and gynecologists would go get bodies from the morgue so they could study the uterus, and so forth. It is not just us in the eye department who benefited from Kasr el Aini morgue.[6] The ear, nose, throat department downstairs used to go to it so that they could take a piece of the ear for ear patching. It is not just *us* who benefited from Kasr el Aini morgue.

Somewhat taken by Shadi's ability to argue both cases so persuasively, I clarified, "But you still think it is *haram*?" He quickly answered,

> Yes, yes. This was *haram*. It's stealing. It's theft. And [the famous eye doctor] would say, "You aren't stealing and putting something in your

own pocket, are you?" I felt guilty, but I had no choice *[kan ghasbin 'anni]*; this was an official order. When I would say, "I refuse this work," he [the doctor] would say, "It's not up to you to decide. You don't work at your own whim *['ala mazagak]*." This was an order, not what I wanted to do. "Find someone else," I would tell him. "No, *you* are going to go," he would order. It was just like a military order.

Shadi related how he used to carry a tremendous sense of guilt and fear, the same as if he were smuggling heroine or hashish across cities. He described shaking from head to foot until he reached his own hospital and released "the package" to the doctors. He knew how vulnerable his situation was. Even though he had been ordered to go, "like a military order," if he had been caught, the doctors would have denied having sent him. The full burden of the crime would fall on him.

Because Shadi was taking the "samples" illicitly for another hospital in another city, and he himself was not a trained medical specialist or ophthalmologist, he was sent to procure the entire eye globe (without screening against diseases), to travel the distance back to the Delta province, and deliver the sample to the doctors, who would extract the actual cornea from it. He explained that he used to find the dead bodies of patients who were under fifty years of age, because after that age, the cornea tends toward opacity. He would then take the eye globes, put them in a solution, put in drops of antibiotics, then tape it all up, "so nothing gets inside," and put it on ice in a cooler, "because the weather is so hot, and to come all the way from Cairo to here it would get spoiled, so it has to be on ice." He would look for anyone who had come out "clean," such as those who died in surgery, "not those with diabetes or any other kind of disease that affects the eyes."

Another male worker, not Shadi, was eventually caught. The deceased "donor" involved was yet another young woman, whose family wanted to take her back to their *balad* (homeland) to wash her ritually. "No, no wash her here," the doctors had tried to persuade the family. But the family insisted on taking her. And when they opened her eyes, they discovered that the hollowed sockets were stuffed with cotton. This theft had occurred around 1995 in Kasr el Aini. The police arrived, investigated, and arrested the worker and the doctors, the latter of whom, of course, easily got themselves off the hook. As for the worker, he was able to come up with the ten thousand pounds to get himself out of jail. After having been compelled to perform an illegal and risky procedure and one that he was ethically opposed to, Shadi was relieved that the thieving of cadaveric eyeballs had finally been put to a stop, even though he realized that cornea opacity patients' chances at sight had also been shut down.

All of the ophthalmologists with whom I spoke adamantly opposed the closing of the public eye banks. They especially scoffed at the idea that the shutdown was prompted by a moral defense of the poor, because they felt that they were the ones who were best serving the poor by keeping the eye banks functioning. As I sat with Dr. Mustafa, an ophthalmologist at a large private eye hospital in the old wealthy Duqqi Quarter of Cairo, he shook his head, in frustration, about the closure of the public eye banks. He told me:

> This is a very simple operation; we performed it with a lot of success since the early 1960s. Now there are problems because of religious views. . . . The first lab was [opened] around 1987; the Arabs [i.e., Saudis] had come and donated refrigerators and other equipment.[7]
>
> Then in 1996, there was the big problem in Ain Shams. Some relatives came and saw the eyes were missing. They complained; the district attorneys came and investigated. They grilled the head of the eye department, Dr. Muhammad Ibrahim, a very respected and well-known ophthalmologist, one of the pioneers in Egyptian ophthalmology. At the end of it all, he told them to write down in their report: "*I now renounce my Egyptian nationality,*" because he was so furious, so disgusted with what they did.

Dr. Mustafa's account related the indignation that many ophthalmologists expressed to me over the shift in focus that now made *them* the objects of legal scrutiny. The ability of any poor, uneducated patient to file a complaint that upsets the authority of the medical physician in charge is a clear disturbance in power relations.[8] The eye doctors emphasized that these operations were done for no profit and at very little cost to the patient. Arguing in terms of the betterment of society, many noted that they had taken disabled people whose loss of sight precluded them from working and supporting their families and returned these patients to society as "full-functioning citizens." The doctors working in the public hospitals often worked with very limited resources and made triage decisions about what they believed was best for the majority. The issue of cornea transplantation exploded into a public scandal that upended the professional authority of medical professionals in the name of the rights and dignity of poor families of the dead. Both sides of the debate equally mobilized discourses of "service to the poor." The physicians' narrative inverted that of the corrupt medical institutions exploiting the poor. In many ophthalmologists' accounts, it was the selfless physicians who labored day and night in public facilities under egregious circumstances, serving the poor and getting underpaid or not paid at all, and who struggled to help their fellow Egyptians, particularly the victims of poverty, ignorance, and blindness.[9] This made the physicians vulnerable, as they saw it, to selfish members of the underclasses who aimed to "make noise" and to invert the social order by allowing the police to investigate and hold the *doctors* under suspicion. This narrative echoed themes from many of the more famous and popular Egyptian films and television serials studied by Walter Armbrust (1996) and Lila Abu-Lughod (2005), of the vulgar underclasses turned nouveau-riche who bully the noble educated classes and thereby threaten Egypt's path toward enlightenment.[10] Common story lines in Egyptian popular culture about the uneducated underclass seizing power from the educated nobles played directly into the outrage many felt that an unschooled family member could file suit against the medical profession for eye theft.[11] With cornea transplantation and with numerous other procedures that physicians must carry out with meager resources and under difficult circumstances, eye doctors worked with a triage mindset. That is, they often had to sort out those patients who needed critical attention, because resources were inadequate to treat all. Restoring sight to the living blind was a clear priority for them above seeking consent from the surviving family of the dead.[12]

For many of these ophthalmologists, cornea transfer could not possibly be *haram*, because it involves such a materially insignificant tissue from a person who is "truly" dead and because it will result in dramatic benefit to the recipient.[13] This conclusion led them to decide then that because it is not *haram* and the public benefit is overwhelmingly clear, there should be no requirement for obtaining consent, because this would only impede the process. As Dr. Mustafa said about the issue of consent for corneas, "Well, the person won't be walking around with the consent form in his pocket, and how will the person know when he is going to die? It is 90 percent water, 10 percent proteins and collagen. It is no big deal; it is nothing; it will totally disintegrate." The material insignificance of the cornea, as eye doctors saw it, renders an insistence on consent incongruous and irrational. Dr. Mustafa further argued that the requirement of consent was impractical, because the cornea must be procured within six hours after death.

Physicians, journalists, and state officials are not the only ones who find this "cultural attachment to the dead" frustrating to medical progress. Virtually all cornea opacity patients with whom I spoke argued that the rights of the living come before the rights of the dead. 'Aziz, for example, argued that people should agree to donate their eyes after death if others are in need. But he also said that it would be criminal to take the cornea without explicit consent of the donor: "Otherwise it would be theft." Many patients in need of grafts hold on to the idea that people *will* donate corneas to help others when awareness is raised and that there could be a proper way to do this. But most of the eye doctors I interviewed were so certain that the benefits were obvious that they did not see why consent was necessary, because it would only impede a potential good.

BACKWARDNESS AND STRUCTURAL INEQUALITY

After the eye banks were ordered to be closed by the district attorney, physicians expressed their frustration in the media that they now had low supplies. They knew that they could help more patients if more corneas were available. They solicited support from Shaykh Tantawi, then the grand mufti, blaming what they called the "religious obstacle" as an impediment to restoring sight to desperately blind patients, many of whom were poor. Tantawi eagerly took on this role. In addition to repeated performances on state television, he also publicly donated his own body and organs. In a national public health campaign that began in the late 1990s to promote cornea donation, Tantawi's donor card—with "#1" on it to show that he was the very first Egyptian citizen to sign up—was reproduced and published in the state newspapers.

The Egyptian state has for the past half century effectively used television as a pedagogical tool in regard to its citizens (Abu-Lughod 2005). The government pushed mass media for citizen education, introducing television on July 21, 1960. Nasser's government invested heavily in television, under a mandate to educate and reform, and even subsidized television sets for cooperatives and village councils to promote television access in rural areas, with a major part of the programming including shows with developmental and educational themes (Abu-Lughod 2005: 10). Promotional programs for public health messages through television were most notably used for family planning campaigns, as well as for vaccination programs that continue today. Thus, the Ministry of Health's attempt to solve the problem of the eye bank incident and the availability of cornea grafts by turning to television was fitting. Medical doctors, Islamic legal scholars, including Shaykh Tantawi, the Coptic patriarch Baba Shenouda, and the minister of health all congregated on various television programs to discuss the importance of cornea transplantation in the mid-1990s.

In the nationwide media campaign, state officials and doctors argued that cornea procurement requires the extraction of something as insignificant as "a fish scale" or "the peel of the onion," images that effectively dehumanized the substance. Describing the cornea as a common food or a kitchen substance rendered it something easily transferrable among people, taken in without altering the body or sense of self. As one of the administrators of the eye hospital in Tanta University explained to me, "I saw it all on the television. The cornea is just a small tiny thing, like a fish scale. . . . It was a man from the Ministry of Health explaining it on television: they were talking about how they do it and about the National Eye Bank. Now that there is television, there is nothing called 'ignorance' anymore."

Indeed, even the illiterate peasants whom I met in their villages were able to reiterate the arguments that they had heard about cornea transplants on television. Another accountant in the eye hospital whose job it was to file hospital records also told me, "The Dar al-Ifta' says that if it is for the sake of knowledge, then it is not *haram*. . . . I saw this all on television. The other muftis said that it is permissable. There are people who say, 'I don't know; I have to ask people.' But why would they say this, if the media outlets are all there in front of them?" This administrator suggested that people were now more informed because of these types of television programs and that you don't even have to go out of your way to seek a fatwa from a learned Islamic scholar when the opinions are delivered on-screen in your own home.[14]

The language of scientific and civilizational progress in which ophthalmologists tend to speak saturated this campaign, as did earlier arguments to legitimate the opening of the national eye banks after the foreign donations were made in 1989. A newspaper article from that year in *Al-Wafd* quotes an ophthalmologist who makes the following typical assertion:

> Some advanced countries in Europe and America have special documents like driver's licenses for donating organs after death, but we unfortunately have not reached this sophisticated level of thought or culture, and that is why we need constant awareness campaigns for citizens to stop their wrong ideas.
>
> Even though trachoma is so high in Egypt and nearly every family has an affected member, there are still a lot of obstacles to donating. This could be the religious obstacle, but Shaykh Tantawi said that God created illnesses and cures and that as long as the doctors say that this is a cure, then it is not forbidden/sinful *(fa la tujid hurma)* to take from the dead.[15]

The ophthalmologist points to the *perception* among people that their reservations are due to religious principles. But in citing Shaykh Tantawi, he dismisses these religious positions as ignorant and backward thoughts that need to be eradicated through education.

Many patients and physicians have internalized this discourse. They told me that Egyptian culture does not easily allow for turning over the dead, despite pronouncements from religious scholars such as Tantawi,

:ffered his own body for use in medical practice. Most cornea opacity
.......s waiting for cornea transplants agreed with this sentiment. Several
rural patients, internalizing the dominant rhetoric, readily admitted to me
that they were backward and that they knew that they or anyone else in
their *balad* could not accept giving away a part of the dead. Yet they also
desperately wished to be able to see again. While some associated themselves with this "backward culture," others separated themselves from the
communities to which they belonged. As Samah, a young rural girl of fifteen in need of a cornea, told me, "People think wrongly. They think that
if you take the eyes of the dead, then they can't be resurrected [whole].
This is backward thinking, because of course people who die in accidents
and in pieces will also be resurrected. If a man is dying, he should think to
donate, because what use will he get out of it? If they had any awareness
and knew that the person who donated could get rewards from God, it might
happen. But there is no awareness. Especially here among the peasants *[fil
fellahin]*." Even though some considered positions against "tampering with
the dead" to be "superstitious" and "backward" in the context of cornea
transplantation, many other Egyptians with whom I spoke seemed to imply
that *any* tampering with the dead body unacceptably violates the sanctity
of the dead.

   In my conversations with them, many ophthalmologists mocked what
they imagined to be the superstitious beliefs of their ignorant patients who
feared that "the spirit of the corpse would demand his eyes back." In fact,
I never heard a patient articulate this particular fear; patients were more
concerned about medical mistreatment. Physicians' assumptions that "the
poor" hold on to "ignorant beliefs" were often based on very little social
contact with their poor patients outside the clinical encounter.

   Dr. Fadil, a major figure in eye banking in Egypt, now long retired,
spoke with me about the need for education so that the "Egyptian masses"
(al-ʿawwam) could be convinced that Islam is a practical religion *(al-din
al-muʿamila)*. "They need to have the backward part of religion taken out
of them and reeducated so that they learn that this [donating the cornea]
would be a continuous spiritual reward even after death *[sadaqa gariyya]*.
The man who receives the cornea will be, with every step he can now take,
praying for this donor to enter Paradise." At the same time, wealthier
patients in private practice and their surviving kin are themselves never
approached about donation upon death. When pressed, even the eye doctors admitted to me their personal uneasiness with bequeathing the eyes
of their own dead kin.[16] Dr. Fadil, now at a mature age, reflected honestly
on this point:

My wife died of a heart attack in 1995. We were sitting together drinking tea. She had a heart attack at 9:50 A.M. She died at 10:10 A.M. in hospital. I never, never thought of taking her corneas.

And I was the head of the Department of Ophthalmology and director of [a major Cairo] eye bank. For me, when I think back on this, I think, "Why, that was just stupid—why didn't I take those two fresh corneas?"

This is a problem everywhere, the religious issue. In Turkey they quietly take the corneas, Bulgaria the same. In Israel, the Jews there have a "negative eye bank": they import but do not export.

I was the head of the Department of Ophthalmology and one of the founders of eye banking in Egypt; I was the major figure in charge of cornea transplantation at that time. And before me were *two fresh eyes, like ripe apples waiting for me to pluck them!* But I never thought of it at the time. All I wanted to do was to run to my two daughters and cry with them that their mother was gone.

This physician on one occasion spoke distantly of "the Egyptians" as a mass of poor, ignorant people constrained by religious traditionalism. Yet on another occasion, he admitted that, despite his own high status and education, he was like other Egyptians, unwilling to turn over corneas when his own wife died. In his astonishingly frank account of his experience with the death of a loved one, he brings up the well-known fact that people of means are treated with far more respect when their kin die in private hospitals. This doctor could embrace his daughters in grief, and no one pressed him about the donation of his wife's eyes or dared take them without his consent. The poor, who are treated in public hospitals, have far less autonomy over their bodies and are given far less information about their treatment procedures and fewer choices in the treatment of the bodies of their loved ones if they should die in the public facilities. This great disparity in treatment among different social classes was continually collapsed into a civilizing discourse of cultural inferiority mobilized by the state television campaign.

The contradictory messages—between trying to solicit consent and minimizing its importance—have left medical professionals divided. On the one side are the more powerful, established, and older physicians who think that the families of the dead should not be consulted because corneas should be seen as a common good. And on the other side are the younger physicians, fewer in number, who think that a massive educational campaign could convince people to consent. During the mid-1990s, some hospitals attempted to present entering patients with forms asking them to bequeath their corneas in the event of death. These slips of paper, in the absence of any earlier system resembling interest in anything like "informed consent," were anomalous in patients' experiences and the object of grave suspicion. I spoke with several hospital administrators and medical practitioners who had witnessed the distribution of these slips of paper as pilot programs that were launched to gauge patients' willingness to consent to donating their corneas after death. According to the administrators, nurses, and doctors, the patients, when faced with papers to sign, had exclaimed, "They will make mincemeat out of us [*hayy bashsharu fina*]!"[17]

The public campaign launched in the mid-1990s did nothing to increase the cornea supply, given the lack of a formalized system for obtaining consent and the new emphasis on its importance. And to further exacerbate the distinctions between the treatment of the poor and that of the better off, cornea transplants became available only in private clinics after the shutdown of the eye banks. Private clinics imported cornea grafts from other countries and performed the operations, but only at a high cost. Access to cornea transplantation was thus narrowed to those few who could afford the private procedure. Furthermore, according to many ophthalmologists in private practice, the imported cornea grafts were of much lower quality than those previously procured locally. The ophthalmologists complained that the nonprofit international eye banks sent them their poor-quality "leftovers," which significantly diminished the outcome of the operations. Meanwhile, patients suspected that a black market in illegally obtained Egyptian corneas was what was actually fueling these private clinics, given the high cost and the fact that the private physicians now monopolized the source of (supposedly imported) cornea grafts.[18] In this context of suspicion and mistrust, launching a campaign to promote donation "for the public good" became even more difficult when both the idea of "benefit" and the notion of who constituted "the public" continued to marginalize the poor.

FROM SECRET TO SCANDAL

The "pioneering" eye surgeons, such as Dr. Fadil, who practiced in the early years of cornea transplantation in Egypt, went abroad for training, mostly to England or Spain, before bringing the skills and techniques back to Egypt. I tracked down some of these older retired ophthalmologists and asked them to tell me about the early transplant years.[19] Dr. Mohamed Ibrahim, known as one of the founders of cornea transplantation and eye banking in Egypt, described his experiences as a fellow training in England in his youth.[20] The year was 1961:

The secretary [in the English Eye Institute] would tell me: "We have a Mrs. Smith on the telephone. She has eyes to donate."

I would get on the telephone and [an old English lady] would say: "My husband has just died and he bequeathed his eyes to the eye bank. You may come pick them up."

And so I would go immediately to the [dead person's] house, with a nurse and my sterile equipment, in an ambulance. People would be sitting around the living room, all dressed in black.

[*Mimics his younger formal self, shaking hands*] "Hello, Mrs. Smith. I am very sorry to hear of your loss." [And she would say,] "Hello, Doctor, he is in the back room. Oh please just don't disfigure him too much."

I would go in with my equipment and take out the eye globes. I'd replace the sockets with an artificial shell with a cover to replace the eye. I would close the eyelids and that was it. I'd come back to the hospital and put the eyes in the fridge, with a note to my seniors saying that there were two new corneas ready for transplant. See how simple it all was!

To imagine such a scene in Egypt—the whole situation is completely reversed. I couldn't even dare to ask [family members]!

In London, the apparent lack of attachment to the whole body, what Dr. Ibrahim described as an "easy-going attitude" among some English families, was simply impossible for this doctor to imagine in an Egyptian context. He knew well that in Egyptian society, the dead body plays an important role in ritual funerary practices. Dr. Ibrahim had gone to London to learn everything he could about techniques as they were honed in a relatively well-functioning medical system. Unlike the political postcolonial sensibilities that Shaykh 'Ali Guma'a voiced in the previous chapter, Dr. Ibrahim was a member of the old-guard elite who did not contextualize England's medical system in terms of its status as a wealthier nation. Much less did he contextualize England as a former imperial power whose wealth was ill gained from the colonial exploitation of countries like Egypt. Dr. Ibrahim did not particularize the cultural attitudes of the English, nor did he criticize them. He did not think of his own culture's treatment of the dead as equally or more valid. And he did not wonder whether London's medical context was, in ethical terms, applicable to an Egyptian context.

Dr. Ibrahim, like other elite professional colleagues of his generation, held that "science has no homeland" (Gershoni and Jankowski 1995). For him, Egypt's postcolonial role is to "catch up" to Western medical science; in his youth, this meant working to prove that being Egyptian did not preclude being a medical scientist. He saw the superiority of London's medical system as owing, in part, to a superior cultural system in which advancement

[margin, handwritten: have the resources from deep past of exploitation]

to science has been privileged over adherence to ritual practice. The ophthalmologist recounted how impressed he was with the English for offering the body parts of their dead to medicine and contrasted this to an unyielding attachment to the dead among Egyptians: "For Egyptians? The entire eye globe?!" He exclaimed, "There is no way!"[21]

Ophthalmologists of Dr. Ibrahim's generation generally explained the noncompliance of their Egyptian patients in terms of cultural inferiority. They labeled beliefs and practices of Egyptians that differ from modern European attitudes as "ignorant." Further, they identified ignorance as the major impediment to medical treatment and advancement (El-Mehairy 1984).[22] Particularly offensive to modernist Muslim sensibilities are notions that the dead can hear, smell, and feel what is around them and that *awliya'* Allah (friends of God, also often called "saints") can intercede, upon request, on behalf of the living. These beliefs are questioned not only on the basis of modern science but also on the basis of the arguments of Islamic reformers following in the wake of Muhammad 'Abduh, who emphasized that God alone can intercede on behalf of the living. Today, Salafis in particular hold that appealing to the *baraka* (blessings) of saints is akin to denying the ultimate and unique omnipotence of God (a denial that is referred to as *al-shirk*), which is the gravest sin in Islam. Poor patients, knowing that their strongly held convictions are generally disrespected, have often avoided hospital care out of fear that the hospitals are places where dead bodies will be desecrated. These fears have been derided as "ignorant" and "unfounded" by physicians, journalists, and public health campaigns.

The prevailing sentiment that occurred in the early years of cornea transplantation and that continues among many ophthalmologists today is that if they were to attempt to reason or consult with common (poor) patients, there would simply be no advancement in medicine. Physicians told me that in order to help patients, they must keep details of procedures from them, lest they protest and refuse to cooperate. In the practice of cornea transplantation, more specifically, ophthalmologists have simply proceeded without informing the public or even those directly involved, knowing full well that no surviving kin would willingly abdicate the body parts of their dead. In this way the details of cornea transplantation remained, for decades, a professional secret.

ADAPTING IGNORANCE

The only medium that introduced a large Egyptian audience to the term *cornea transplantation* in this period took a decidedly pro-biomedical approach. It was a 1968 film adaptation of *The Lamp of Umm Hashim,* a classic piece of modern Arabic literature, written by the Egyptian nationalist, diplomat, cultural critic, and novelist Yahya Haqqi in 1944.[23] Produced in the wake of the devastating defeat of the 1967 Arab-Israeli War, the film adaptation promotes an unquestioning faith in modern science and technology to serve the aims of the modern state. In contrast to the novel, the film allows no space for ambiguity or self-questioning.

Following the novel's plot, the film details the life of Ismail, whose family migrated to Cairo from their rural village, bringing with them their peasant attitudes, religious practices, and provincial worldview. They set up their new home in a poor, popular quarter of the city near the shrine of Umm Hashim, a term of endearment for Sayyida Zaynab, the granddaughter of the Prophet Muhammad. The family sacrifices everything for the future of Ismail, the youngest son, who, they pray, is destined to become a doctor and bring the family into upward mobility and urban prestige. His parents sell their land, furniture, and possessions to support Ismail's medical education in Europe; meanwhile, Ismail frolics in European parks and romances blond women. When Ismail returns to Egypt, he is disgusted by the filth and disorder around him and can no longer relate to his fellow countrymen. His family expects him to marry his orphaned cousin Fatima, whom he now perceives as a backward peasant girl.

On the first night of his arrival, Ismail happens to find his mother anointing Fatima's diseased eyes with oil from the lamp of the shrine of Sayyida Zaynab, such that divine light—emanating from the Prophet and his family—might reach Fatima's blinded eyes. His mother's "superstitious" healing method irrevocably offends Ismail's newly honed biomedical sensibilities. In outrage, Ismail jumps to his feet, screams, "Ignorance!" at everyone, and runs to the shrine, where he smashes the mosque lamp to pieces. He is immediately attacked by a mass of devotees of the shrine who are depicted as the ignorant inhabitants of the popular urban quarter. They beat him unconscious. When he awakes and recovers, he treats Fatima with his own modern medicine, which ends up blinding her completely.

In the original novel, Ismail eventually realizes that he cannot repudiate an integral aspect of himself: he comes to respect the popular devotion to Sayyida Zaynab and combines the healing practice of the oil with his own modern biomedicine. It is this mixture of old and new, of traditional and modern, combined with his repentance, that enables Fatima to see again. In the end, they marry and have many children, and Ismail opens a medical clinic for the poor.

The film adaptation, however, changes the ending dramatically. After smashing the lamp to pieces, Ismail is far from repentant. When his medical

> powerful story w/t agenda

treatment blinds Fatima, he takes her to a clinic to consult with his Egyptian medical colleagues. They decide together that Fatima is suffering from "hysterical blindness" as a result of Ismail's harsh treatment. She also has infected trachoma. Her only hope for sight now is surgery.

Knowing that neither his own mother nor Fatima would agree to subjecting Fatima's eyes to surgical knives, Ismail and his medical colleagues devise a plan in the film version. Ismail collects the oil from the lamp only to please Fatima and his mother, and then he surreptitiously replaces it with the "real" medicine, which is used to prepare Fatima for her course of treatment. Ismail clandestinely prepares Fatima for surgery—a cornea transplant operation—and it is through this high-biotechnological achievement that Fatima's sight is ultimately restored. The film ends with a scene in which Ismail gifts Fatima a European dress and hat and exclaims, once she is properly dressed, that she is every bit as attractive as the European women he knew when studying abroad.

As cinema is the primary medium through which most Egyptians "read" their classic literary texts, many Egyptians with whom I spoke during my fieldwork were familiar with *The Lamp of Umm Hashim* from having watched the 1968 black-and-white film played and replayed on Egyptian television.[24] Those with whom I spoke about it simply did not believe me when I tried to tell them that the original literary work describes Ismail coming to believe in the powers of the lamp oil. As the film relates, the development of science and technology, which includes the acquisition of its related European sensibilities, is the only legitimate path toward restoring sight, literal and figurative, to Egypt's masses. The message of the film is that popular religiohealing practices—including asking favors from Sayyida Zaynab, or others among the dead, to impart her *baraka* to inanimate objects such as lamp oil—are deplorable on a number of levels: (1) they exacerbate disease; (2) they are heretical in that they call on intermediaries between humans and God *(al-shirk)*; and (3) they are a subset of the neglect that characterizes Egyptians' relationships to their own bodies.[25]

Significantly, the film never mentions the source of corneas—that is, that they come from the dead or, more specifically, from fresh corpses in the hospital morgue. Although the "scientific" process remains mystified, any objection to it is cast as ignorant and backward. The masses, including Ismail's own family, cannot know the truth about their treatment because they are too ignorant to reason. This premise justifies their deception by the elite class, including physicians, public health specialists, and filmmakers, all of whom readily depict "cornea transplantation" as a miraculous cure, the details of which ordinary Egyptians need not know.

ACTIONS ACCORDING TO THEIR INTENTIONS

On the very first page of *The Lamp of Umm Hashim*, Yahya Haqqi alludes to a simple truth of Islam that opens fields of argumentation about morality, ethics, and religious authenticity. The novel's opening scene details the peasants, reeking of soil, sweat, and fenugreek, as they arrive in the city and prostrate themselves in sincere devotion at the steps of the shrine of Sayyida Zaynab. They bump against the pedantic theologians of official Islamic scholarship, who scorn these acts, denouncing their heresy and *shirk*. Haqqi, in the voice of the narrator, offers a well-known saying of the Prophet Muhammad's without further comment: *"inna al-'amal bilniyyat"* ([God judges people's] actions according to their intentions). The peasants, Haqqi implies, their hearts full of love for God, the Prophet, and his family, cannot but be rewarded for their pure intentions.

This sentiment—that the *intention* of an act morally outweighs the form or even the consequences of that act—was often evoked by my informants in Egypt in regard to various social and political arguments. In Haqqi's novel, the statement seems deceptively clear in its interpretation: the action itself, here prostration in devotion at the steps of a shrine, may or may not be blameworthy. But the intentions, one's love of God and the Prophet, are certain to be rewarded. A problem with this simple interpretation, however, emerges upon further inquiry. What if the peasants hold that their devotion toward Sayyida Zaynab (the enactment of their faith) is a *necessary condition* for cultivating their love of God (their intention)?[26] If this were the case, God would reward them not *despite* their actions but *because* of them.

Like the trope of "service to the poor," the question about "intentions and actions" has been evoked by people on all sides of the debate about cornea donation in Egypt. The doctors and official religious scholars have all said that God will reward the donor whose intention is to donate and help others. Whether the physical body is still intact, they argue, is relatively insignificant. Their argument makes several analytical moves in one stroke. In defining spiritual merit in terms of intention, they simultaneously divorce *spirit* (the spiritual rewards) from *matter* (the dead body). Additionally, they separate the *intention* of an act (helping another person) from its *form* (the extraction of tissues from the dead). They argue that the relationship between the two is arbitrary and unnecessary. Further, they attribute importance to the spiritual rewards (the intention) while belittling the significance of the dead body (the form).[27]

Shaykh Tantawi in particular was known for promoting this view. In October 2002, at a public conference on eye health in Cairo, I sat in a large audience, mesmerized by Tantawi's role in presenting the "religious view" toward promoting cornea donation.[28] As he spoke, his voice shifted from its regular soft tenor to a more forceful tone:

> The issue of cornea transfer has caused a lot of debate and dispute and controversy, and I get asked a lot about it. Among those who have spoken are people who know and people who do not know, people who understand and people who do not understand. All talk about it, just as they speak about organ transplantation in general. There are those who like to talk outside their specialty.
>
> When I was asked about it, I had to know what it was first [before answering]. So I asked [experts] about it. There is no shame for the shaykh of al-Azhar to be the student of Dr. Mohammad 'Awad [the minister of health] in his specialty, just as there is no shame for him to be my student in my specialty.[29]
>
> So I asked [about cornea donation], and I was taught what it is and how it is done. And when I understood, I said, "What is greater than this? This is at the door of *al-sadaqa al-gariyya*" [the continual accrual of spiritual rewards after death].
>
> So I said, "Take from my own eyes!" *[applause in the audience]*
>
> You seated before me are my witnesses. I say to this good doctor [Dr. 'Awad]: take from my body what you will after I die! Because this is your specialty. *[big applause]*
>
> As for those who say this will only open the door to bad things, that there are people who mistreat and deal wrongly with bodies . . . this is a very weak argument. If a doctor does wrong, then hold that one accountable, not all of them. If five doctors in a hospital have done wrong, then take those five to account, not the entire hospital. Give the criminal his due punishment.
>
> If the mufti did something wrong, then make him accountable. You are a coward, you who say, "If we open this door then such and such bad will happen"![30] Why not just say, "I am a coward"? If someone does wrong, then hold him accountable. . . .
>
> Those who talk about organ transplants, who worry what will happen—God made the world with good and evil: those in charge must take the evil doers to task for what they do. Those against organ transfer say it is wrong because it belongs to God [*innahu milk Allah*]. This is a lack of understanding. *Everything* belongs to God. The earth belongs to God: this doesn't mean that we can't plant or irrigate it. God allowed us to deal with what we can—properly. But how? On the road to what brings beneficence [*al-nafa'a*]. The entire planet is God's possession, we are meant to build it with goodness, good deeds, good words, planting, but with limits [prescribed in divine law]. . . .
>
> God, most exalted and high, knows what is in the womb and what will happen tomorrow. The body after a few days turns to dust. God

will give you what you will, He will reward you when you present good things in your life, good deeds and good work.[31]

Not only is cornea donation permissible, Tantawi argues, it is also commendable in Islam as an act of charity. Tantawi marvels that cornea donation is a *sadaqa jariyya*, or perpetual charity, which is one of the three ways that the Prophet Muhammad specified that a dead person can continue to accrue spiritual rewards in the afterlife by remaining socially beneficial in this world. In the saying of the Prophet related in Sahih al-Muslim: "When a human dies, his good deeds stop, with three exceptions: a *sadaqa jariyya* (perennial charity), beneficial knowledge, and a righteous child who prays for him."[32] Familiar examples of the ways in which people have historically interpreted a *sadaqa jariyya* are the digging of a well and the building of a public water fountain, mosque, school, hospital, or orphanage. If a person creates this perennial charity in her lifetime, then, even in her death, she will be rewarded spiritually by God each time a living person benefits from the charity. Or a person can perform a *sadaqa jariyya* in the name of a loved one who has already died, with the intention *(niyya)* that all benefit and rewards be channeled into that person's spiritual account. In these terms, if someone donates her cornea in death, every time the recipient of this cornea uses it (that is, everytime the recipient sees) the donor is spiritually rewarded. Not only Tantawi but also many other Muslims in Egypt have explained tissue or organ donation upon death in terms of a *sadaqa jariyya*. This resignification of *sadaqa jariyya* is in line with the many other ways in which contemporary Muslims see Islam as a dynamic living tradition that provides guidance in all places and times, such that novel practices can be framed in familiar ethical terms.

Notably, people who have disagreed with Tantawi's position have *not* refuted the premise that donated tissue or organ can be interpreted as a *sadaqa jariyya*. Yet Tantawi's passionate speeches—continually published in the print media—had little effect in convincing the larger Egyptian population make arrangements to donate their corneas. If people do not disagree with his notion of *sadaqa jariyya*, what, then, has remained problematic about Tantawi's stance?

It is not what Tantawi said in the quoted speech that has been controversial, but what he did *not* say. Tantawi elided people's social relationships with and obligations to the dead. By refusing to engage with the dead in material terms, Tantawi effectively promoted a complete divorce between matter and spirit, such that the "spirit" of the person is connected not to the body but to the intangible accrual of the rewards of her charity. As for the materiality of the dead body, Tantawi told us that it will "turn to dust in a matter of days." This stance not only diminishes the body's materiality—it generally takes longer than a few days for a human corpse to disintegrate—but also dismisses its social and religious significance. The limitation of Tantawi's stance is not the rendering of bodily donation as charity; it is the elision of the bodily sacrifice that is necessary to materialize this charity.[33] By refusing to acknowledge the value of the material body in death, Tantawi's stance has further alienated many Egyptians for whom bodily donation is not an easy thing to do, despite the potential for spiritual rewards.

Muslims in Egypt relate socially in multiple ways to the bodily materiality of their dead. Tantawi's interpretation may be justifiable within the terms of Islamic tradition, but less justifiable is the presentation of his position as the *only* correct, true interpretation or the dismissal of all other engagements with the dead as "ignorant."[34] Like the filmic version of *The Lamp of Umm Hashim*, Tantawi delegitimates rich popular traditions that recognize the dead (and their tombs and shrines) as sources of *baraka* (blessings or grace). Shaykh Tantawi argues that to focus on minutiae, such as the holism of the body or mortuary rituals, leads to a narrow-minded and ignorant interpretation of the shari'a, which holds that God, the omnipotent, can will anything. Surely, he argues, God can transition the soul to the afterlife with or without the corneas! And surely, he insists, God can resurrect the body again intact.

If we are attentive to some of the objections that people raise to "tampering" with the dead, however, they are both more general and more specific than Tantawi's position suggests. As Charles Hirschkind has shown, many Egyptians, some of whom are more or less self-consciously enlisted in a larger project of Islamic revivalism, believe that "an experiential knowledge of death is a condition of moral agency" and that "the task of acquiring this agency has been rendered increasingly difficult by the gradual effacement of death—in all its sensory dimensions—from public life within the modern metropolis and by the assumption of ever more responsibility for the dying by secular bureaucracies of medical expertise" (Hirschkind 2006: 174). People feel a moral responsibility to wash the body carefully—right side and then left, as in washing for ablutions before prayer—and to perfume, wrap, shroud, bury, and ritually pray for the dead.[35] In these duties, family and community members are understood to enact their respect for the dead and to experience moral edification for their own lives. The Muslim traditions, including the Prophetic example, teach that remaining attentive socially and bodily to the dead can bring people closer to an embodied recognition of their own mortality and to God's final accounting. This recognition is understood to be essential to leading a virtuous life.

There are also more mundane approaches to the dead. Many health practitioners as well as patients I spoke with described the dead as yet another segment of society especially vulnerable to exploitation and mistreatment. As one nurse in Tanta University's Eye Department put it:

> By God, I think this [human body] is a trust [amana] from God. It's not up to me to deal in it and cut it up. It's not right for someone to take the body and just go in and take his cornea. It's not right to say that just because he is dead, now he does not feel. You know, when we wash the body, even if a single hair comes off we take it and gently put it back with the body to be buried.
>
> It's not right for us to go and take the corneas and put them in someone else. . . . If I am alive and I want to give my kidney to someone so he can get better, then this is fine. But it is not right for them to take it from us just because I'm now dead. This is wrong. To take the body and cut it up and to take from it what they want is wrong.

This nurse articulated a sentiment that many others expressed as well. God will reward the family members, they believe, for their intentions of enacting their duties to the dead, so how can others deem their beliefs "ignorant"? One hospital administrator, Hala, who worked in a public eye hospital told me:

> The family is not going to let the eye be taken. While they stand by the dead person, they won't let a tiny piece of the pinky finger be touched. You should see how it is at the morgue. Egyptians are always like that. They are always afraid that they [the hospital workers] are going to steal their bodies.
>
> And they did! They used to steal the corneas. They used to take them out, just hideous. They showed us the cornea [on television]; it's like the scale of a fish. . . . If the family saw them taking an eye, they would slaughter them. They were stealing part of the body, when all the while the most important thing for the family members is for him to be buried properly.

Hala points out that if anyone touches or mistreats the dead body, this form of personal injury will not only hurt but also enrage the surviving family members. The dead, many of whom suffered illnesses, devastation, or accidents, can now finally rest in peace—but only if properly taken care of. Family members describe their duty to remain vigilant, to care for the body, to prevent any more unnecessary suffering. In this understanding, mishandling of the dead by hospital staff represents an egregious attack on the most vulnerable members of society. I remember clearly an overworked laborer, raising four young girls, who answered my questions about cornea donation with a look of utter weariness: "When I die? Even after I die, they still want to take from me?!" There was an underlying exhaustion in his remarks, hoping for a more restful and peaceful afterlife but apprehensive that this aim would be disrupted, presumably by the same forces rendering his life on this earth so arduous. These remarks recall anthropologists Julie Chu and Jean Langford's suggestions of a bare *after*life, a phrase that takes from but adds to Agamben's notion of "bare life." Bare afterlife refers to the stripping of political and material rights from the dead, denying them the social and material debts of the living (Langford 2009; Chu 2010).

BREAKING THE BONES OF THE DEAD

Dr. Safwat Lotfy, the anesthesiologist described in chapter 2 who agitated against procuring organs from the brain dead, was also reluctant to accept the procurement of organs from those whom he understood to be "really" dead. In his pamphlets, he had raised the following points:

> The Prophet of God, may God's blessings and peace be upon him, has left us with instructions for our duty of dealing with the dead in utmost detail, even specifying that the temperature that we use to bathe the dead [ritually] be neither too cold nor too hot, so as not to abuse the dead.
>
> Then the Prophet specified that we shroud the dead, pray for them, and bury them properly, and the Prophet warned us against any mistreatment of the dead body as in his noble hadith "Breaking the bones of the dead is like breaking the bones of the living." Do we not perform ritual funerary prayers [*salat al-janaza*] only for those things that are sacred?

Reported traditions of the Prophet include instructions to bathe the dead gently in tepid water: the dead should be treated as carefully as they would be treated in life. The reason for this, whether it is that the dead are in fact sentient beings who would be harmed by mishandling or that this ritual act is to instantiate one's own disposition of respect toward the dead and awe before God, is subject to interpretation.[36] But there is a rich Muslim tradition, both within and outside Egypt, that elaborates on the dead as sentient—as able to hear, feel, and sense what is around them (Smith and Haddad 2002; Hirschkind 2006; Kugle 2007). And throughout my fieldwork, doctors, patients, and religious scholars, such as Dr. Lotfy, referenced the Prophetic saying that condemns breaking the bones of the dead (see also al-Ghumari 1987; Krawietz 1991; and Moosa 1999). According to the narration, the Prophet Muhammad said this to express his displeasure with a gravedigger whom he chanced upon as the man was breaking up dirt, and along with it old bones, in order to make space for a new grave.[37]

The first fatwa in Egypt to respond to the notion of cornea transplantation also alluded to this hadith. In 1959, although cornea transplantation was not yet a subject of public debate, a charitable organization for the blind that had heard about the idea of "eye banking" solicited a fatwa from the grand mufti, Shaykh Hasan Ma'mun, to find out if this procedure is permissible in Islam. Unlike the subsequent fatwas and public performances by later muftis, including Tantawi, the 1959 fatwa was a private answer to a private question, still on record at Dar al-Ifta' but not published in the newspapers. The question was as follows:

> The Light and Hope Foundation asks for a fatwa on the taking of eyes from the dead after their death and preserving them in a bank to be called "the Eye Bank," similar to the preservation of blood of the living in a blood bank. [38]
>
> Is this *haram* or *halal*? The eyes are to be used by putting them into those who have recently damaged their corneas, as is the current practice of physicians to restore the eyesight of the visually impaired.
>
> Does the religion prevent the issuance of a law that would allow for taking the eyes of the dead for use in the medical treatment of the living?

The question implies that if a problem exists, it would pertain to transgressing the dignity *(hurma)* of the dead. The mufti's answer immediately addresses this exact point:

> We have researched this matter and found that the human being, after his death, requires care and preservation, his burial, his treatment with dignity, and a lack of disrespect.
>
> The Prophet—peace and blessings be upon him—forbade breaking the bones of the dead, for it is akin to breaking the bones of the living.
>
> The meaning of this hadith is that the dead deserve respect and dignity as do the living . . . and extracting the eye of the dead is like extracting the eye of the living; it is considered an attack on him and is not allowed legally unless it is in a situation of dire necessity in which there is a benefit *[maslaha]* that is greater than the harm that would befall the dead, because the laws of the Islamic religion are built on the preservation of benefits that take precedence over a lesser harm.
>
> If taking the eye of the dead is done in order to use the cornea for the visually impaired, then *maslaha* would be realized; this benefit would take precedence over the preservation of the dead, and in this case it would be permissible. The harm that would befall this living person who

is in need of this treatment is greater [without intervention] than the harm that would befall the dead whose eyes will be taken after his death.

Furthermore, this is not disrespect toward the dead and not an attack on his dignity that the *shariʿa* bestows upon him. The prohibition [against transgressing the dead] was made in the absence of a dire necessity or purpose. And we have already permitted this for the case of dissecting the corpses of those without [surviving] family members before their burial in [charity] graves, to realize the public benefit [*maslaha ʿama*] that takes precedence, in saving lives or treating the ill or determining the cause of crime if under investigation, as we have clarified [in an earlier fatwa on autopsy].

The Prophet's narration about "breaking the bones" is often asserted as evidence that any type of tampering or cutting into the dead is forbidden. But Mufti Maʾmun's fatwa asserts two reasons for why this hadith should not be interpreted as a *universal* prohibition of the procurement of eyes. First, he argues that the Prophetic tradition teaches a general rule—to respect the dead—in the absence of a situation of dire need *(darura)*. Second, the mufti argues that intentions matter. If the intention of removing eyes from the corpse is desecration of the dead, it is not allowed. If the intention is to benefit the life of another, then it is permissible. When weighing benefits and harms, the mufti concludes that the benefit of allowing a blind person to see is greater than the benefit of leaving a dead body preserved. And he argues that the harm of leaving a blind person untreated is greater than the harm of removing eyes from a dead body.

Few doctors of the period knew about or paid much attention to Mufti Maʾmun's very specific stipulations about what he deemed to be the conditional permissibility of eye extraction. In 1959, physicians were simply less interested in obtaining official religious guidance for their clinical practice. Although many considered themselves Muslims, this period of Egyptian history was marked by the politics of technological achievement. Professional elites in medicine have largely considered Islamic law *(fiqh)* to be an esoteric and irrelevant field of expertise, with little to offer in relation to medical knowledge. In the fatwa, Maʾmun stipulated three conditions: (1) the eyes must be procured under a condition of dire necessity *(darura)* for the potential recipient of the graft; (2) the ideal "donor" is someone who died with no surviving family members to claim his body; and (3) in the event that the need for grafts supersedes the number of donors without surviving family, then the eyes must be procured with the consent of surviving family members.[39] These stipulations were never met. There is no overall system to ensure that these and other ethical guidelines are followed, including the fair distribution of corneas. Furthermore, the practice of extracting eyes without consent of surviving family members was a clear transgression that occurred with impunity. Fatwas are, after all, not legally binding.

Ma'mun's fatwa, like Tantawi's, permits cornea donation. Yet I want to draw attention to the different logics, premises, and reasoning employed by the two muftis. The problem with Tantawi's stance, I have argued, is that it effaces the sacrifice of the dead donor. Tantawi never addressed the issue of the dignity of the dead, and he did not confirm views about the importance of bodily integrity. He minimized the significance of the dead body by focusing on the spiritual rewards that would accrue from the donation.

In contrast, Ma'mun argued that the permissibility of cornea extraction is *conditional* upon the intention and care of the procurement. He argued that the (presumably beneficial) medical extraction of eyes from the dead body is substantively different from the case of someone interfering with a dead body carelessly, without feeling or purpose or in order to cause deliberate harm. For Ma'mun, the burden of "pure intention" falls on the medical procurer, not on the donor. And even if the medical practitioners have the noblest of intentions in extracting the eyes of the dead to restore sight to blinded patients, the rights of the dead cannot be totally offset. Ma'mun delivered his 1959 fatwa on the basis of a hypothetical situation—an eye bank in Egypt that was to procure eyes from the dead for the benefit of the living. The assumption in 1959 was that the medical staff would be faced with a dead body with potential medical value (eyes). Ma'mun's fatwa sought to guide these medical practitioners on how to face such a situation in a context in which there was no public awareness of the issue. Ma'mun's fatwa made room for the permissibility of cornea extraction without dismissing the importance of carefully treating the dead and without denying what is largely regarded as a *necessary* connection between the spirit of the person and her body.

In contrast, by the time Tantawi took the public stage on the cornea debate, he sought to quell the public outcry following the media scandal of 1996 that had exposed rampant eye theft in public hospitals. Tantawi did not try to convince the public that respect for the dead would still be guaranteed in hospitals. He argued instead that it does not really matter how the dead body is treated, given the great spiritual rewards that the donor would accrue. After failing to garner support for a public awareness campaign launched in the mid-1990s for the donation of corneas, he ultimately began to eschew the question of consent altogether in his speeches.[40] Tantawi proceeded from the assumption that cornea donation results in

[handwritten marginalia: Egypt struggles in this way w/ corruption]

overwhelming public benefit, but he did not offer an explanation for why he thought so. Nor did he offer guidance on how to guarantee that overall benefit would be realized; again, he assumed this is the responsibility of medical practitioners, whom he believed are working for the benefit of the Egyptian population, including the poor. Shaykh Tantawi was obviously aware that abuses occur in the practice of transplantation and that to maintain credibility he had to address them. But, unlike those on the opposing side of the argument, he argued that nothing inherent in the practice itself leads to the abuse. The guilty individuals, he maintained, should be held accountable. This presumes the existence of just administrative and legal systems that can hold such individuals accountable, if in fact individuals are at fault and not the entire system of transplantation itself. Those who have argued against transplantation in all its permutations have had much more critical views of the workings of public hospitals, malpractice, and the Egyptian legal system.

Tantawi ultimately premised his fatwa on unacknowledged contradictions. The thrust of his argument is that the donor would be rewarded for a *sadaqa jariyya*, a perennial charity, for having helped another person through bodily sacrifice. Yet if the body is inconsequential, then there is no real sacrifice entailed and nothing of value to donate charitably. And more important, if the donor is to receive spiritual rewards for perpetual charity, she presumably *had that intention,* meaning that she must have consented to the donation.[41] Tantawi left the issue of consent exceedingly vague in his public speeches, and newspaper reports of his fatwas indicate that he authorized the physicians to extract corneas from the dead with no mention of donor or family consent. For Tantawi, the "crisis" of blinded cornea opacity patients, unable to see, work, or support themselves, renders excessive attachment to the dead both impractical and unethical.

CONCLUSIONS

The 1996 media scandal involving stolen eyes proved disastrous to the future of cornea grafting in Egypt. The exposure of the procurement of eyes from the public morgues scandalized a public by prompting long unresolved questions: What rights and dignity can poor patients expect? Will their autonomy and consent be respected? What is the state of equity and justice within Egyptian medical institutions? And, finally, how should access to medical resources allocated? The debate over Egypt's national eye banks has also evoked larger problems about the marketing of the body

within the greater context of the increased commercialization of l
itself. The lack of a local cornea supply has had severe repercussio₁
lives of cornea opacity patients, particularly the poor who cann₁
treatment in private clinics or abroad.

Public health campaigns in the late 1990s aimed to rectify the lack of
corneas by convincing people to make arrangements for donation after
death. Given the longstanding association of infectious eye disease with
"Egyptian ignorance," the language of the campaigns was saturated with
a civilizing discourse that ignored the issues of how to attain consent and
respect patient autonomy. The campaigns featured both religious and medical authorities who complained that opposition to donating eyes to the dead
is "ignorant" of both medical science and "true" religious doctrine. The
campaign launched two contradictory tactics: First, it rendered the cornea
both ordinary and insignificant, so that any reasonable person *would consent* to its being used to "restore sight to the blind." Second, it implied that
because so little is needed to contribute to so overwhelming a benefit, *no
one should have the right to refuse* donation.

Ultimately, doctors, public health specialists, legislators, and religious
scholars have all been unable to resolve this tangle of questions: (1) How can
proper treatment and respect of the dead, particularly of the poor's dead, be
ensured?[42] (2) Should doctors be required to obtain consent from donors or
their family members? (3) What system will guarantee that corneas are distributed fairly? (4) And, finally, who will assess and maintain standards of
the "public benefit" of eye banking? These questions, as well as the cost and
efficacy of the operations, have all factored into considerations of whether
or not this procedure is ultimately beneficial. And its benefit has been a basis
for evaluating whether it is ethically and religiously permissible.

In this setting where the poor are marginalized for being poor, the
materiality of death affords an important reminder that God alone ultimately issues the final judgment. People's most immediate obligations are
to their family members, and it is upon them that they depend for care,
both in life and in death. Given that the public medical system disap-
points more than it delivers, its demands for bodily sacrifice in the name of
"generosity" have compelled little action. One might imagine a system in
which eye tissues are procured only with people's knowledge and explicit
consent and a system that benefits poor and wealthy alike in restoring
their sight. With such a system in place, Shaykh Tantawi's arguments that
gifting eyes constitutes a *sadaqa jariyya* would likely sound much more
compelling. But in the context of medical institutions that do not accord
much respect to the poor, family members have asserted the importance of

caring properly for their dead and protecting them from further mistreatment *(bahdala)*.

Ophthalmologists and cornea opacity patients have collectively agreed that the rights of the living should be prioritized over the rights of the dead. Unlike other aspects of organ transplantation, physicians involved with cornea transplantation and patients who hope to be the recipients of the transplants agree on the benefits, and they have agitated over the urgency and necessity of cornea transplantations for Egypt's blind. Even if some have admitted uneasiness in tampering with the bodies of their own loved ones, they have all agreed in principle that cornea donation is a necessary and commendable act. In the next chapters, we will see that, in contrast, the benefits of kidney transplantation have been much more contested by religious scholars, patients in need, and transplant surgeons themselves. Again, questions about the ethics of transferring body parts from one person to another necessarily take on different meanings when one considers specifics such as the materiality and symbolic associations of the body part, its procurement method, the efficacy of its transplantation, and the postsurgical repercussions for patients.

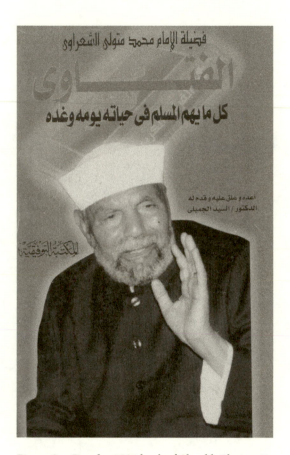

Figure 9. Popular 1996 book of Shaykh Sha'rawi's
fatwas: "Everything that pertains to a Muslim's life,
today and tomorrow."

4. Shaykh of the People

Genealogy of an Utterance

As we have seen so far, questions that we might classify as "bioethical" have been vigorously debated in Egypt by official muftis and doctors. These have included questions about whether procurement of organs from the dead is appropriate, who counts as dead, and whether (and how) to obtain consent from surviving family members. With the diversification of media outlets, these debates have entered into a larger public domain, in which nonexperts, including patients and family members, have become more familiar with a wide array of expert opinion. Meanwhile, amid the scandals of eye theft and mistreatment of the dead, a larger, more troubling debate has taken place in Egypt about the ethics of procuring organs from *living* donors, the realities of which—sometimes uplifting and other times horrifying—have been made increasingly visible in opposition-party and state-aligned newspapers and, more important, on television.

In fact, it was a television star, not a doctor or a state-appointed mufti, who stood at the center of the debate about organ transplantation in Egypt. As scholars of Egypt have noted, television plays a particularly important role in the country (Abu-Lughod 2005), and this remains true for public engagement with bioethical debates as well. Muhammad Mutwalli Sha'rawi (1911–98), a popular and enormously influential figure who hosted his own religious television show, was the first to argue against organ transplantation with the statement "the body belongs to God," a statement that has been repeated more than any other on the topic of transplantation. Those who have struggled to come to terms with the complicated ethical dimensions of organ transplantation have often referenced Sha'rawi by confirming, resignifying, or outright refuting the idea that organ transplantation is directly prohibited simply because the body belongs to God.[1]

Understanding Sha'rawi's statement—that is, the context in which it was uttered, delivered, and received—is an important step in understanding how debates in Egypt have ensued over the practice of extracting vital organs from living donors and transplanting them into dying patients. Outside Egypt, commentators on the ethics and laws of organ transplantation in the Arab world have often missed Sha'rawi's importance. And within Egypt, commentators and ordinary people have generally elided the depths of Sha'rawi's statement and the different arguments, positions, and modes of reasoning that inspired it. This has much to do with the tendency in dominant narratives to polarize debates into "progressive versus traditional trends" or "medical versus religious views." In fact, Sha'rawi's statement, I argue in later chapters, has been resonant in part because it bears medical significance; that is, it raises important questions about medical risk, futility, and efficacy. In chapters 5 and 6, I detail the ways in which patients in kidney failure and their family members make sense of their conviction that the body belongs to God, both when they decide to seek transplantation as a medical treatment and when they refuse it. But first, this chapter outlines who Sha'rawi was, why his statement has come to matter, what his defenders and detractors have interpreted from it, and how his reasoning fit into his larger public role.

FIRM IN THE MIDST OF SOCIAL UPHEAVAL

As Egypt pivoted in the 1970s from Nasser's brand of secularist socialism, allied with the Soviet Union, to Sadat's "Open Door" economic policy, aligned with the United States, Sha'rawi was a central public figure. Amid the jolting political-economic transformation that occurred simultaneously with mass immigration to the petro-rich Gulf states and the related social changes of the Islamic revival *(al-sahwa al-islamiyya)*, he was a constant, familiar, and comforting presence to many Egyptians. During Nasser's regime, Sha'rawi had spoken out in disagreement with it and was subsequently exiled from Egypt.[2] Upon Nasser's death, Sadat took office, seeking legitimacy by bolstering support for his stance against leftist Nasserists by appealing to the Islamist movement, which Nasser had violently repressed.[3] Toward this end, Sadat welcomed Sha'rawi back to Egypt and appointed him as minister of *awqaf* (religious endowments) from 1976 to 1978. During this time, Sadat also granted Sha'rawi his own slot on Egyptian state television to host *Nur 'ala Nur* (Light upon Light), which would become his famous Qur'anic commentary show, the vehicle for his popular ascendance.[4]

Overestimating Sha'rawi's influence throughout Egyptian society would be difficult. His later show, *Khawatir Imaniyya* (Steps of Faith) showcased his linguistic genius. His popularity rested on the perception among the Egyptian public that he "spoke the truth," as someone firmly rooted in the Islamic tradition, even if this involved speaking out against those in power. In his self-presentation, he always remained a simple, humble figure. His admirers did not forget his years in political exile and that his candor had once cost him access to his home and family. In this respect, Sha'rawi's renewed links to the state seemed insignificant to his admirers, perhaps because they held him to be incorruptible by political or financial interests. His devotees often contrasted him with state-appointed muftis, whom they described as government employees who went so far as to "sell the religion" in order to facilitate the aims of the government.[5]

At the time of my fieldwork, nearly a decade after his death, his television program was still replayed every Friday after communal prayers and rerun regularly during the month of Ramadan. Sha'rawi's popularity has generally been attributed to his charismatic personality and his ability to connect with the "common people." He has been perceived as one who would "reawaken the people" to the call to Islam and reinvigorate society with a devotion to faith that would cure all contemporary ills: corruption, crime, dishonesty, greed, the disintegration of the family, godlessness, political instability. To these ills Sha'rawi consistently offered exceedingly simple solutions: turn to the Qur'an, devote yourself to God, follow the teachings of the Prophet. Sha'rawi's books of religious lessons, cassette tapes, CDs, and summaries of key religious teachings continue to saturate bookshops, street bookstalls, and even high-end grocery stores throughout Egypt's cities. The Danish social historian Jakob Skovgaard-Petersen once remarked that the Qur'an and Sha'rawi's book of fatwas were often the only two books that he saw in Egyptian friends' homes (Skovgaard-Petersen 1997: 12).[6]

On his famous television shows, at times filmed in a studio and at other times in a mosque, Sha'rawi, simply dressed in a *galabiyya* and his trademark white cap, interpreted the Qur'an in everyday, accessible language— that is, in colloquial Egyptian Arabic—to the rhythm of his inimitable bodily movements and gestures. Through his exegesis, he demonstrated the Qur'an's relevance to all aspects of everyday life. At the same time, he was not interested in apologizing for the incompatibilities he saw between fast-paced urban modernity and religious devotion, nor was he interested in reconciling them. His critics, particularly members of a Western-educated elite, perceived Sha'rawi as a throwback to the past, an "anti-modern" irrational figure. But even as these critics' voices seemed loud in their columns in the major newspapers, they were in the minority in regard to perceptions of Sha'rawi. When I began my field research in Egypt, I was surprised to learn of the near unanimous respect for Sha'rawi that people of various classes, professional roles, and dispositions expressed to me. Having read negative accounts of him in the Egyptian press and having heard cynical and sarcastic personal attacks on him from Egyptian intellectuals living in the United States, I was unprepared to hear doctors, surgeons, nurses, medical students, pathologists, bus passengers, taxi drivers, rural patients, and urban businesspeople in Egypt speak fondly of Sha'rawi and refer respectfully to the depths of his knowledge of the Qur'an. Even if they did not agree with Sha'rawi's specific stance on contemporary topics like organ donation, they recognized that he had an unparalleled role in transforming their worldviews and the social and religious landscape of Egypt more generally.

In this sense, it seemed paradoxical that the state, in its moment of political and economic alignment with the United States and Western Europe, would have promoted such a figure. Yet Sha'rawi was not oppositional toward the political regimes of Sadat or Mubarak, as were the leaders of politicized Islamist groups such as the Muslim Brotherhood. His disinclination to embrace modern life helped him to appear unthreatening. By promoting Sha'rawi's religious programming, Sadat's administration, and later that of Mubarak, wagered that it could co-opt his religious popularity yet be certain that he operated in a distinct realm, speaking a different language and addressing different concerns that did not directly challenge state authority.[7] As political scientist Carrie Wickham (2002) argues, both Sadat and Mubarak miscalculated the extent to which the social and pietistic strands of the Islamic revival would have political import.

Sha'rawi's stated agenda was to "reawaken" Egyptians with a call to piety. His immediate accessibility made him a lovable figure. While he did not speak in terms of Islamic jurisprudence or formal legal reasoning, he had a solid foundation in traditional Islamic learning, and his exegesis was universally respected by scholars of Islam. At the lessons that I attended in jurisprudence at al-Azhar, the teacher Shaykh 'Amr fondly recalled that in the early mornings the late Sha'rawi would walk from the *masjid* of Sayyidna al-Hussayn to that of al-Azhar with a team of schoolboys, who would admiringly tag after him as he walked. He would begin a chant, to which the schoolboys would accompany him in rhythm: "Hadhir, Nadhir, ya Ikhwani, / Amma al Ghafla, da shay' Tani!" Shaykh 'Amr would recall that the effect was a melodic sound, to which women on the balconies of the old city would weep with emotion. The chant's rhythmic qualities cannot be rendered in translation, but the meaning evoked is: God is ever-watchful, O brothers, [so let us steer away from] a state of negligence that would render us heedless of divine ever-presence.

As a "common" religious figure from a humble rural background, Sha'rawi symbolized to many the purity of a pristine, rural, devout Egypt: the moral center and fiber of a society that was now in decline.[8] Unlike the state-appointed muftis or those who specialized in legal scholarship, Sha'rawi was not particularly interested in reinvigorating modes of Islamic legal reasoning that would render the tradition flexible and adaptable to modern society.[9] As he saw it, modern society turns people away from devotion to God. His main stated interest was to reinvigorate a firm faith that would bring Muslim society out of a state of moral and social degradation.

Sha'rawi thus came into direct conflict with those who worked at shaping Egypt as a modernizing, liberalizing nation: a secular country of development, a technologically and scientifically advanced nation of experts, and a center of high culture and the fine arts.[10] His position on organ transplantation offers one concrete example of what "developmentalist" and "liberal" Egyptian intellectuals have found most worrisome: that traditionalism and literalist religious interpretations would stand as obstacles to Egypt's progress. Further problematic for many of these Egyptian intellectuals who voiced their criticism in the press was that a man from a poor rural background who specialized only in traditional Islamic studies would presume to speak authoritatively about other fields of expertise, such as modern science, politics, medicine, international conflict, and biotechnology.

Sha'rawi's stance against particular types of medical interventions was formed within his larger role of urging believing, pious Muslims not to fear death and reminding them that the Qur'an bears the ultimate truth. In one of the compendia of Sha'rawi's teachings, he responded to the question: "How is it that the Qur'an claims that God alone knows what is in mothers' wombs, when we today have ultrasound technology?" His reply was that the ultrasound might reveal physical, anatomical features, but only God knows the fate of the child-to-come. In responding to another questioner, he explained that in "making test-tube babies" scientists were not creating life but rather were only facilitating a process that God, the sole Creator, had already begun.[11] He constantly spoke against the assumption that new technologies make Islamic teachings outdated or irrelevant.

DEPRIVING POOR PATIENTS

In a break from his usual appearance as the host of his own television series, in December 1988, Shaykh Sha'rawi appeared as a guest on a social commentary program called *Min al-alif ila al-ya'* (From A to Z).[12] When Tariq Habib, the host of the show, asked him what he thought about organ transplantation, Sha'rawi replied that it is *haram* because the body belongs to God.[13] He further remarked that costly and extraordinary medical measures should be avoided in the case of terminal illness, as true believers should embrace their final meeting with God. These televised remarks set off a major controversy and much adversity in the Egyptian press. As one of Sha'rawi's biographers put it: "Among the fatwas of the shaykh that caused a huge shock and commotion in public space was the fatwa that the shaykh uttered on the television program hosted by Mr. Tariq Habib over four consecutive episodes. The shaykh spoke on it spontaneously, simply and from his heart. Perhaps the reader knows now from this description to what I am referring: the fatwa that exposed the honorable shaykh to a media attack that was utterly baseless, all because of his opinion on the issue of organ transplantation" (Hasan 1990: 84).[14] Journalists and physicians soon vociferously condemned Sha'rawi in the press for taking a position that was perceived and depicted as extreme and nonsensical. Newspapers reported that Sha'rawi was against medical treatment and thus breaking with the Prophetic tradition that encourages the pursuit of healing in illness. Rumors circulated about his personal and moral integrity. On many occasions I heard his critics caustically remark that although Sha'rawi had forbidden blood transfusions (which was untrue), he received numerous transfusions himself when he was ill. And I was told on more than one occasion that although Sha'rawi forbade transplants, he himself received a cornea transplant when he was sick. This was also untrue; he did, however, undergo a cataract operation.[15] One example of such caustic criticism is an article published in the state newspaper and titled: "Shaykh Sha'rawi Made Permissible for Himself What He Declared to Be Forbidden to Others!"[16]

The controversy over Sha'rawi's position on transplants has been about different powers vying over who can legitimately speak for "the Egyptian people."[17] Self-described "progressive" journalists with whom I spoke further complained that his version of Islam is backward and, more dangerous, that he was the leader of a largely ignorant mass of devotees who would blindly follow whatever he preached. His critics' vigorous media campaign against his position was passionately carried out in the name of defending poor ignorant patients whom Sha'rawi had "deprived" of potential treatment. A typical example is this piece by columnist Sulayman Guda in the Egyptian newspaper *Al-Misry al-Yawm*:

> The real problem is that most of the Shaykh's followers who keenly attended his lessons, who followed him from one mosque to another, and who watched all his recorded shows used to completely stop thinking in his presence. They used to accept the Shaykh's interpretations, right or wrong, with no one daring to question or discuss his interpretations with him.
>
> . . . The Shaykh's interpretations were based on his own perspective and point of view, from which he interpreted the meanings of verses. And it's natural that there would be differences of opinion from one interpreter to another and from one historical context to another and from one particular social situation to another.
>
> When he for example, objected to blood transfusions and organ transplantation, saying that they were impermissible in religion, he was wrong, and he should have been questioned on this, because his position was against the interests of many patients. . . .
>
> . . . The Honorable Shaykh was—and still is—a member of the [fallible] human race, and his words need be subject to scrutiny. Saying this does not belittle his importance. All that has been said does not stop us from deeply respecting the great *mujtahid* Shaykh Sha'rawi. (Guda 2008)

The idea that shaykhs like Sha'rawi wield enormous influence among "blind devotees" is a part of the cultural imagining that has played into larger debates about Islamic authority and its relevance to bioethical questions. None of these commentators ever actually examined or scrutinized how, precisely, Sha'rawi's words influenced the lives of patients. As the next chapters detail, my own fieldwork shows no evidence that people in fact "closed their minds" and acted against their own interests in their "blind" emulation of Sha'rawi. The contention that people wrongly elevated Sha'rawi to the status of someone "holy" even though there should be no such figures in Islam, reflects a long legalistically oriented prejudice against more popular Sufi-oriented Muslim practices in which a spiritual hierarchy indeed elevates particular figures, both in life and in death. Because these popular practices are said to be "backward," they are faulted for not allowing for rational thought. Critics of Sha'rawi often framed their larger arguments in nationalist discourse that stresses the importance of Egyptians acting as "citizens" rather than as members of particular family or ethnic groups or as followers of unofficial religious figures, thereby helping to bolster the legal-ethical authority of the modern state.

Indeed, Sha'rawi's remarks were most explosive when uttered on television, a medium accessible to the largest swath of Egyptians, including illiterate peasants. When Sha'rawi made similar statements earlier, recorded in print newspapers or issued verbally to medical professionals since the mid-1970s, there was no public outcry. When the personal attacks against Sha'rawi intensified, columnist Salah Muntassar provided a full transcript of Sha'rawi's televised remarks, contextualizing and explicating them, in an effort to clarify the terms of the debate (Muntassar 1989). And more than a year before his controversial televised appearance, a more detailed explication of his argument was published in a government-produced newspaper, *Al-Liwa' al-Islami*. I turn to an analysis of this text below.[18]

AS GOD'S PROPERTY

Sha'rawi's stance against organ transplantation was based on the premise that the human body is the exclusive property of God. The caption under his huge image in the article read: "The Honorable Shaykh Sha'rawi says that the human being does not own his body, so how could he donate or sell a part of it?" From this premise, he makes two corollary arguments: (1) In our duties to help our fellow beings, we need to distinguish between the body's capabilities and the body's physical parts; and, most controversially, (2) There is divine wisdom behind disease and bodily incapacity.

Sha'rawi drew on the explicit Qur'anic forbiddance of suicide as evidence of his premise that the human body belongs to God.[19] As he put it, "The person does not own his own self; the self is owned by God, most exalted and high. And from here we come to understand the punishment of suicide, which is to remain in hellfire, for the human in such a case destroyed a being that belonged to God and not to him." Sha'rawi thus argues that there are limits to what a person can rightly do to his or her own body, and that these limits—God's command—are inscribed in the divine revelation. In his first corollary argument, Sha'rawi is responding to his followers' questions about their duty to save the life of another. If someone were in a burning building, would it not be incumbent upon Muslims to save potential victims, even if doing so might endanger their own lives? Sha'rawi's response to this is to assert a distinction between one's bodily capabilities, what he calls the body's effects *(athar al-jasad)*, and the physical body parts. In his words:

> Just as there is a difference between donating the whole body and
> donating its parts, so is there a difference between donating the *effects*
> of the body and the *effects* of the parts. For me to donate the effects, this

is permitted and commanded in the religion. For example, even if I were
to lose a body part [in saving a person from a fire], the goal here was for
me to donate my *abilities* of movement to save a person from the dangers of burning, and in any case this all could not happen without the
will of God.[20]

Sha'rawi thus reasoned that even if he were to lose a part of his body in the
process of running into the fire and rescuing another person, this would
be permitted, even commanded by religion, because the intention would
not be to give a part of the body but to give the effects of one's bodily
abilities. This is different from deciding a priori that the body parts that
God has created would be better placed in the body of someone else. This
distinction allowed Sha'rawi to justify his view on the permissibility of
blood donation. As he explained: "[My position on organ donation] does
not nullify the permissibility of blood donation. Blood is regenerated and
is regarded as an effect of the self rather than a part of it. The blood cells
are continually renewed and regenerated when the person loses some of
it."[21] For Sha'rawi, the distinction between the body's capabilities and the
body's material parts was commonsensical, yet his critics, who did not
share this view of the body, saw his different stances on blood and organ
donation as hypocritical.

Sha'rawi's second corollary argument was particularly provocative. He
disputed the presumption that illness is an abhorrence to be rectified and
instead stated that affliction and disability are among the signs of God's
perfect wisdom. He believed that God tries some of His servants by depriv-
ing them of certain bodily functions, and that this in turn heightens the
awareness that the body is ultimately controlled by divine will. Sha'rawi
contested the notion that the body is something that we should seek to
control, arguing that this is an arrogant imposition on God's creation and
on the fact of God's total and ultimate power. As he stated:

The human owns neither the existence of his self nor parts of this self.
All of the parts of the human body function by the will of God alone.
It is not for the person to interfere in this. The heart beats by the will
of God. And the stomach and the intestines and the liver all function in
their roles without the interference of human will. Air is inspired and
expired through and out of the two lungs without us even realizing
that we are breathing and without our will. The human being does not
govern the organ functions of his own body.

[A person] cannot order his own heart to beat if it stops. . . . [A per-
son] cannot interfere with many [minute] functions and movements
of his own body parts, like the kidney, the liver, the lungs, the intestines, et cetera. Even those body parts that do submit outwardly to the

human will, such as the hand and the foot and the eye and the tongue, they still [ultimately] submit to human will only by the will of God.

The mute person has a tongue, and yet he cannot speak. A paralyzed person may have two feet and two hands, but he cannot move them, even if these body parts work with the will of the self. . . . it is the will of God that ultimately gave it movement and submitted it to the will of the human. And if it is the will of God for [this movement] to slip away, then the movement will be lost.[22]

Sha'rawi explicated that devout humans should be conscious at every moment that it is God who owns and wills each intricate mechanism and function of their bodies. The involuntary cellular mechanisms of the body—that which humans do not actively control—are signs that reflect God's ultimate will. Humans' voluntary movements, such as our ability to will our arms to move, are reminders that humans are morally responsible for their actions, even as it is God who ultimately controls and judges them.

In this argument, Sha'rawi articulated a position that struck at the very heart of biomedical philosophy and at strands of its Western Christian antecedents. As Bryan Turner writes, "At least in the West (during the classical and Christian eras) the body has been seen to be a threatening and dangerous phenomenon, if not adequately controlled and regulated by cultural processes" (Turner 1997: 20). For Sha'rawi, who took a position that can be traced to a long tradition of Muslim philosophical thought and who was often associated with a particularly Sufi disposition, it is a state of heedlessness of divine omnipotence *(ghafla)* that distances people from the ontological reality that God, not us, is in control of every infinitesimal bodily process. Turner, following Erving Goffman notes, "Any loss of control over our bodies is socially embarrassing, implying a loss of control over ourselves" (Turner 1997: 19). In contrast, Sha'rawi suggested that loss of immediate control—as in a paralyzed person's lack of control over limb movement or a blind person's loss of visual control—brings the afflicted person closer to the ontological reality of the body as belonging to God and ultimately subject to divine omnipotence.[23]

Sha'rawi aimed to challenge the notion that humans should presume to control or own their bodies, that humans can prolong life or thwart death. For Sha'rawi, our inability to tell our hearts when to beat or stop beating is among the divine signs meant to remind humans to cultivate the proper disposition of utter submission and gratitude to God. In the Islamic tradition, it is not the flesh of the human body that is the source of sin or evil; rather, the fallibility of the human being is the tendency to forget and neglect God. Thus the path to salvation in Islam is the constant remembrance *(al-dhikr)* of God, the appreciation of God's mercy, the under-standing that all of creation is a reflection of God's signs to which humans should submit in gratitude *(al-shukr)*. This is not disputed among Muslims.

However, what is contentious is Sha'rawi's implication that the impera-tive to treat an affliction nullifies the opportunity to view the affliction nonetheless as a sign from God. Many physicians and patients have coun-tered that medicine, too, is a divine sign, a point that Sha'rawi himself readily admitted. The questions then became: At which point does medical treatment pull us away from a disposition of God-awareness and piety? Why do *particular* medical treatments endanger such a disposition while others do not? Why does organ transplantation, in particular, turn us away from God's will, obscuring its status as "treatment"?

Rather than answering these nagging questions, Sha'rawi's response was to shun the practice altogether:

> One cannot donate something that one does not own; in that case the donation would be invalid. The human being does not own his whole self and does not own some or parts of his self [*dhatihi*]. The human being does not own his body. Rather, this body is the property of God, most exalted and high. He is the One who created it. No one can claim otherwise. It is God who gives the gift of life [*huwa aladhi wahhabahu al-hayat*].
>
> So a person, no matter who he is or what he has accomplished, can never claim to have given the gift of life. Or to have created life. God is the One who makes [a person] die whenever He wills it, and no one on this earth could supersede His will by preventing death or by making a person on the verge of death live a single second beyond his final time.[24]

In another instance, he said,

> Those who have permitted organ donation do not have the justification to say that they are "saving the life" of another. Saving life is an imper-ative owned by God alone. . . . My plea to those scholars and doctors for whom the humanitarian spirit and love has dominated their work is for them to stay far away from arrogance and rebelliousness toward God's creation. They have issued a new opinion that says this is "saving life." My response to such an opinion is: don't denigrate the religions in order to "save life."
>
> Now this does not mean that we do not take precautions or cures or that we do not take medicine for illness, for it is God who created ill-ness and God who created its medicine.[25]

In keeping with his general message and his role to "reawaken" Egyptian society, Sha'rawi was interested in asserting a particular disposition that humans should have toward their Maker and toward their bodies as God's creation. Shaʿrawi acted within his role as a *daʿiya* to stress that God is the sole dealer in life and death. He argued that the discursive field of a "gift of life" that has surrounded organ transplantation is an arrogant imposition on the correct relationship that worshipers should cultivate toward their Creator. While he clarified that his stance against organ donation was not a stance against biomedical intervention writ large, he also refused to engage in the myriad questions raised by this seeming contradiction.

NOT A FATWA

Specialists in Islamic jurisprudence, including Shaʿrawi's defenders, have argued that his position was not wrong but that it was simply "not a fatwa." Unlike state muftis, Shaʿrawi did not employ legal reasoning or tools of legal theory to make his case. Several religious scholars condemned the media for having mistaken Shaʿrawi's statement about piety by wrongly rendering it a legal judgment. As one religious scholar told me in frustration, the state-oriented media often treats a figure like Shaʿrawi or a mufti as if he were "the pope of Islam," knowing full well, of course, that no such figure exists. The state-oriented journalists then deride these figures for not, in actuality, having such authority by arguing that (Sunni) Islam has no official clergy.

Shaykh ʿAli Gumaʿa, the current grand mufti, has held a more nuanced position on the complexities of the question of organ transplantation in Muslim legal ethics but still appreciates Shaʿrawi's position. In a private interview, Gumaʿa explained to me that Shaʿrawi's response to organ transplantation in the statement "the body belongs to God" represents a *"madhhab,"* a particular way of seeing things.[26] This should not be confused with a fatwa, he clarified, which is a legal opinion or answer to a question. Nor should Shaʿrawi's *madhhab* be seen as a recommendation, let alone a prescription for someone's particular case. According to Gumaʿa, Shaʿrawi's *madhhab* does not answer the question of whether or not a particular person can receive a transplant in a particular way. ʿAli Gumaʿa argued that for the media to have seized upon Shaʿrawi's position and read it as a prohibition against anyone ever having a transplant is a misapplication and misunderstanding of how Islamic legal ethics works.

Shaykh ʿAli Gumaʿa offered the following case. Consider, he said, a healthy mother desperate to donate her kidney to her sick child, who would benefit from the operation. Did that not pose an entirely different set of ethical questions than would the case of a poor man trying to sell his kidney to alleviate his debts, or the case of a heartbeating brain-dead donor who is prematurely declared dead in order for his organs to be procured? The role of the legal scholar or mufti, according to Guma'a, is to be able to apply the tenets of Islam to the different particulars of each case. Shaykh Guma'a further insisted that two hundred years ago (i.e., before the devastating effects colonialism had on traditional institutions of learning), ordinary people *(al-'awwam)* knew the difference between a fatwa and a *hukm* (a general rule), and he argued that it is the irresponsible media and "entertainment-style journalism" of today that distort people's understandings of how Islamic legal ethics should be applied.[27]

Many other scholars have pointed out that difference of opinion in Islamic scholarship has long been encouraged and understood to be one of the strengths of Islamic law (Muntasar 1989). In saying this, they are referring to a principle found in some narrations of the Prophet, in which he is reported to have said, "Verily my companions are like the stars in the sky. Whichever one you choose and follow, you will be guided. The differences of companions for you are a mercy [*ikhtilafu ummati rahma*]."[28] However, in the contemporary period, scholars have lamented that traditional institutes of Islamic learning and scholarship have been displaced and are expected to conform to modern-state codification of law, a consequence of which is that nonspecialists expect religious scholars always to issue only a *single* opinion on a new or complex topic. As Mufti Guma'a complained when explaining his stance on brain death, the mainstream media consider "difference in opinion" *(ikhtilaf)* among scholars to be evidence that "Islamic experts" cannot adequately answer the question at hand. The larger problem is that state discourses have given very little space to the casuistic workings of Islamic scholarship, rendering the various genres, disciplines, approaches, and fields of expertise as one catchall category, religion. Further, they seem to have precluded the possibility of multiple legitimate perspectives.

Sha'rawi's biographers have offered similar arguments about the validity of differing opinions and why Sha'rawi's position should not be considered a legal fatwa.[29] In one biography, Abdul Mu'ti 'Imran, the editor-in-chief of *Al-Liwa' al-Islami*, stated, "His Honor Shaykh Sha'rawi decided to take the road of caution in his interpretation [*ijtihad*] of this issue, and difference of opinion is by all means allowed. His words were issued forth out of deep spiritual sentiments that one should never challenge the trials of God. And he is a special case. Muslims should understand him before they whisper evil about him."[30] Sha'rawi's colleagues and supporters were deeply hurt and offended by the vicious tenor taken against him, holding that he was, indeed, a "special case" who spoke out of deep spiritual sentiment, as a way of holding him above the rank of those who had attacked him. Significantly, his defenders have not generally agreed with his position on organ transplantation. Rather, they have contended that Sha'rawi, who uttered this opinion, was above reproach and that Muslims should defer to the high spiritual level that he achieved. As the dean of al-Azhar, Dr. Ra'uf Shalabi, further stated,

> This is not a defense of Shaykh Sha'rawi, because he is not in need of anyone defending him. The words of his honor about seeking treatment and organ transplantation were not legal fatwas. Rather, they were the expressions of deep spiritual sentiment that God's servants should never challenge what God tries them with. If people wish to seek treatment, then it is legally allowed, and there is nothing wrong with this. . . .
>
> From the perspective of Islamic jurisprudence, Shaykh Sha'rawi is deeply knowledgeable in legal matters, and if he had been speaking in this vein, then he would have spoken correctly. But he was speaking from a personal, spiritual perspective regarding God's trials. This is an issue about which there are differences of opinion: taking treatment is permissible, and neither human reason nor divine law denies this. Healing comes from God, not from the medicine, not from the doctor.[31] Shaykh Sha'rawi did not say that seeking treatment is forbidden.[32]

Sha'rawi, on numerous occasions, responded to his critics and opponents.[33] He made clear in his rebuttal that his major aim was to encourage people to cultivate proper dispositions toward death, toward the divine decree, and toward all aspects of life, including the abilities and functions of the material body. Muslims, he argued, should not fear death; they should welcome all trials and illnesses as God's command and submit themselves to the recognition that we all belong ultimately to God. Sha'rawi elaborated:

> I never asked anyone not to pursue treatment. God is the most compassionate toward His servants, more compassionate than they are toward themselves.
>
> There was a huge commotion caused by what I said about organ transplantation and end-of-life care. And words that I never said were put into my mouth. I did not oppose treatment, nor did I oppose patients seeking medical care. . . . Islam does not forbid treatment, nor does it oppose medicine. I personally go to doctors when I fall ill.
>
> I also spoke about death. I said: We must not look at it with fear. Death is the encounter with God, and whoever loves to meet God, God loves to meet him.
>
> I spoke about intensive care units. And how in many cases a person could remain on an artificial mechanism that artificially continues life that no longer could proceed [on its own]. So if the electricity is stopped

for one minute, the person would die. . . . Umm Kulthum was left in such a state for more than a week.[34]

I said: This is [prolonging] suffering. . . . I said: Be merciful upon such people [i.e., let them die]. They have suffered enough. And do not be afraid of death, because it is the meeting of God. This is what I said, and I clarify it again. All success is with God.[35]

Sha'rawi thus argued that if the Muslim community is truly focused on God consciousness and piety, then it will embrace all events, catastrophes, illnesses, and trials as signs of God's infinite justice and ultimate mercy. This cultivation of a pious disposition *(al-ta'addub bi'adab al-'abudiyya)* requires working on the self through acts of devotion, a goal for which Sha'rawi uniquely and truly excelled at striving, according to his defenders. Yet it is a goal that Sha'rawi called for *all* Muslims to realize.

TANTAWI'S COUNTERFATWA: ANOTHER WAY TO BELONG TO GOD

Although Sha'rawi may have spoken from "personal conviction" in his newspaper interview with *al-Liwa' al-Islami* in 1987 and in his televised interview in 1988, he also went beyond the personal in counseling and cautioning others against pursuing a transplant and advised doctors not to work in organ transplantation. His position, then, was not simply a disinclination that he felt he should apply to his own life. Further, even if it was true that Sha'rawi was known as a *da'iya* and that he had not spoken in the genre of legal reasoning, Sha'rawi's followers routinely gathered his answers to questions posed by his audience and followers in compendia of "Sha'rawi's fatwas," which were then widely disseminated. By restoring the generic meaning of *fatwa* to refer simply to responses that scholars offer to questions posed to them, his followers decentered the authority of *ifta'* (fatwa giving) from the state. As I describe in the next chapter, many physicians, including Egypt's top surgeons, solicited fatwas from Sha'rawi. His response to them, about the permissibility of organ transplantation, was an unyielding "no."

In response to Sha'rawi's influence, Shaykh Tantawi, during his tenure as Egypt's grand mufti, issued his own counterfatwa soon afterward, which referenced Sha'rawi's arguments (Muntasar 1989). This shows the sometimes unexpected channels of influence in the production of Islamic legal knowledge and bioethical norms in Egypt: a television star with millions of followers and devotees shaped the logic and contours of the official fatwas issued by the state bureaucratic office of fatwa giving (Dar al-Ifta').

Tantawi's counterfatwa began with an elaborate explanation of the human body as being owned solely by God and of its elevated stature in Islamic belief. Like Sha'rawi, he referred to the prohibition of suicide as evidence that one cannot do what one wishes with one's body but rather that a Muslim must abide by the command of the Creator, who endowed humans with their bodies as a trust. After an elaborate discussion that read much like Sha'rawi's arguments, Tantawi remarked that God's ownership of our bodies is evidence of the prohibition of the *sale* or *commodification* of any body part. Tantawi then noted that "unlike other scholars," he distinguished between selling an organ and donating it out of love or concern for the welfare of the recipient, which he stated is surely a noble act that God will generously reward. Tantawi ultimately permitted living organ donation under the conditions of the dire need of the recipient, the clear overall benefit, and the avoidance of undue harm to the donor, which must be assessed by a "doctor of confidence." Tantawi asserted that the shari'a honored the human being in life and in death and aimed to lessen suffering and that the doctors of confidence, who were the experts in the field, were ultimately responsible before God and before others for working toward attaining these goals. Throughout his fatwa, Tantawi made many implicit references to the words of Sha'rawi, using Sha'rawi's arguments to prohibit organ *selling* rather than organ transplantation more generally.

As Tantawi put it:

> Organ donation comes up only in situations of dire need, for someone dear to the donor. And the motivation for doing this is to do a great favor to the person in need, [for no other reward than] to please God. We don't say [in this case], "The human body does not belong to him but belongs to God," and that since this is the case it is not right for the person to deal with what he does not own, either by selling or by donating."
>
> What we say instead is, "There is no doubt that being motivated by trying to alleviate suffering for another person is one of the supreme ways of pleasing God, and may such persons be rewarded greatly for their deeds."
>
> Under this rule, the selling or commodification of any part of a human, organ, or blood is prohibited, for this is void in the shari'a.

By including stipulations of permissibility, these types of fatwas appealed to the logic and rationalism embedded within Islamic legal reasoning.[36] If the aim of the shari'a is to uphold the ultimate spiritual and material benefits of the Muslim community at large, then a practice aimed at medical treatment or the improvement of quality of life would, by this logic, be permissible as long as it does not contradict any current religious principles.

This leads us back to the thorny question of how "benefit" is to be determined and who is to determine it. Muslim legal reasoning, fatwas, and the use of criteria such as *maslaha* (public benefit, or social good) must be studied within their specific social contexts, taking into account the particular worldview, political persuasions, education, and outlook of the particular muftis (Skovgaard-Petersen 1997; Opwis 2005). Here again it becomes evident that religious scholars' differing positions on a practice such as organ transplantation may have less to do with their different approaches to Islamic legal tenets than with their views of the practice at hand and its relationship to state institutions.

While the official and popular press sought to draw a contrast between Sha'rawi as a "backward extremist" and Tantawi as "forward-thinking" in their approach to religion, their different understandings of the medical procedure itself and whether it causes more benefit than harm were left unexamined. We should not be surprised that those more likely to benefit from medical treatment have encouraged religious arguments for it, whereas those who have more reason to fear mistreatment and exploitation have appealed to the logic of keeping the body to oneself and to God. Aside from the two shaykhs' different roles in society—Tantawi as an official mufti, and Sha'rawi as a popular *da'iya*—they also had different attitudes about modern medical practices and whether or not these lead to "benefit." Tantawi assumed that benefit is the leading motivation of the medical profession; he was less apt to interrogate directly the medical justification of the procedure, leaving this task to the "trustworthy" medical experts.[37] In contrast, Sha'rawi generally doubted the "salvific" promises of modern scientific "breakthroughs." With organ transplantation in particular, he often spoke of the negative effects that he had witnessed or heard about in Egypt and particularly the black market in human organs. In his rebuttal argument to his critics, he stated, "I spoke about organ transplantation and I said: it is *haram*. And I have [a right to] my opinion. Because the human being does not own his own body. . . . And most cases of organ transplantation fail anyway and do not succeed in their goals. The one who receives a transplant remains seriously ill and suffers for the two or three months that he lives."[38]

His "clarification" of his position reveals what he has witnessed or heard about transplants: that most fail and those that "succeed" do not end the patients' suffering. For Sha'rawi, the high failure rates of organ transplants (in its early years) is further evidence that transplantation does not constitute suitable "treatment" (morally or scientifically). However, Sha'rawi did not state that these reasons formed the *basis* of his position. Rather, he cited the detrimental effects of transplants as *evidence* that his position was correct. [39]

Sha'rawi remained one of the few voices among public religious figures who have opposed organ transplantation and other interventionist medical technologies. His argument that the body belongs to God is in fact a truism in Islam, and no Muslim scholar would argue against it. But when legal scholars have employed the legal tools of necessity *(darura)* and overall benefit *(maslaha)*, the majority has come to judge organ transplantation to be permissible under several conditions—consent of donor, benefit to recipient, no harm to donor, no financial transaction. Because Sha'rawi had so successfully linked the idea of organ transplantation to the body as God's property, these scholars have had to reconcile their legal judgments with the premise that the body does, indeed, belong to God. The international Islamic legal conference (Majma' al-Fiqh al-Islami), for example, in a publication that ultimately judges organ transplantation to be permissible, titled their study "What It Means for the Body to Belong to God."[40]

Other opponents of organ transplantation have invoked the legal tool of *sadd al-dhara'i'* (or "blocking the means"), used to forbid something that is not itself forbidden *(haram li-dhatihi)* but which leads to things that are forbidden *(haram li-ghayrihi)*.[41] For example, in another article in *al-Liwa' al-Islami*, Dr. 'Abd al-Salam al-Sukari, a professor of Islamic law, argues that organ transplantation's capacity to lead to such clearly horrific practices as a black market in human organs and bodily exploitation should be the basis of its prohibition, according to the tenet of *sadd al-dhara'i'*.[42]

Still others have argued that, prior to issuing a fatwa, the mufti's role is to research, rather than assume, the extent to which organ transplantation is a safe and efficacious procedure. This latter group of muftis, such as Shaykh 'Ali Guma'a, solicited information about graft survival, patient well-being, and other indications to help judge the "social welfare" *(maslaha 'amma)* of this medical procedure. Shar'awi's evident disbelief that this medical procedure benefits organ recipients must have contributed to the position that he took. Yet, throughout his lifetime, Sha'rawi insisted that his position was merely based on divine properties: omnipotence, perfection in creation, and infinite wisdom.

WEIGHING THE BENEFITS

While we may on one level of analysis point to distinct modes of ethical reasoning used throughout Islamic legal history to analyze different positions toward organ transplantation, we must also at another level remain attuned to the contextual social factors that inform each person's position toward this issue (see Opwis 2005). As Skovgaard-Petersen notes, while scholars supposedly consult traditional sources of jurisprudence *(fiqh)* to answer new questions, they are just as likely also to apply "the political knowledge, values, and common sense of their day" (1997: 29). Similarly, Felicitas Opwis argues, "The way in which jurists employ the principle of *maslaha* is not random but rather is influenced by education, personal position, and historical environment" (2005: 182).

The social history and context of Sha'rawi's medical knowledge help explain his distinction between bodily effects and bodily parts, and why he regarded organ transplantation to be sinful, whereas he considered blood transfusion to be religiously recommended.[43] During Sha'rawi's lifetime, blood banks were readily available in Egypt, and obtaining a blood transfusion from a relative was thought to cause little or no harm to the donor. In fact, many, including Sha'rawi, argued that it *benefits* the donor to give blood by instigating the generation of new blood cells.[44] To argue that blood donation is beneficial followed the logic of a long tradition of blood cupping (known as *higama* or *hajim*) within the traditional medical sciences that flourished throughout the Muslim world. There were even reported narratives of *higama* being used at the time of the Prophet and of the Prophet himself using and approving of this method of treatment.[45] The enthusiasm with which many devout Muslims and Islamic scholars have encouraged blood transfusion as a practice may be partly explained by the tradition of *higama*. This explains why many religious scholars, and not just Sha'rawi, have considered blood transfusion not only permissible but also commendable and yet have disapproved of kidney transplants. Sha'rawi, like many of the Azhari Islamic scholars with whom I spoke, argued that blood is not a part of the body but, rather, is a renewable resource whose regeneration is healthful and ultimately strengthens bodily processes.[46]

Yet for Dr. Walid, a nephrologist in Cairo who had worked in kidney transplantation for over thirteen years at the time of my conversations with him, this argument poses an unacceptable contradiction. When discussing this issue, Dr. Walid shook his head and said to me, "No, this makes no sense. The red blood cells are an organ, and the kidney is an organ, and the liver is an organ. What is different about the red blood cell? Is it because it's small, microscopic? I have two kidneys and their cells are constantly regenerating."

The idea that organ cells are also continually regenerating has allowed proponents of organ donation to argue for its permissibility by drawing its equivalence to blood where others have drawn a contrast between blood and body part. For example, in Tantawi's fatwa, he wrote, again apparently referencing Shaʿrawi's words: "[Organ] donation is permitted, because the experts say that it is the effects of the self rather than parts of the self, as evidenced by the fact that [the cells' functions] change and regenerate and the body compensates for what it lost." This type of reasoning demonstrates how crucial medical knowledge is to the religious scholar as he formulates his opinion about the ethics of the procedure. Shaʿrawi claimed to find the question of medical benefit irrelevant to his reasoning, although he clearly believed that organ transplantation did more harm than good. Tantawi, in contrast, was briefed by physicians who stressed that no harm comes to the donor because the body regenerates cells lost and compensates for lost function of the kidney or liver.

But Dr. Walid was unsatisfied with either logic. Responding to the idea that with blood donation no harm comes to the donor while it might to the kidney donor, Dr. Walid answered:

> No, if you take the kidney from the donor [too], the donor is fine. If he doesn't have any problems and he's healthy, he'll be fine. If he was already predisposed to a problem that would have affected both of his kidneys, then he'll have a problem with the one he has left . . . but I can't think like this [in terms of risks].
>
> The real question should be: Do I, as the one created by God, have the right to donate [God's creation] or not? Then I would think it is *all haram*, even blood donation. You see, in our religion, a major principle is no harm can be inflicted or tolerated *[la darar wa la dirar]*. It doesn't say, "Only a little bit of harm is better." It says *no* harm *[la darar]*. So it's not as if I can drink a tiny bit of beer or whisky and this is okay, and only if I drink a lot is it *haram*. It's not allowed at all.[47]
>
> It's not about risks and harms, because there is nothing that doesn't have harm in it. The vitamins we take have chemicals in them, the vegetables we eat have been genetically engineered, and the meat we eat comes from cows that could be fed with animal parts! And something that we don't yet know the harm of may later prove to be harmful—even blood donation.

For Dr. Walid, rationalist objectivism, the belief that divine law is discernible by the human intellect, is flawed. He argued that the criteria upon which we judge whether acts are beneficial or harmful are constantly evolving and can be subjectively argued. Instead, like Shaʿrawi, he took the position of a theistic subjectivist, arguing that we can know divine law only from the revelatory scripture.[48] The obvious problem here is that there is no clear divine revelatory text about organ transplantation. Dr. Walid thus argued that we must then look to revelation for what is relevant to the question of transplants: that God is the one who creates and thus owns our bodies. Yet Dr. Walid was reluctant to argue that organ transplantation is *haram* because God is both Creator and Owner. He remained uncertain as to whether this theological attribute necessarily leads to a legal-ethical judgment forbidding transplantation. Like many other physicians with whom I spoke, Dr. Walid respected Sha'rawi's position and agreed whole-heartedly with the tenet that God is Creator and Owner of human bodies. Yet he did not see why this should necessarily render organ transplantation impermissible.

Dr. Walid's position then, like that of many other physicians working in transplantation, hung ambivalently, with no clear position in regard to a practice within his own medical specialty. He recognized that he helped many patients, and yet he worried about the spiritual consequences of his actions. As another devout transplant surgeon, Dr. Kotb, once said to me, the problem with arguments that rely on consideration of social benefit *(maslaha)* or necessity *(darura)* is that one can then argue anything: "Even the thief who steals will argue that he had to do it, because he was starving."

With the increasing institutionalization of *ifta'* (fatwa giving) within the confines of the modern nation-state, state-appointed muftis have been expected to assess new questions on the basis of finding the utmost "public benefit" *(maslaha)* for the entire nation, if not the Muslim community *(umma)* at large (Skovgaard-Petersen 1997). As many scholars of modern Islamic thought have argued, the reinvigoration of tools like *maslaha* by nineteenth-century Muslim reformers has been crucial to scholars' own projects of increasing flexibility in the Islamic legal tradition and its adaptation to the contemporary needs of Muslim societies (Kerr 1966; Krawietz 1997; Dallal 2000; Kurzman 2002; Opwis 2005).[49]

The association of *maslaha* with legitimating modern practices has also caused some unease about its overuse and the integrity of the tradition. As Birgit Krawietz puts it, "The question is whether we can go so far as to regard *maslaha* as a sort of universal means whereby all kinds of modernization are sanctioned. Some authors seem to regard *maslaha* as a dangerous opening of human value judgments or as the principal weak point within the Islamic legal system. Not seldomly they accuse the 'modernists' of its abuse" (1997: 186). The fear is that the overuse of *maslaha* as a source of law will reduce the position of Divine law to that of man-made laws.[50]

Sha'rawi was reluctant to appeal to the legal tools of reasoning, such as *maslaha*, which were the most familiar modes of reasoning for approaching a novel medical procedure such as organ transplantation (Krawietz 1997).[51]

That is why his position was unrecognizable as a fatwa and also why he was open to such a virulent attack from his critics. At the same time, many have expressed misgivings about the overuse of *maslaha* to legitimate all "modern" practices (Krawietz 1997). Sha'rawi's refusal to do so fit with his popular role as someone who was "firm in the tradition." Further, his elicitation of such basic tenets of Islam, with the suggestion that invasive medical technologies threaten these beliefs, has struck at particular vulnerabilities in Egyptian society: the distrust and mismanagement of biomedical institutions, concerns about the desacralization of the body and life processes, and the poor's subjection to bodily exploitation.

CONCLUSIONS

Sha'rawi, unquestionably the most well-known of the emergent religious figures in Egypt, was near the last decade of his life when he was at the center of the organ transplant controversy. His opposition to organ transplantation was at once controversial and influential, both in his life and after his death.[52] Many of the biographies and hagiographies on Sha'rawi include his famous statement on organ transplantation, as do his obituaries and a biographical television serial, *Imam al Dua'* (Leader of the Preachers), which aired during Ramadan in 2002. Unlike many religious scholars and state muftis who have relied on scholarly language in their arguments, Sha'rawi rose to fame because of his ability to speak to "the common people" *(al-'awwam)* and to make classical learning accessible. Before Sha'rawi's death, some of the Egyptian intelligentsia, particularly journalists writing in the mainstream press, considered him to be one of those "hard-headed extremists," but the vast majority of middle-class Egyptians, including religious scholars, had a tremendous amount of respect for Sha'rawi and credited him with reawakening Muslims with a sense of spiritual awareness and piety.

Many "progressive" journalists in the mainstream media, in attempts to dismiss Sha'rawi's position, singled him out as having a minority voice against organ transplantation. They pointed out that he explained his initial antipathy toward the idea of transplanting human body parts in terms of a general aversion to medical intervention in natural processes. The idea that the ill should be left alone because God willed their illness can hardly in and of itself make sense to religiously observant surgeons, whose everyday practices are aimed at treating disease. Nor is it consistent with a long-standing tradition of Islamic medical sciences, in which medicine itself is understood to be God's creation. Sha'rawi's critics argued that he could not deny the duty to receive medical treatment when the Prophet Muhammad himself encouraged it.[53]

This criticism of Sha'rawi has not, in the end, diminished his popularity or influence. His followers have generally understood that no authoritative Islamic scholar, including Sha'rawi himself, would ever make a blanket statement against medicine in general, because abundant Islamic sources support the prevention and treatment of illness. As we will see in the next chapter, Sha'rawi's iteration has resonated among patients and doctors as a broad theological statement, not as a particular prescription. Although Sha'rawi himself would not contextualize his position via Islamic legal tools, his stance against organ transplantation has been made meaningful in a social context in which it is widely perceived that this particular medical intervention does not necessarily lead to overall social benefit.

In contrast to the position taken by the state-appointed muftis, Sha'rawi's call reflects a different understanding of the ontology of the body, its relation to the Creator, and its potential for affliction. His position also reflects how much power he felt individuals can and should attempt to exert over terminal disease, which he conflated with divine will. As I argue in forthcoming chapters, the theological question about the limits of human will is necessarily tangled with that of how much autonomy people can exert within available political-economic systems of medical care.

Sha'rawi's defenders have argued that a "media attack" took place against him, imagining those critical voices to be dominant and oppressive, even when Sha'rawi himself was a central media figure. And his defenders have also located him as outside state interests, even when his position and popularity depended on state support. Different positions on organ transplantation have also reflected religious scholars' varying views about how Islamic ethical and moral positions should be determined. Tantawi, the former grand mufti, also used the statement that the body belongs to God but, in his case, to legitimate the altruistic donation of organs and to declare the buying and selling of organs to be *haram*. Tantawi argued that clear harm is done to a person who sells his kidney, yet he did not seem to believe that harm is inflicted upon the person who *donates* his kidney, as did Sha'rawi. Equally if not more important is considering their differing views about the nature of the body, the dispositions we should have toward illness, and the medical risks and benefits of organ transplantation.

As I show in the next chapters, very few people in Egypt have had ethical quandaries about parents donating organs to their own children, as the idea that life passes from parent to child does not contradict, for them, the premise that our bodies belong to God. However, Sha'rawi himself, during his lifetime, never made allowances for particular cases, and several of his critics have exploited this point, highlighting his insistence that even a mother does not have the right to donate a kidney to her young child.[54] Yet if some in the print media were hostile to Sha'rawi's stringency, admiration of him among the majority of Egyptians has not waned. While other muftis have worked to make Islam appear a simple religion, easily applicable to daily life, through appeals to its rationalism (Skovgaard-Petersen 1997), Sha'rawi, as a *da'iya*, made religion appear accessible and simple by drawing stark black-and-white contrasts of what is right and what is wrong. In the end, however, the idea that organ transplantation is forbidden or sinful in religion because God is all powerful and owns everything involves a tenuous connection. Sha'rawi could not make it applicable to particular situations on the strength of his own argument. There have to be other reasons why his statement has been so resonant, so powerful among doctors, patients, family members, and even transplant surgeons. In the coming chapters, I demonstrate how Sha'rawi's statement that our bodies belong to God has been richly (re)interpreted as it has circulated in the experiences and imaginations of those most intimately involved with kidney transplantation in Egypt.

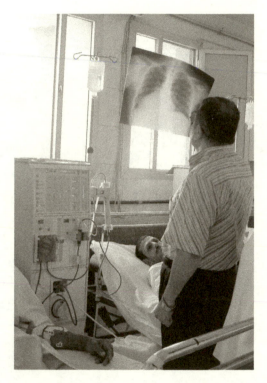

Figure 10.   Nephrologist assesses X-ray of dialysis patient in acute renal failure.

5. Transplanting God's Property

The Ethics of Scale

In 1976, medical teams in Cairo and Mansoura competed to perform the first kidney transplant in Egypt. While the Mansoura team officially won the "race," to much fanfare in the Egyptian press, Cairo surgeons followed only two months later with their own successful transplant. Dr. Abdel Kader Kotb, a vascular surgeon who was a recent medical graduate at the time, performed all the essential elements of the first Cairo surgery. As a young no-name doctor, he would be the one blamed by the "big doctors" if anything went wrong. The operation was purposely scheduled on the weekend of a national holiday: the third-year anniversary of the October 1973 War.[1] That way, the doctors reasoned, the press would be distracted with other news if it was a failure, and they could hail it as yet another national victory if it was a success. They invited Dr. Mohamed Ghoneim, who had led the Mansoura team to the first operation two months earlier, to come and watch. In May 2004, Dr. Kotb recalled this historic affair to me as we sat together in the waiting room of a private hospital in the Cairo suburb of Maʿadi:

> We got the [donor's] kidney ready. We worked on the donor vessels and got them ready. They made me do everything, so if anything happened to the vessels, it would be *me* who was responsible. Then I got the recipient ready, the stitches and everything.
>
> And from the time of taking the kidney from the donor and [putting it] into the recipient and getting an output of urine—how long do you think this took? Guess—for the first operation in all of Cairo?
>
> Twenty-four minutes! And five of those minutes were for perfusion,[2] so *nineteen minutes it took* for the work to do the transplant. The blood went to the kidney, and we got an output of urine. They announced it: "The kidney has urine in it." Mohamed Ghoneim was completely shocked. He had taken about *an hour* in the first Mansoura operation.

I sat in my seat, puzzled, while Dr. Kotb excitedly relayed to me the important events of the history of transplantation in Egypt. I had wanted to meet Dr. Kotb, because I had heard from other surgeons that although he had performed the first successful kidney transplant in Cairo, he was now convinced that it was *haram* and no longer worked in transplantation. He had even gone on national television and had outlined why he felt that organ transplantation is both unethical and improper medical science. If he indeed held this conviction, it was hard to recognize now. I took copious notes, although not always following his surgical terminology, and tried unsuccessfully to intervene to ask him if it was true that he now thought that organ transplantation is *haram*. But there was no stopping Dr. Kotb. He bubbled with excitement over past accomplishments. He pulled out a big file filled with awards and certifications he had received for initiating transplant centers in other medical facilities in Cairo, including al-Azhar Faculty of Medicine. And he began to tell me about a life-long career in medicine, through which he has been guided by God's infinite wisdom and compassion.

SEEKING COUNSEL FROM YOUR OWN HEART

When I asked Dr. Kotb how he knew what to do in the first transplant operation with no previous experience, he pointed upward to God. He also explained that, since he had been a small child, he knew that he wanted to be a surgeon. Having scored in the top percentile in the national college entrance exams, he could choose to go into any field. Back then, he said, there were only two professors of vascular surgery, and there wasn't much clinical work. So they would finish their work in the clinic and go out to find stray dogs in the alleys on which to experiment. He explained that in those days they worked until they perfected their skills; they were good at surgery because they loved it and they loved to learn; they didn't rely on just studying but spent much of their time on experimental medicine as well. Then, he continued, the war began in 1973, and he worked in the emergency room of the Kasr el Aini medical school, where he performed numerous surgeries on the injured victims of the war.[3] They could perform amazing surgeries, in those days, Dr. Kotb reflected. Pulling out an Egyptian newspaper article featuring a picture of himself on its cover, Dr. Kotb recounted the story of an American petroleum engineer who had been treated in Boston for an aneurism in his leg. In Boston they were able to use only two-thirds of his great saphenous vein for a bypass, and so they supplemented it with a bovine graft.[4] But while the American engineer was working in Egypt, the graft failed. The American Embassy wanted to evacuate him. Embassy officials consulted Dr. Kotb, who told them, "If you evacuate him, he will lose his leg over the Atlantic." So, after a short investigation to find out what they could about this young Egyptian surgeon, the embassy officials agreed to let him perform the operation. Dr. Kotb opened the leg and found the remaining third of the great saphenous vein that the Boston surgeons had been unable to use and made a new bypass with it. When the engineer traveled back to America, the surgeons there were amazed, Dr. Kotb said, at how an *Egyptian* surgeon could perform such an operation.

"Amazing things we did," he said. So when the opportunity for carrying out the first transplant came, Dr. Kotb fearlessly took it up. A kidney transplant would be a simple and easy operation, he implied, compared with other surgeries in which he had excelled during his clinical training.

"But Dr. Kotb," I finally got a word in edgewise, "what changed your mind, then? What made you think transplants are *haram*?"

He looked at me, confused: "I didn't change my mind. Praise to God, I was always a devout Muslim."

"But you said on *Sabah al-Khayr ya Misr* [Good Morning, Egypt—a TV program] that organ transplantation is *haram*; you said that it was not a good solution."

"It's not," he shrugged. "Let me tell you why." Now turning to the very sheet of paper from which he had prepared his televised remarks, he explained in great detail why he thought transplants are *haram*:

> Now, organ transplantation from living donors—this is not supposed to happen. Why? What does God, most exalted, say? In the [Qur'anic] chapter "The Fig," God says, "We created the human in the finest state."[5] So nothing is superfluous and nothing is deficient in the human. There are two kidneys, just like there are two eyes. Why do we have two eyes? Because this gives us a full field of vision, so I can bring two things close together—see? If I close one eye, I can't do this. That's why someone with uni-ocular vision can't drive, for example; he would hit the cars in front of him. So God gave us two eyes. Why did he give us two ears? So that we can have 360 degrees of hearing. . . . Why did God give us two kidneys? Just as there are two eyes for the function of complete sight and two ears to hear all 360 degrees around us, so are the two kidneys essential to filter toxins throughout the body.
>
> With two kidneys, there is extra energy for us to absorb exposure to external or internal insults to the body. When we take out one of the kidneys, there is inflation in the remaining kidney, proving that the function rises. Sometimes a kidney donor will need occasional dialysis,

because both kidneys are necessary. Like the fibers in our muscles—most of the time, they compensate for one another. Each takes turns working; they don't all work at the same time. It is like the alternating keys on the piano.

God created humans in this way. Each kidney has one million neph-rons, and only 10 percent work at a time, taking turns. Why? Why did God give us so much function? The function of the kidneys is to make the toxins in the urine stay under a particular level in the blood. . . . Because the kidneys carry out such a huge important task, there has to be *two* of them. And there's a relationship between them; they compen-sate for one another. They call this *counterbalance*.

Like the liver, you take a piece of it, a lobe, and transplant it into someone else. And this small lobe will grow to the size of a normal liver, and then it stops. Why doesn't it keep on growing? How does it know which size to grow? The cells have a memory; these are divine signs that no one understands exactly. Now when you take a piece of this liver from the donor, there are great risks involved. He could die, the donor. When we go on a car journey, we carry a spare tire in the car. And life is an eternal journey, [so] we need the reserves that God gave us.

This is why organ transplantation from living donors creates harm to the donors. And we have a legal-ethical principle in Islam: *la darar wa la dirar* [no harm can be inflicted or tolerated]. And that prevention of harm takes precedence over taking a benefit.

This is why it is not acceptable to expose someone to such risk, to take from someone else. First of all, this is not a certain treatment: the kidney could be rejected, and the donor could be harmed. So this is not for *maslaha* [the realization of public benefit]. As long as there is harm to the donor, then taking from donors is *haram*. It is also illogical, and it is uncivilized [*ghayr hadari*].[6] That is why in the Qur'an suicide is strictly prohibited; you cannot cause harm to yourself.

Dr. Kotb handed me the sheet on which he had bulleted these points, saying, "A lot of people liked what I had to say, but a lot of doctors became very angry with me."

I was confused. How did he reconcile this detailed, ethical rejection of transplantation with his excitement about the actual transplants he had performed? Nowhere did his story suggest that he thought he was doing something good in medicine, like saving his patients' lives—that evocative "gift of life" phrase so ubiquitous in North American discussions of organ transplantation. And I was still waiting for some sort of "turning point" in the narrative: the epiphany that led him to think that organ transplants are *haram*. After all, Renée Fox and Judith Swazey, who pioneered the sociolog-ical study of organ transplantation in North America with their book *The Courage to Fail* (1974), themselves explain why they had been enthusiasts of the promise of transplants and then, after decades of studying it (as described in their follow up book *Spare Parts* [1992]), they grew disillusioned with this technology, the excessive ardor to prolong life and the move toward financial incentives. Renée Fox (1996) wrote that she hoped her public decision would serve as a moral lesson about the perversion of a technology she had initially believed in. I wanted to know when, how, and why Dr. Kotb, too, had come to reject it. But he offered me no such story. Organ transplantation had *never*, in his mind, offered a "gift of life." For surely, he said, we all know that only God wills and gives life. I pressed him on this. Dr. Kotb shook his head:

> No, all along, from the very beginning, I felt like this was *haram*. And then, at the time, a group of us doctors went to Shaykh Shaʿrawi, may God have mercy on his soul, to ask his opinion. He was completely adamant about this. He saw this as *haram*. Shaʿrawi said to us, "Are you afraid of death? Are you doing all this to prevent death? If we are God-fearing Muslims, what do we have to be afraid of? Death will go on no matter what you do! [*Al-mawt lazim yimshi!*]"
>
> We said to him, "Now, wait here, and we'll go and get you a kidney-failure patient who is dying, who could be helped with this. So you can see for yourself." But it was no use. Shaʿrawi said that a person cannot give away a part of his body that God gave him to have.
>
> So I went to hear the opinion of another shaykh. He said, "As long as your intentions are pure, and you are doing this to help humanity and the sick, then it is permissible; you can do this." So I used this fatwa as my permission. Then that same shaykh several years later got very sick. He fell into a coma. He was treated in the Cleveland Clinic in America. He came out of it, and he could no longer speak or anything. But God preserved his knowledge.
>
> [After he had returned], we used to go to him and understand what he was saying from his signs and gestures. One day we asked him again about organ transplantation. He said, "No, I changed my mind. I take back my fatwa [permitting it]." So I didn't have one to work with anymore.

I had never heard anyone in such a context speak frankly about having "shopped around" for a fatwa to suit one's needs, which is technically frowned upon. Neither had I ever heard of anyone changing his own life decisions after having a fatwa rescinded—in this case, abandoning a medical practice he had excelled in. The dominant way that Cairo professionals argue that their modern practices are in complete alignment with Islamic values is through understanding their efforts to work toward attaining the most benefit for society *(maslaha)*, which they take to be a key religious guiding principle. This echoes the dominant state discourse on Islam. It was much more common to hear highly educated Cairenes speak of looking into their own conscience, asking God for direct guidance, seeking counsel from their own hearts, than to hear of their seeking advice from a religious authority, much less one from humble peasant origins. So I asked, "But Dr. Kotb, why ask around for a fatwa if you yourself saw it as *haram?* Didn't the Prophet say to seek the fatwa from your own heart *[istafti qalbak]?*"

"Exactly!" he exclaimed, "*Istafti qalbak*—that's exactly right! Deep down inside I knew that this was *haram.*"

Dr. Kotb's strong ethical reservations about organ transplantation had persisted throughout his career, but the push to strive in what was universally defined as "surgical excellence" was too great. As he described it, the intellectual and professional impetus thrust him forward, and he temporarily ignored what he would later call "the troubles in his heart," that is, toward the irreverence and hubris that come with transplanting "God's creation." He was still proud of his own professional and medical accomplishments. The immediacy of the patient suffering in kidney failure was so compelling to him that he thought if he could somehow show Sha'rawi these clinical realities, the shaykh's opinion might change. His excitement at being able to end his patients' suffering through his hard-earned surgical skills impelled him to enter the field of transplant medicine.

But years later, when widening the scope of the problem, he came to see not just the immediate situation of his own patients' decline but also larger questions about transplantation's benefits and costs to others, including the lives of the donors. In an ambivalent mixture of pride and remorse, ambition and conscientiousness, Dr. Kotb particularly regretted that the first operation he participated in had involved an "unrelated living donor," a euphemism for donors who sell their organs for money. As a long-term practitioner in Cairo's deeply classed medical landscape, he saw the poor selling their kidneys to the rich as an inevitable and predictable outcome of transplant medicine. He came to hold grave reservations about the overall benefit of kidney transplantation and no longer worked in this field.

The question is about more than what Sha'rawi had posed, which was whether organ transplantation entails an attempt to cheat death. For Dr. Kotb, it also entailed the potential of extending one person's life at the expense of another's. Again, the ideal type, that "doctor of confidence," is one who not only looks at the immediate benefit of his own patients but always has the wider Egyptian society's interests at heart as well. In emotive medical television dramas, popular in both the United States and the Middle East, the immediacy of one person's life-or-death plight is spotlighted—a tendency that bioethics as a field has replicated. The immediacy of the individual's plight is an important and powerful way that an outsider can connect to the suffering of another; in this case, it compelled Dr. Kotb to act. But too often in bioethics the plight of one individual is highlighted to the exclusion of other social relations, consequences, and ramifications. Depending on how the scale and scope of the problem are defined, different risk-benefit analyses will inform ethical decisions. In the logic of caring for his patients, Dr. Kotb could not continue to turn to the rubric of "individual choice" to justify the fact that poor donors were making unsafe medical decisions, such as selling their body parts for fast cash.[7]

Rhetoric establishing the incommensurabilities between medicine and religion shaped Dr. Kotb's narrative. He maintained that his fatwa seeking was what had led to his differing views of kidney transplantation. But in my analysis of patients, doctors, and religious scholars, I have discerned a pattern that better explains Dr. Kotb's change of heart. Ethical decisions shift, but not along the lines of religiosity or stringency in religious interpretation. Rather, ethical decisions differ depending on how the scale and scope of kidney transplantation are defined. The picture looks different when cost-benefit analyses are made on the basis of the life of one patient in renal failure, or the larger social relations in which he is embedded, or the larger national context in which inequalities are exacerbated between the rich and the poor. Dr. Kotb's religious views were not irreconcilable with those of biomedical science; rather, his integration of biomedical science and religion, together with an awareness of the complicating social factors such as the market and donor-recipient relations, offered compelling arguments against the logics of organ transplantation.[8] His ambivalence reveals the shifting and inconclusive risk-benefit calculations that vary depending on the scope of the case and who is included in the ethical decision-making process.

CONSIDERING TRANSPLANTATION— THE CONTEXT OF DECISIONS

Like Dr. Kotb, many patients in end-stage kidney failure expressed to me their ambivalence about undergoing a kidney transplant both in religious terms and by questioning whether it provides a "medical solution" when considering its larger social consequences. Sometimes doctors and medical staff tried to convince dialysis patients that transplantation was their only chance at returning to a semblance of normalcy. If transplantation were a treatment that affected only one individual patient at a time, the decision would be easier to make. Medically, life with a transplanted kidney should be much improved over life on dialysis. But patients were concerned about the familial and social relations in which they were embedded; the financial cost of the surgery and the biological cost of a donated organ were tremendous. Procuring the transplant was a burden shared by many people in the family. Further, the entrenchment and seeming inevitability of the organ trade in transplantation, in which patients in need pay "donors" to part with their kidneys, have colored doctors' and patients' distaste of the practice. Those who questioned the ethics of kidney transplantation, argued, among other things, that the medical harm posed to the living donor is unacceptable.

The majority of kidney transplants in Egypt have been carried out in public and private hospitals in Cairo, and unrelated, paid donors have been the major source of the organs. Thus, for the vast majority of end-stage renal patients, obtaining a kidney transplant has required a prohibitive sum of money for the related medical services, for the kidney itself, and for follow-up pharmaceuticals.[9] Most of Egypt's poor cannot afford to consider transplantation as a possibility. In any case, many patients I spoke with were unconvinced that a transplant would result in more benefit than harm, considering the financial costs, the sacrifice of the kidney donor, and the management of postoperative complications. They continued to endure difficult and, at times, unreliable treatment and to manage the symptoms of chronic kidney failure and the side effects of medications and hemodialysis, including dietary restrictions and unpredictable episodes of sharp pain, dizziness, weakness, nausea, muscle cramps, and fatigue. Most dialysis patients have been forced to discontinue work and experience emotional, financial, and family strains.[10] At the time of my research, only a relatively small number of patients (eighty to one hundred per year) could undergo a fully subsidized transplantation and receive excellent follow-up care free of charge at the public facility of the Mansoura Kidney Center. The few who can attain a spot for a transplant operation at Mansoura's public facilities have family members able and willing to donate medically compatible kidneys to them, and both donor and recipient have to pass through strict medical screening to ensure the highest success rates (Afifi and Abdel Karim 1996; Afifi 2000). The number of public transplant facilities was simply insufficient for the tens of thousands of dialysis patients in Egypt, and none at all existed for those patients who could never meet the strict screening standards imposed by Mansoura's facility and who could not pay the exorbitant out-of-pocket sums for private care.

Throughout Egypt, over thirty thousand patients with end-stage kidney failure received hemodialysis in the mid-2000s, and the number is steadily increasing each year. But fewer than 3 percent of dialysis patients received a kidney transplant in Egypt—approximately seven hundred to eight hundred kidney transplants were performed every year in Egypt in the mid-2000s from living donors.[11] Many proponents of kidney transplantation argue for its cost-effectiveness as compared to long-term care with hemodialysis. A single kidney transplant requires a large amount of cash upfront, but in the long run, it is less expensive than the cumulative cost of hemodialysis treatment over five to ten years.[12] Patients who can navigate the difficult bureaucratic maze and persist in obtaining the right connections can bill their dialysis sessions to the Ministry of Health if they can demonstrate their dire need for a life-saving treatment and if they can find a local parliamentarian to "sponsor" their application.[13] Some could also receive compensation from the Ministry of Health to offset the cost of a kidney transplant at any major hospital, minus the cost of the kidney itself. Thus, it is in the interest of the Ministry of Health to promote organ transplantation, given its overall cost effectiveness, but there is no way to ensure a supply of altruistically donated kidneys, and surgical outcomes are widely variable. Thus, even when cost-benefit analyses on a national level are reduced to economic factors that exclude social and emotional issues, the calculation still does not yield straightforward answers to the question: how much risk should be tolerated and at what cost?

THE COSTS OF A TRANSPLANT

Shadya, a college student I met who at the age of twenty had kidney failure due to lupus, an autoimmune disease, had been continually encouraged by the physician in charge of the dialysis unit to seek transplantation, as were all the young patients with whom I spoke. Whereas in the United States, patients in need of kidneys tend to pressure medical professionals to put them on waiting lists; the demand for kidney transplants in dialysis clinics in Egypt has often been *created* by medical staff, who consider transplantation to be the only way the patients can return to a "normal" life (Crowley-Matoka 2005). Because most Egyptians in kidney failure generally do not think of a transplant as a realistic possibility, they do not initiate requests to be considered for transplantation; in any case, a waiting list for kidneys does not exist in Egypt because there is no national program or registry in effect.

Shadya considered transplantation something that could happen "naturally" within the family. She told me, "A mother gives *everything* to her child. Why would she not also give a kidney?" Yet it was her bad luck that neither of her distraught parents had her same blood type. Her siblings were also ruled out as possible donors because they were under ten years of age, and furthermore one of them was ill with a heart condition.

A bright and lively person, Shadya "lit up the room," the nurses would say, even when confined to a bed during her dialysis sessions. She had been receiving dialysis treatments for the past four years. Before her treatments began, she had suffered severe pain in her joints, high fevers, and red swollen feet. Her family had taken her to numerous dermatologists, thinking that she had a skin condition. When the problem worsened, they went to a private hospital in Tanta, where she was told that she had rheumatism in her heart and was prescribed penicillin and given other shots. Only during another hospital admission in Cairo was she diagnosed with lupus and acute renal failure. She was told that she needed dialysis immediately. Her first year of dialysis was spent commuting between Tanta and Cairo, before Shadya's mother found a dialysis unit in Tanta, closer to home.

Shadya confided in me that she had not told any of her college friends or professors about her disease or about being on dialysis. She scheduled her classes for the same days as her dialysis sessions so that she could have the other days to rest and recuperate at home from the exhaustion. She underwent dialysis treatment beside her fellow patient and friend Tamir, a twenty-four-year-old who had received a transplant from his father at the age of fourteen and experienced acute rejection three years later. Tamir also took classes during the day, and the two kept each other company discussing school, politics, religion, and family life during their sessions. Shadya's educational training was through a Tanta branch of the Islamic al-Azhar schools, and she was specializing in Islamic studies at the university level as well. When we began our discussions, I asked her if she knew what the Islamic scholars who taught her at her university thought about organ transplantation. She told me that she did not want to ask, because she never wanted to be identified or treated differently by revealing her illness.

But Shadya had her own ideas. She told me matter-of-factly, the first time I met her, that she did not agree with the concept of organ transplantation at all. She said, "I have my ideas, but I am not enacting them in practice ['andi nazariyya bas mish mashya ma'ha]. I think it is all *haram.* Because God gave each person a part for him to live with. Once he is dead, then it is okay [to donate organs]; in that case the donor would be worthy of continual spiritual rewards after death [sadaqa gariyya]. If God gave me kidneys, and they failed, well then that was God's will. Each person should be pleased with his fate from God, and that's it."

When I asked her how she came to have this view, she elaborated:

I asked myself: the other person who has to donate, why does he have to do this [*zanbuh ay*]? It's like someone with cancer—is he going to go and get [healthy] tissues from another person? Then why is it different for the kidney failure patient? Each person should remain content with his fate. But once he dies, it [donating an organ] is *sadaqa gariyya,* because the dead person won't benefit from it anymore, but the living person will. So it would be like almsgiving [*zakat*] or prayer. Then there wouldn't be a market.

I have this idea, but I'm not following it. I go to labs for tests, then the lab calls up and says they have a donor, and this gets my hopes up. Then we go each time, and every time they get a sample and do the cross-matching, and each time it does not work—because of my lupus.

The truth is, I want a donor. And when one appears, and [the tissue match] doesn't work, I get upset.

I told Shadya that some religious scholars have permitted organ transplant, as long as the recipient will benefit and the donor will not be hurt. She replied, "How can the donor *not* be hurt? Why did God give him two kidneys then? Why didn't God also give people two pancreases for all the people with diabetes? God wouldn't create anything in vain. It *must* be there for a reason. And it *must* hurt the person to take it out."

The question of whether or not each person should remain content with his fate (that is, with falling ill) was for Shadya inextricably bound up with the idea that overcoming her illness would come at the expense of another person's body. Rather than disputing the terms of ethics or scriptural interpretation by which some religious scholars deem transplantation to be permissible, Shadya questioned the *medical* bases for such opinions. She also questioned the scale on which she should be basing her decision; that is, unlike her own physicians, she did not want to think only of the medical consequences to her own body. She agonized over whether the transplant would in fact entail a safe operation for the donor and whether the donor would be harmed by a nephrectomy.

The physicians in the ward who advocated transplantation for their young patients were constantly frustrated by what they saw as the interference of their patients' misguided religious beliefs with medical care. But their understanding of religion as a "constraint" to medical treatment did not adequately capture the ways in which patients' religious beliefs were embodied and embedded in medical discourse. "Religion" cannot be adequately analyzed as a category separate from and effectively constraining other aspects of social life. For Shadya, religion was an integral part of who she was, of how she saw the world. Shadya was articulate about her views that transplantation, the only alternative to dialysis, was itself a constraint that impinged upon her beliefs. Further, Shadya did not draw on religious symbolism or imagery instrumentally to justify her course of action or to gain social prestige. Rather, much like Dr. Kotb, in frustration she felt that her only option to treatment constrained her genuine religious and commonsense beliefs. Her ethical troubles increased when she thought of the larger social consequences of a transplant beyond the potential medical benefits that it would bring to her own body.

For Shadya's parents, who were deeply religious and pious people, the question of doing all that they could to save their daughter was not as fraught as this decision for Shadya herself. Her family desperately wanted her to go through with the transplant, and Shadya wanted to be better and free from dialysis. She privately questioned the ethics of the surgery, but more than anything else, she wanted to be in agreement with her parents. She wanted to end their suffering in seeing their daughter ill, to ease her own pain and to follow the steps that they were taking to offer her the best chance at survival. Here again, the ethical struggle was in part due to the shifting scale of the problem: when Shadya thought of her own survival, she resisted what she saw as the selfishness required to end her own pain and suffering at the expense of someone else, but when she thought in terms of her larger family unit, she followed her parents' decision, knowing that their distress would be alleviated by her recovery.

In the end, Shadya's family found her a donor. Excluded from the possibility of donating their own kidneys to Shadya because of their mismatched blood type, her parents' sacrifice was to liquidate all their assets and raise enough funds to buy their daughter a kidney. They found a young man who was eager to sell his kidney in Cairo and whose tissues matched. Shadya was carried along by the force of their will and by the force of their insistence on making every sacrifice so that their daughter could survive. After a rigorous and grueling number of tests conducted at the Mansoura Kidney Center, Shadya and her donor were admitted for the operation. According to the surgeons, after the operation, her graft appeared to be doing well and produced a good amount of urine. Yet, two and a half hours later, in a sad twist of fate, Shadya suddenly and unexpectedly took ill and died. The surgeons were mystified.[14]

The other patients in the unit, though shielded by the nurses from the truth for as long as possible, finally found out and were shocked and pained by the news. Shadya's sudden death, and those of others before her, confirmed to many of the patients that "God is the one who takes and gives," reiterating the Qur'anic message that God is the sole dealer in life and death. Her death influenced her fellow patients' attitudes toward organ transplantation and their future decisions about whether to pursue the promises of a new kidney.

No one told Tamir, Shadya's friend in the dialysis unit, what had happened to her. The entire medical staff at the dialysis unit agreed to keep her death from him for fear that he would not be able to handle the devastation. The nurses constantly feared that the patients would lose all hope for recovery when hearing about a death among their fellow patients, especially a young and lively one like Shadya.

Everyone knew that Tamir was especially devoted to Shadya. He himself had been through a transplant procedure and had reassured Shadya before hers. They had encouraged one another, holding on to the hope that their families might find them kidneys to transplant, even when they worried about the necessary medical and spiritual gamble that they would have to take. Nearly nine months passed after Shadya's death before I was able to meet again with Tamir, who was now receiving dialysis treatment at another center. He told me, "You know, death has its rights over us. We cannot be upset when God wills death to happen; God, most exalted and high, is the one who gave us life to begin with. Shadya only died in body. But her spirit is still here; it's with me all the time. And I believe that on the Day of Judgment we will see each other again."

He looked at me and said quietly,

> You know, I considered Shadya to be one of my dearest and closest friends. You know that we used to do dialysis together. When she died, everyone hid it from me. My parents even went to give condolences to her parents without telling me. Everyone in the hospital knew except for me.
>
> I finally found out a month later. And I finally went to give condolences to her parents. It was really awkward, although they are wonderful and very good people, because the mom wears *niqab* [the face veil], and I wasn't sure what to say to her. And here I was coming a whole month after it happened. But they all knew that it was because I didn't know.

Tamir's arms were so badly bruised and scarred from the dialysis and his fistula operations that I found myself trying to avoid looking at them. A year before, when I had first talked to him, he told me that he was hoping to receive another transplant to be able to get off dialysis. But after Shadya's death, he seemed much less hopeful:

> A transplant now would be very difficult. I had a transplant before, from my father, and it didn't work out that well. And I also have a heart condition, and now I have hepatitis C in my liver, which I got from the dialysis. Also I had to get my thyroid removed because of a goiter.

I went to get tested in Cairo, in Maʿadi Hospital, to have the goiter operation, and they told me that my blood pressure was too high to do the operation, and they had to find the cause of it. So they did a number of X-rays, and one of the doctors said that I had a swelling in my stomach causing it. I became so upset, I didn't even know where to begin: with my goiter, my stomach, my heart, my kidney. So we went to get more opinions.

We went to a doctor—she was a really great person, a really humane person—and she saw all of the scars on my body, and she was really concerned about my case and tried to help me as best as she could. She gave me a kind of treatment and told me to be very careful about what I ate. I followed it [the diet], and then they did X-rays, and there was no more swelling there. So then I did the goiter operation.

Tamir told me that it would be very difficult to think about transplantation now, when he had all these conditions and also worried about the harm it might cause. "Anyway," he said gravely, "My fate [*nasib*] is my fate."[15] The costs of transplantation were high. And the burden of these costs was never confined to a single individual. For Shadya, they included her commitment to her convictions and ultimately her life. For Tamir, the costs included his best friend, the fear of hurting someone else, and despair over how much more his ailing body could take.

NOT IDEAL

In Cairo, Dr. Badr's private dialysis unit was full of patients who adored him. Throughout my work, I had never seen a more affable or popular physician, nor one who was able to connect on so many levels with all his patients, from rural peasants to high-powered urban professionals. Aside from his private clinic in Tanta, he was also affiliated with a number of private hospitals in Cairo. For the few of his patients who could afford it and who decided to pursue transplantation, Dr. Badr arranged for the operations and continued to follow their posttransplant care.

One of these patients, Hani, was a businessman whose work demanded continual travel but whose life was now completely disrupted by his dialysis regime. He decided to find a donor and pay for a kidney, reasoning that he would lose much valuable time with all the tissue typing and other tests to determine whether his wife could be a donor, and that he wanted to spare her from all that anyway.[16] Dr. Badr encouraged him to turn to a Cairo hospital analysis lab, where he could find a stranger who had already signed up to have his tissue and blood data available. The lab, in a public university in Cairo, had only to match the test results of willing "donors" with those of potential patients. He also reasoned that he would be helping a poor person. Some of these commercial donors even came knocking at Dr. Badr's dialysis clinic doors, offering to sell their kidneys to the sick patients lying in beds connected to dialysis tubes. In contrast to the "shortage of organs" discourse that pervades U.S. and European transplant programs, in which procurement from brain-dead donors is dominant, in many poor countries the supply of organs from eager, willing, living sellers outweighs the demand (Cohen 1999, 2001; Scheper-Hughes 2000, 2003; Lock 2002b; Crowley-Matoka 2005; Budiani and Shibly 2006; Crowley-Matoka and Lock 2006; Sharp 2006; Budiani 2007; Budiani-Saberi and Delmonico 2008). It is an exchange characterized by desperation: commercial donors want the alleviation of the suffocating grip of debt; organ failure patients want to be free from their machines and from the exhaustion of chronic terminal illness.

Dr. Badr witnessed much anguish in his daily clinical practice: poor rural peasants who could barely afford the transportation to his dialysis clinic for their treatments and potential organ donors who came knocking at his door, offering their organs for cash. He made clinical assessments of exhausted, ill patients who had traveled long distances carrying X-rays of their failed kidneys under their arms, some of whom had scraped together all their savings to make deals with seller-donors. He treated patients who could not afford expensive dialysis solvents and patients who unwittingly bought "unguaranteed" counterfeit medications on the black market. He received phone calls from lab analysts at public hospitals offering the names of seller-donors whose tissues matched those of his patients and inquiries from brokers offering him unofficial loans to keep his clinic running at lower interest rates than those of the government banks. In between patients, Dr. Badr met with sales representatives from multinational pharmaceutical companies, promoting new lines of dialysis solvent, equipment, and medication. Dr. Badr traveled frequently to international conferences, kept himself updated, and, shaking his head, dismissed his medical colleagues who had "made a lot of noise" against organ transplantation. He was especially cynical toward those colleagues who had not been interested in acquiring the skills for or knowledge about new transplant procedures, those who had no financial or personal interests in transplantation but much to lose from it, and those who, he said, hid their own motivations of personal greed and professional jealousy in "ethical" talk about avoiding a market in organs.

On several occasions he said to me,

Look, I'm not defending the selling of organs. But what is the alternative? This is the reality we live in. These people who come up with
lines like 'No to transplant because of a market'—have they experienced what these patients go through? Have they themselves tried
dialysis, so that they can tell a person that the rest of his life he should
remain on it?

   Dialysis makes you feel like a sock that's been pulled inside out. This
isn't hard to live on? Why don't we ask people after transplantation
which life was better?

   I have to be honest with myself: I work hard and I have built a family, a home, I send my kids to good schools with money that could come
from the sales of organs. But my conscience is fine. Why? Because for
my own sake I did a study on these donors, I follow up with them, and
they are fine years later.

He shrugged at the same time, remarking that the donor faces known
hazards. When I asked if poor people, who are more likely to feel that they
must sell their organs, are more vulnerable to disease and risks after having a kidney removed, he answered, "Well, he has another one." Then he
told me, "God will forgive him. Like someone who can't go to hajj because
he's poor, God gives him other things to compensate: he can pray and fast
more. When I go to hajj, I can go with a five-star luxury hotel because of
[the money I make from] working hard here. I can perform the hajj in ten
days; other people—it takes them thirty days. [And if I were sick] I [would]
have the money to buy a kidney." Dr. Badr's frankness was striking to
me and forced me to realize that in my own social circles, I have become
accustomed to hearing people either condemn social inequalities or ignore
them; I was not used to hearing people acknowledge their entrenchment.
But this is exactly what physicians and organ recipients who had bought
kidneys in Egypt did. "This is how the world works," Dr. Badr told me. He
emphasized that in the end it is God who will judge what people do with
their different resources; it is God who will judge the decisions they had to
make, including those for survival.

   It is interesting to note here that Dr. Badr was not, and could never be,
considered a "doctor of confidence." He had attained his medical degree
abroad, in a post-Soviet republic. Because he was not trained in any of
Egypt's national teaching hospitals, he could never receive a faculty position there. All of his social prestige and standing came from the work in his
private clinics. He had no medical students to mentor, and he was not indoctrinated in the ideologies of an older generation of physicians who believed
in the nationalist, Muslim-oriented, and socialist ideals of the physician's
responsibility to serve the community at large.

His patient Hani was nervous about his upcoming transplant operation. The Mansoura Kidney Center, which more strictly controls for patients receiving kidneys from relatives, would never have taken Hani's case because of the complicated nature of his disease, one that resulted from a congenital abnormality. Dr. Badr was faced with many such patients: those excluded by strict Mansoura criteria, those who had no willing relatives to donate, and those who were able and willing to pay potential donors. "It is not an ideal situation," Dr. Badr said. On the one hand, as the physician, he felt that he should not have to investigate or know about the origin of the donor kidney and what transactions had gone on. His job was to assure that the operations went well. On the other hand, he told me that he could not live with himself unless he was assured somehow that what he was doing brought more benefit than harm. He requested that the donors, most of whom were paid, continue to come to him for follow-up visits free of charge, to ensure that they were still well with one kidney. It is not uncommon for physicians in private practices to come to such informal agreements with their patients. In this case, Dr. Badr had decided to settle in his mind the scope of the problem for which he felt responsible: Was he causing the donors medical harm?

His follow-up observations of the donors, including a survey he conducted on them, gave him a satisfactory response: he was not. The other problems—the lack of financial benefit that most donors experienced from the sale, their psychological feelings of inferiority postdonation, their overall regret about the decision—these were issues for which Dr. Badr firmly felt unaccountable, despite his curiosity. He often joked with the donors and even teased them for selling off their body parts. One of the questions on his survey was: "Who do you think benefits the most from such an arrangement?" The donors were supposed to rank all those who participate in a transplant in the order of who benefits most: the patient (the recipient), the doctors, the hospital, the analytic labs, and the donor. Dr. Badr chuckled cynically that the paid donors had *all* ranked themselves as benefiting the least.[17]

By the time I went to visit Hani in the hospital after his transplant operation, his donor had already been discharged. Hani's parents were both there, anxiously firing hundreds of questions at Dr. Badr, who answered them all jovially and reassured them that their son would be fine. Hani was not supposed to have visitors, so his parents lingered in the hallway calling to him, his mother blowing him kisses. She wanted to leave him money so that he could buy drinks and food from the hospital if he wanted, but not wanting him to touch such a filthy thing as Egyptian monetary bills, she entrusted the grimy pound notes to one of the nurses. Dr. Badr joked with the nurse that she was the perfect one to carry out such "dirty work."

I, too, lingered in the hallway calling my greetings out to Hani after his parents had left. Not knowing what to say or do, I awkwardly dug into my purse and fished out a small booklet with the Qur'anic chapter *"Ya Sin"* printed on it. The pages had been pushed into my cab at a traffic light by a disabled street peddler, and I had barely managed to thrust back with a one-pound note before the light changed. Now the pages were wrinkled from having sat in my purse for weeks, and I offered them hesitatingly to Dr. Badr to deliver to Hani. This particular Qur'anic chapter is often recited for the benefit of the ill.

"I don't know," said Dr. Badr turning over the pages and inspecting them, ". . . Has this *Ya Sin* been sterilized?" Dr. Badr laughed at his own arguably impious joke before deciding that the booklet could pass the threshold of Hani's room. When the pages reached Hani, he expressed pure elation and thanked me profusely. Dr. Badr told me that I was allowed to come in, and I walked in hesitantly after putting on a surgical mask and covering my shoes, to find a thin, masked Hani reading and gently turning the pages. I was shocked to find that his room, on the twelfth floor of a private Cairo hospital, had a large balcony opened to the Cairo air: the pollution, dust, and black soot wafted in freely from the busy, honking street below. I edged to the wall as far from Hani as possible, worrying about his immunosuppressed state and my germs, the grimy pound notes, the unsterilized booklet I had brought in, and the heavy, gray air that he was now breathing. I had no way of knowing whether Hani, who was clearly in a much better economic state than most of the patients I had seen, would fare any better, in the end, than the others whom he had left behind, stuck to their dialysis machines.

While he had been making the arrangements for the surgery, Hani justified his pursuit of a paid donor by saying, "I have to live. And I can't live on dialysis. It's ruining me. I can't work or anything. And this way, I am helping a poor person. He needs this money to support his family." At other times, Hani looked a bit more worried. Now in his postoperative hospital room, and into the mask, he repeatedly breathed the supplication: *"Astagh-far Allah*—May God forgive me."

QUEST FOR THE GOOD

Back in the Tanta dialysis unit, after Shadya's death, stories of posttransplantation nightmares circulated among patients. Many patients often repeated that a person cannot "save" someone or "lengthen a life" by donating an organ to someone else. ʿAli, a young patient, often said that you might think doctors can help, but if they can heal, it is only because they are instruments of God's unique healing abilities. Unlike the other patients, who many times seemed completely exhausted by their treatment, ʿAli could successfully fight off the exhaustion, keeping up his energy and making everyone in his session laugh. ʿAli lived with his family in the countryside, but because he had worked in the national army, he had the insurance to cover his treatment. ʿAli stood out not only for his good humor but also for his politicized Muslim identity. The other patients poked fun of his full beard, joking that he would be mistaken for a terrorist, especially in my "American research." ʿAli tended to talk animatedly about the current attack on the *umma* (Muslim community) and about the ways in which we must come closer to God to regain political and moral strength.

According to ʿAli, you might borrow large sums of money to pay a donor to part with his kidney, but you are self-deceived if you think this will guarantee your recovery. God is the sole guarantor who heals whomever He will and the one who decides who will die and when. He once said to me, "What is it, again, that Zewail discovered? A 'femto-sone'? We are less than a 'femto-sone' in God's creation!" ʿAli, like many literate Egyptians, knew well the accomplishments of the Egyptian-American Nobel Prize laureate and chemist Ahmed Zewail and his ability to describe atoms and molecules at the level of the femtosecond (which ʿAli pronounced as "femto-sone" in Egyptian Arabic), a technical term that, through national pride, has entered the Egyptian lexicon. One femtosecond is 10^{-15} of a second, which is to one second what one second is to thirty-two million years.

ʿAli said this to me after I had shown him the back of my U.S. driver's license, where I was designated as an organ donor after death. ʿAli did not approve of organ transplantation, even from dead donors. Echoing Shaykh Shaʿrawi, ʿAli asked me disapprovingly, "How could you give something away that you do not own?" ʿAli further stated that whoever thinks they are "saving" someone by "becoming an organ donor" is presumptuous, as the lives we hold so dear on this earth are only femtoseconds long when compared with divine existence and the hereafter. He shook his head and repeated to me, "God is the only one who saves."

In the hospital dialysis center, ʿAli remained the most outspoken opponent of the idea of organ transplantation—for himself, that is. He never discouraged others. But ʿAli genuinely struggled against the idea that having a transplant would improve his own situation. ʿAli and his young wife had two small children—the youngest born, he told me, after ʿAli "got sick."

owing that my work was focused on transplants, 'Ali spent many hours
th me debating the Islamic stance on donating or receiving body parts.
'Ali was one of the few patients in the ward who could in practical terms
undergo a transplant without too much financial hardship: his wife and his
many siblings had repeatedly offered to donate their kidneys to him, and
his army insurance would cover all costs of the operation in Cairo. Yet 'Ali
was convinced that this was *haram*.

At one point during our discussions, Ruwayda, the nurse attending to
'Ali, herself a Coptic Christian, interceded to argue that transplantation was
not *haram*. Their argument was as follows:

RUWAYDA: If God gave us intellect and advancement of science, then
why not listen to doctors? It is not *haram*, neither in Islam,
nor in Christianity. I saw it on TV; they brought Tantawi
[the shaykh of al-Azhar] and Pope Shenouda [the patriarch
of the Coptic Orthodox Church].

'ALI: Hey, stick to talking about yourself [Christianity], not about
Islam.

RUWAYDA: This [the donor's second kidney] is something extra, so you
can take it.

'ALI: What do you mean "extra"? What if that one also goes bad?

RUWAYDA: Then that's fate.

'ALI: This is also my fate, to just be like this.

RUWAYDA: This is something complicated; doctors do it carefully;
[they're] not just playing around.

'ALI: And how are you guaranteeing that the [donor left] with
one kidney will be okay?

RUWAYDA: Science says that.

'ALI: Says what?

RUWAYDA: Science says you can live for twenty years like that.

'ALI: *No one* lives that long!

RUWAYDA: Well, what's your alternative?

'ALI: Dialysis.

RUWAYDA: That's not a choice; that's a bad alternative. You can't work
or anything. Are you working?

'ALI: No.

RUWAYDA: Why not? Because you are on dialysis!

'ALI: Yes, and if I have a transplant, will that get me my job back?

RUWAYDA: No.

'ALI: Well, then there you are.

RUWAYDA: Are you happy with your life as it is?

'ALI: I thank God.

At this point, 'Ali looked at me and told Ruwayda that they needed to get me a much fatter notebook, because I write everything down. Ruwayda stopped and asked if I had really written down their conversation. I said yes and showed it to her. They both laughed, the tension now broken. Ruwayda went back to her job.

'Ali and I continued for months, though, discussing his situation. One day he told me, "Religion is the only issue that is stopping me. Most people in my situation would say it is *halal* [permissible], because they need it. It is very rare to find someone like me who needs it and still says it is *haram*."[18]

I asked him, "Why are you not convinced by the *shuyukh* [Islamic scholars] who say it is *halal*?"

He answered, "I have nothing to do with them [*ma lish da'wa bihum*]." 'Ali asked me to read to him what I had written so far. After I did, he nodded and continued, "Write this down: If I did a transplant, I would have to pay no money. My wife wants to give me her kidney, and the army will pay for it, and they say that I will get experts from abroad [to perform the operation]. But I am convinced: No."[19]

He pulled out a wrinkled piece of paper that he carries in his wallet and told me, "Look at the date."

The date on the piece of paper was over a year old: April 26, 2002. It was a referral from the army for a fully paid appointment for 'Ali's wife to be tissue-typed with him. 'Ali's wife had been pleading that they go to the appointment, but 'Ali refused, feeling it was not right.

I asked him why he was so convinced, and he told me that God did not make it easy for him to accept the idea of it. I told him, "But you wouldn't have to pay any money, and your wife has offered to give you a kidney; why isn't this [evidence that] God has made it easy for you?" 'Ali shook his head and said, "No, but I prayed *salat al-istikhara*."

The Arabic word *istikhara* means "seeking the good." Many Muslims, when faced with a choice they feel they cannot make, perform a special ritual prayer in which they ask God directly for proper guidance so that they can choose what will be good for them in life and in faith.[20] In Egypt, Muslims often pray *salat al-istikhara* before a marriage choice. They believe that your heart must be neutral, that you cannot be leaning toward one decision or another, and that you must truly be committed to doing what is right. God will then answer by guiding them to make the right choice.

'Ali told me that after praying *salat al-istikhara,* he never felt happy about a decision to go and be tissue-typed. He told me that he did not feel as if the right thing for him to do was to get up and get dressed and say to his wife, "Let's bring the kids and go get tested now." I asked him, perhaps too cynically, if he felt this way about going to the dialysis unit three times a week. Defiant, he said yes. 'Ali explained that he had interpreted his reluctance to follow through with the tests as to be God's answer. He had thus refused the idea of transplant for five years out of fear that it might be *haram.*

Having articulated a deep mistrust of state-appointed Islamic scholars, those who have described organ transplantation as "permissible" on state television and in the newspapers, 'Ali felt that he had only his own heart and conscience to trust. That is why he was deeply committed to seeking God's counsel through prayer. When he sought counsel from his own heart through prayer, he did not find transplant an option that would bring "the good" *(al-khayr).* 'Ali identified religion as the "only thing stopping" him, thus adopting rhetoric that essentialized religion, particularly to explain his defiant stance against Ruwayda's views. But the more I learned from 'Ali's conundrum, the more I realized that his struggle had to do with the way in which the scope and scale of the treatment were defined. Ruwayda had insisted that transplantation was the "better" option: if this was medically true, she reasoned, then it should be religiously true as well, as religion urges proper treatment and caretaking of the body. The problem was that 'Ali could not reduce the decision to his own individual medical state. Larger stakes were involved, ones that he could not shake and that slowly became apparent to me, as I explain below.

A CHANGE OF HEART

'Ali spent hours debating with himself, and with me, about why something like this could not possibly be pleasing to God. He told me, "God is trying me with this disease. When we are tried by God, we remember Him and praise Him for everything. God says, 'He who is not pleased with My will can find another universe to live in!'" So I was surprised when one day I came to the unit and 'Ali announced to me that he was going to seek a transplant. I asked him what had changed his mind. He had gone to Cairo to the military hospital in Ma'adi for a check-up, and the doctor who treated him there had had a transplant operation himself, done in America. He encouraged 'Ali, telling him that God has given us our bodies as a trust *(amana)* and that we are therefore responsible for taking care of ourselves. Dialysis was slowly ruining his body, the doctor told him, and is not a treatment that would ever make him better. But, the doctor reasoned, God had blessed him with the *chance* to have a transplant and the military insurance that would cover it. When I had previously spoken to ʿAli, he told me that his wife pleaded with him daily to accept one of her kidneys but that he flatly refused, not wanting to hurt her in any way. This new doctor's appointment, however, had clearly made an impression on him. Furthermore, he said, one of the patient's sons in the room, a military captain, had watched a television program on which a respected Islamic scholar said that having this procedure done is not *haram* and that God urges us to seek cures. ʿAli explained, "The scholars on television said that it is *haram* to let your body deteriorate, because God tells us [in the Qurʾan] not to throw our selves into destruction [*ma tirmish nafsak fil tahluka*]."

ʿAli was happy and laughing that day, saying, "May God stand by us." He said that he spoke to a lot of doctors when in the Maʿadi hospital and that they said people received transplants there every day and were fine. ʿAli told his wife, Wafiyya, to come to the unit that day so that I could speak with her as well. As we passed by him to go to the waiting room, he winked and gave her a high-five.

ʿAli and Wafiyya, both twenty-eight years old, had been married for seven years and had two young children. Unable and unwilling to separate the consequences of his own bodily intervention from the bodies and lives of his family, ʿAli struggled with what course of action to take. Wafiyya told me,

> Before, ʿAli kept saying it was *haram*, and also he was worried about me because of the children. From the beginning of his sickness, I've been begging him to have a transplant. Dr. Charles, also for the past two to three years has been telling him that he's young and the disease will hurt him. But he kept saying it was *haram*.
>
> Back when we got the *qirar* [authorization for state medical coverage] to be able to do the tests, we were on the path to getting this transplant done, and all of a sudden he said no. But now he's again starting to accept the idea. . . .
>
> I heard Shaykh Shaʿrawi say that God gave [your body] to you, and you can't give away what God has given you. But I said [to ʿAli], "Why can't I give it to you? I'm going to save you." Am I supposed to leave him and let him die? But he kept saying no, because of the children. Back then, our daughter was three and a half years old and the boy was just three or four months old.
>
> I'm still worried about them. [She started to cry.] Where would I leave them? Who will look after them? His brothers and sisters say,

"We'll donate for you. Leave your wife. She's so young." I went and talked to my parents. I told them, "This is my life and he's my husband, and if, God forbid, something happens to him, what am I going to do?" [She started to cry again.]

Wafiyya's parents felt that they had to protect her at all costs. Like many young wives in such a position, Wafiyya's natal family interceded on her behalf, afraid that her husband's family might place unfair expectations on her. What went unstated was the fear that Wafiyya would soon be widowed, regardless of whether she underwent the surgery to donate her kidney to 'Ali. How would she support herself in the event of her husband's death? Would having a nephrectomy hurt her chances of supporting herself, of caring for the children, or of remarriage later in life?

But Wafiyya herself refused to think along these lines. Her main concern was helping her husband get better so that their family life could continue. 'Ali's siblings said that they felt bad letting Wafiyya be the one to donate, but if they were to donate, 'Ali would have to worry about the feelings of his siblings' spouses, a burden he did not want to take on. Wafiyya continued: "Yesterday, the army doctor in Cairo said to him, 'It's been five years on dialysis. That's enough.' The doctor's wife had given him her kidney, but [the operation was performed] in the United States. So 'Ali said to himself, 'After five to six years on dialysis, the body wears out.' He is struggling so hard to get better; he is struggling with his whole heart, his whole body." The other patients' family members in the waiting area nodded and said, "This is right; it is like a spiritual struggle [*jihad*]; the body wears out from dialysis, and the patients must continue their struggle."

Wafiyya was obviously torn about the position she was in. At least when 'Ali had refused to consider transplant, on the grounds that it is *haram*, she had given up feeling responsible. She said, "I just want him to have a transplant so he gets better and so he can get back to his normal self. But he says that he doesn't believe that transplanting will get him back to normal. I tell him, our Lord is with us [*Rabbina mawgud*]."

The patient's son, the captain who had seen the television show, offered: "I saw a shaykh on TV—I don't remember which one—but he said it wasn't *haram*."

Wafiyya nodded and said, "So when 'Ali heard this, he said, 'Well I won't understand the matter better than the shaykhs; if they said it's not *haram*, after they have understood and studied the Qur'an, well . . .'"

The captain added, "But they said it's in specific cases, like if there's no harm to the donor, then it's okay."

Wafiyya looked up at the captain and smiled feebly. Then she continued: "After dialysis, he is so tired. He gets very sick if he misses a session. I talked to my parents, and they said, 'Well it's your life, and he's your husband. They were [by now] not opposed [to her donation of a kidney].' His older brother wants to donate his kidney for him, and they went together to the center in Mansoura, and when they got back, 'Ali got scared for his brother and wouldn't agree to it. And his older sister also wanted to donate her kidney to him, but he said, 'No, if I take one, I'll take it from my wife.' "

Wafiyya had suggested that, since his mother is deceased, 'Ali's father should have offered to donate to his son, but he never did. This would have been the best solution, if it was medically feasible. But neither 'Ali nor his father ever mentioned it.

I continued to think about Wafiyya during the following weeks, wondering what she would do. A few weeks later, I was back at the dialysis center when 'Ali got a phone call. He had been his usual self, joking with Madame Sabah, an older woman in the unit who had taken on a maternal role toward him. Sitting between him and Madame Sabah, I could see 'Ali's face clearly while he was on the phone. The call was from Wafiyya, and she had just received the results of the lab work. 'Ali tried to act calm and unaffected: "Wafiyya heard from the [military] hospital. Let's see what will happen now," he announced to Madame Sabah before returning to Wafiyya on the phone.

There was no tissue match.

'Ali still sounded unimpressed, saying, "Okay, okay, Madame Sabah sends her greetings to you," and hung up, announcing to whomever was interested that Wafiyya's tissues did not match his well enough for the military doctors to proceed with the transplant.[21]

Madame Sabah saw through 'Ali's attempts to be cavalier. She said gently, "Don't be upset, 'Ali; we're better off this way. We won't make other people [i.e., the donors] sick with us. We won't get all swollen [from the postoperative treatment]. We won't be in the hospital day after day, worrying about some kind of infection. The way we are now on dialysis is just better."

Madame Sabah was a widow in her fifties who had never had any children. She was so pleasant and well loved that she had many family members who offered to donate their organs to her, most pressingly her niece. But there was no way Madame Sabah could think of taking this from her. Later, 'Ali told me, "Madame Sabah was just saying those things to make us both feel better, so that we would be able to stay steadfast in the face of this hardship *[tasabbar nafsaha wa tasabbarni]*. But of course she wants a transplant and to get better, just like the rest of us. But what can we do?"

When I had first met Madame Sabah, who was the widow of an army officer and who was now covered by his army insurance, she told me that through her connections, she had made an appointment at the Mansoura Kidney Center just to make sure her dialysis treatment was going well. She was on the waiting list and would have to wait eight months. "And that's with all my connections!" she noted. Insisting that Mansoura was the best, even better than any place in Cairo, she wanted to be assured that she was "moving in the right direction" on dialysis. Her sister and niece were to accompany her. But when the day finally came, shortly after the news of ʿAli's incompatible tissue type, she called me to tell me that she wasn't going after all. She was too tired, she wasn't in the mood, and what would she find out anyway? Months and months on dialysis seemed to deflate the patients' hopes of anything better down the road. And one patient's despair seemed to transfer easily to the next. In the months that followed, however, ʿAli came to accept this news as a gift from God; he eventually said that God had prevented him from doing something potentially *haram*. He continued to thank God for the blessings that he was receiving on dialysis. A year later, the patients in the unit were cheered up by the news that ʿAli's wife, Wafiyya, had given birth to another baby girl, whom ʿAli described as "sweet as honey."

In the hours that I spent talking with ʿAli, I came to appreciate more fully the complex ways in which people embody and live questions about divine will, and how much of their lives they feel they can control, and how much they feel they *should* control. In contrast to the U.S. situation, where kidney-failure patients can be put on a waiting list to receive kidneys from anonymous brain-dead donors, in Egypt, patients have had to "find kidneys" for themselves, bringing to the surface a host of ethical questions and dilemmas. The process has been much more mystifying in the United States, since kidneys are procured through a complex medical industry, the minutiae of procurement rendered less visible to the waiting patients.[22]

Once I asked ʿAli if he were in a medical system in which all he had to do was agree to have his name put on a list and an organ would eventually be procured for him, would he accept it? He hesitated and then said yes, he would, even if he harbored some reservations. A remarkably insightful man, ʿAli realized that his refusal was shaped by and situated in a particular social context in which he had to overcome several obstacles to proceed with a transplant—to find a donor, to be responsible for the donor's tests, and to bear the responsibility for the donor's sacrifice, pain, and side effects.

Already predisposed to mistrust this medical practice, ʿAli lacked the drive to surmount each hurdle, as each of these steps continually raised for him the ethical uncertainties surrounding organ transplantation. He thus recognized that were he in an alternate sociomedical setting in which a kidney was somehow made available to him without such constant reminders, were he able to focus just on himself and not have to face larger ramifications of his treatment, he would likely accept it. In my conversations with Wafiyya, she had noted that if ʿAli had a parent willing and eager to donate an organ to him, this may have solved their problem. It was not that ʿAli had no kin offering to donate; it was that those offering were not the right *kind* of family member to donate to him (more on this in the next chapter). ʿAli could not accept the idea of one of his siblings parting with a kidney for his sake, and he felt ambivalent about using his wife as his donor. ʿAli could not shake his deep reservations about being responsible for his wife's potential illness, suffering, and inability to look after their children. ʿAli insisted that he would rather die and "meet God" than be responsible for causing harm to one of his siblings or his wife or for putting his family in debt to buy a kidney, which he saw as clearly *haram*. Given the reality that he lived in, he turned to God to seek the strength that he needed to remain on dialysis for the rest of his life.

In explaining ʿAli's reluctance to pursue transplantation from his wife in his first five years on dialysis, his physicians in frustration described him as "religiously extreme" or "fatalistic." Indeed, his rhetoric echoed that of Shaykh Shaʿrawi when ʿAli stated that he should merely submit to God's infinite and all-encompassing will. ʿAli's physicians' annoyance with this reasoning resonated with the wider attacks against Shaʿrawi, who had seemed to take a fatalistic and hence nonsensical position, since Islamic teachings encourage seeking treatment, good health, and care of the body. But careful study of the social patterns and people's courses of action reveals that Shaʿrawi's logic resonates only in very specific situations and that these situations shift, even in the same person's case, depending on a number of factors, including how the scope of the intervention is defined. Whether and when to submit to divine will is contingent upon how much control patients feel they have in the face of illness and other trials and on whether they have any options that will actually provide an accessible and appropriate "solution" that they can live with medically, financially, socially, and spiritually.

But what are we to make of ʿAli's sudden change of heart? In considering a competing moral discourse about the meaning of the "body belongs to God," he had allowed himself to be convinced to pursue transplantation as a means to respect and care for the body that God had given him. And how are we to understand then ʿAli's ultimate acceptance of the news of the incompatible tissue type as a divine sign not to pursue the transplant? The doctor at the military hospital and hearsay from a fellow patient's son about the proclamations of a television shaykh—of the type ʿAli had earlier claimed not to trust—were suddenly able to convince ʿAli that it was part of his religious duty to pursue transplantation to protect the body as a divine trust. The key here is that ʿAli heard these arguments in a new context in which he was also shown the fruits of successful transplant surgeries and the routinization of transplantation in a large military hospital in Cairo. His thrice-weekly routine of hemodialysis in a less-than-ideal hospital setting in Tanta had made him wary of medical services and practices. But the state-of-the-art facilities in Cairo made a different impression on him, particularly hearing from a doctor who himself was a posttransplantation survivor, promising him that a return to normal daily activities was well within his reach.

His excitement at seeing the impressive facilities in the Cairo military hospital soon wore off as he returned to the drudgery of the commute to Tanta, the dialysis regimen, and the poverty of his rural village in Minufiya. And his return to his family life reminded him that this was not a decision that would affect his body alone but would necessarily pose a burden on those whose welfare was his primary responsibility. When a slim window of hope had opened and transplantation looked like it might be a beneficial solution to his illness, ʿAli not only saw it as religiously permissible but agreed with the doctor that it would be a religious *duty* to pursue it if it meant restoring his health. This hope was fragile and rapidly crushed with the news of an incompatible tissue match with his wife and with the reminders of the costs that his transplant would impose on other family members.

Here, too, ethical positions shifted depending on how the scale of the transplant was defined. When ʿAli felt that he could focus on his individual body, transplantation seemed like a course of action that he should pursue. But transplantation seemed more complicated when he broadened the scale of the transplant beyond his own suffering body, imagining himself as one small part in his valuable social relations and imagining the scale of his life to be no longer than a femtosecond compared with the eternity of the hereafter. This is why patients who, like ʿAli, at times seemed very resolute in their positions often changed their minds. Their clinical encounters and their family lives compelled them to frame the problem differently. A change of heart did not make their religious convictions any less strong or meaningful. In Egypt, some physicians and interlocutors I encountered interpreted ʿAli's shifting belief—that transplantation was permissible when his wife was still potentially a donor for him and later that it was forbidden or sinful when his wife's tissues were not a match—to be a manipulation of the religion to suit his circumstances.

But such interpretations miss the point. Religion was not an object external to ʿAli's self that he manipulated to suit his needs. Devout patients like ʿAli embody a religious tradition in which they struggle to cultivate within themselves the disposition of *rida,* or contentment with God's will. ʿAli believed strongly that true submission to God maintains that God's will transcends everything, and the purpose of worship and remembrance is to bring oneself in utter closeness to God: "God is with you wherever you are" (the Qurʾan, Al-Hadid 57:4) and "Wheresoever you turn, there is the Face of God" (the Qurʾan, Al-Baqara 2:115). That is to say, in ʿAli's devotion to God, when he felt that he had the opportunity for transplantation, he felt that God had willed him to seize this opportunity. When there was no such potential, after news of his wife's incompatible tissue type, he read God's will favorably as well: that God had prevented him from pursuing something potentially harmful or sinful.

We should not assume that patients foreclose all treatment options out of "fatalism," nor should we assume that they appeal to God only to comfort themselves, after the fact, in their lack of access to treatment.[23] People embody and experience religion to varying effects. In the case of ʿAli, he continually invoked God to allow him to understand each turn of events as part of God's overall plan of benevolence and compassion *(al-rahma).* In the words of an oft-cited Prophetic tradition, "How remarkable is the case of the believer! There is good for him in everything, and this is the case for no one else except for the believer. When the believer receives any good, he is thankful to God, and is rewarded. And when some misfortune befalls him, he is also rewarded for enduring it patiently."[24] As ʿAli and many patients reiterated to me, the Prophet Muhammad indeed told his believers to seek counsel from their own hearts. This had led many to the conviction that behind their specific illnesses lay divine wisdom. In ʿAli's struggles to cultivate dispositions of fortitude, he worked on himself to embody the sentiment that his body indeed belonged to God.

CONCLUSIONS

In Egypt, as elsewhere, medical decisions about life and death are never merely individual decisions; instead, they are bound up in the lives and bodies of others as well. This is particularly the case when the medical treatment necessitates the extraction of a vital body part from one person and its transfer to another. Patients, their family members, and their doctors come to their religious ethical positions through the rubric of cost-benefit analysis, factoring in medical risk, efficacy, and social, familial, and financial costs. This rubric constricts and expands according to how the scope of the problem is defined. As the scale of the medical intervention widens or narrows in people's deliberations, they sometimes come to contradictory, conflicting, or fluctuating positions.

Dr. Kotb, throughout his long career as a Cairo transplant surgeon, revealed moral ambivalence about his own surgical accomplishments as he struggled with whether transplantation, when calculated from a societal perspective, constitutes good medical and scientific practice. When focusing on the immediacy of his dying patient, Dr. Kotb's mission, in his early years, seemed clear. But as time passed and as he realized that his medical responsibilities included a wider portion of society, the question of whether transplantation is "beneficial" was more nebulous. Kotb described this not as a change in priorities or as a turn to greater religiosity, for he had always been, he said, a devout Muslim. Rather, what shifted was his move from the ontogenetic focus of biomedicine to a concern with its broader social consequences; he felt responsible for a wider swath of society than just his own patients. He was initially surprised that Sha'rawi had seemed unmoved to change his stance toward organ transplantation, even when confronted by the suffering of a particular patient. Yet eventually Dr. Kotb, too, came to see the immediate crisis of a dying patient in need of surgical intervention as a distraction from the greater social suffering that can be exacerbated, not remedied, by organ transplantation.

While Sha'rawi was initially unable, or perhaps unwilling, to articulate what precise aspect of organ transplantation he found distasteful, his position that it is *haram* ultimately resonated with many Egyptians, even among transplant surgeons and terminally ill kidney-failure patients. Sha'rawi himself refused to engage with the questions of whether it is realistic to portray transplantation as a medical miracle that can ultimately restore patients to their normal lives and whether it can do so at a reasonable cost. But these were exactly the questions that troubled the physicians and doctors I interviewed when they referenced his statement. Here ethics does not map onto some external codified set of commandments or scripture, nor does ethical reasoning merely mirror the authoritative words of a religious figure, even when he is directly cited. For patients and their family members as well, their cost-benefit analyses necessarily depend on whom and what is included in the calculation. Patients' ethical and medical assessments of whether to seek transplantation depend on their family relations and resources. The burden on the family is in many instances too high to undergo transplantation. The family can also find it unbearable if their devoted child refuses the transplant.

Taking a firm or consistent ethical position requires rigid boundary work in defining the scope of the problem. Dr. Badr, for example, took comfort in knowing that his medical work resulted in "more benefit than harm." He had taken steps to circumscribe for himself the scope of the problems associated with kidney transplantation to include only the surgical outcome, deciding that he was personally responsible for this alone. But for others, the scale of the intervention shifted, from a narrow focus on "fixing" a failed organ to a broader concern with what might fully rehabilitate the person and wider society, bearing in mind the potential disruption of vital kin relations, the potential harm to another living donor, the potential heedlessness that could come with a direct challenge to God's will, and the probable exacerbation of social inequalities. Shadya, Tamir, ʿAli, and other patients I spoke with struggled with their ethical stances when they shifted the scope of the procedure beyond its costs and benefits with respect to their own individual bodies and brought their social contexts into account as well. If Shaʿrawi himself never based his anti-transplant stance on practical concerns, patients and doctors for whom Shaʿrawi's stance is meaningful, question whether kidney transplantation provides a "solution," because it brings with it a host of stresses on kinship ties, financial resources, moral certainty, and bodily health. Organ failure cannot be medically treated on an individual scale, with the treatments and costs borne by the patient alone. Many patients, unwilling to burden their family members, turn to their individual responsibility before God, limiting the overwhelming scale of the problem to something manageable: surviving one day at a time and trusting God to do the rest. The next chapter looks at how different types of risk weigh on the ethical decisions that people make within the rubric of kinship and the realities of scarce resources.

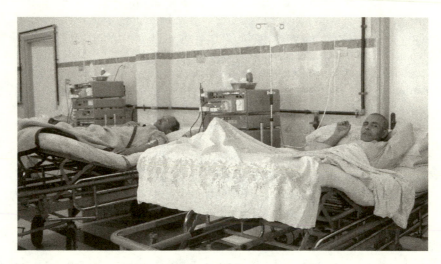

Figure 11.   Patients in a Tanta dialysis ward.

6. Only One Kidney to Give

Ethics and Risk

There was some commotion in the transplant ward of a public Cairo teaching hospital over a young patient who had just received a kidney from his mother. Another patient in the unit explained to me what was going on:

> This poor young man—he has a younger brother who also has kidney failure. While he was in the operating room he heard that his younger brother was upset that the mother had given the older brother her kidney.
>
> You see, the mother had reasoned that her older son was already married and had a child. She thought to give it to him so that he could support his family. But the younger son now will never get one. When the older one heard that his younger brother was upset, he was so distressed that he almost rejected his [new] kidney. The doctors had to give him extra attention, and we all tried to make him feel better about the situation. . . . That poor mother—two sons in need, but only one kidney to give!

The mother's body, with two kidneys and two sons in kidney failure, symbolized in a sense the bodies of everyone there in the hospital ward. There was a clear limit to the available resources that could be garnered to fight off disease. As the only viable donor in the family, the mother was expected to "choose" between her two sons, and she chose the one who was in a better position to secure his own family—his wife and child.[1] But the son who received the kidney faced not only the medical and surgical risks associated with the transplant but also the social risks of familial disruption, guilt, and strained relations with his brother. In the face of life-threatening illness, people are forced to make decisions valuing some lives over others, always with uneasy consequences.

Questions about whether to transplant a kidney are informed by various categories of risk that affects the donor and recipient. As we saw in the last chapter, the majority of patients in renal failure see kidney transplantation as holding a promise far beyond their reach, and they also question whether it will deliver on its promise. Both physicians and patients hold misgivings about transplantation: whether it is ethically responsible to put the living donor at risk, and whether, in the end, it will be efficacious. Different types of risk factor into the ethical decision making of patients and their family members. These include the *physical and environmental* risks predisposing patients and their family members to disease, the *iatrogenic* risks of medical mistreatment, the *financial* risk of extraordinary debt and bankruptcy, the *spiritual* risk of doing something that can potentially be displeasing to God, and the significant *social* risks that come from the pressures that a transplant bears on kin relations. The degree to which an organ donation within the family poses stress on familial relations depends on who within the family gifts the kidney and at the expense of whom. As with the above ethnographic account, the different categories of risk are often interrelated; given the older son's financial inability to procure another kidney, the familial disruption caused by his mother's choice threatened the medical outcome of his transplant.

Aware of the different risks involved in pursuing a transplant operation, many patients I spoke with described it as a high-stakes gamble. One young patient, Muhammad, explained that in contrast, he experienced his dialysis sessions as more certain, the outcome knowable, and his life made bearable. As he put it:

> Getting a transplant isn't guaranteed. I know that my kidney is ruined, so I come here for dialysis three days a week. Only God knows if I would die trying to get a transplant. Some people get sick with the transplant—the body rejects it, or they end up with other diseases. So I need just to be content with what I have. If I tried to have a transplant, I could die the next morning. So what would I have gotten out of it—just having myself opened up and stitched back together? Sometimes the operation can last five to six hours; only God knows what could happen during that time. So I need to stick with what is guaranteed. I come here to dialysis and can go home after four hours. And that's it.

Knowing full well that dialysis is not really treatment and that transplantation was the only way out of his chronic condition, Muhammad still questioned whether transplantation was a viable option. Given the significant resources that he would have had to amass in order to pursue a transplant, he knew that he would be taking a chance, one that would ultimately cost him on many levels. Life on dialysis, however difficult, was a safer route that enabled his survival.[2]

Complex ethical decisions cannot be reduced to a single factor, such as medical access or religious stringency. Patients and clinicians weigh different types of risks against the potential benefit of healthy life. Patients and their family members struggle with what to do when they do not have the "right" kin to donate, when their families will be making tremendous financial sacrifices to afford the operation, and when they feel that they might be putting vulnerable family members at risk with organ extraction. Against these risks, they see the medical outcome as uncertain, given the two necessarily invasive surgical procedures—one to procure a kidney from a healthy living person, and the other to receive the kidney transplant and subsequently fight the body's impulse to reject it.

At the time of my research in Egypt, the country's economic situation rocked precariously; the cost of living skyrocketed while salaries and livelihoods fell. Social services in hospitals and clinics dwindled, as did the medical ethos of caring for the poor. Further, news commentaries, television reports, and people's direct experiences with toxic waste, pollutants, and the shortage of clean water highlighted the threats to bodily health through regular activities such as eating, drinking, and breathing, and arduous and unregulated labor practices posed yet more hazards. In this situation, in which economic, medical, and environmental risks pose significant threats to everyday life, people most often turn to family and religious faith for safety and protection. But here, too, organ transplantation poses its threats. Even while holding out the promise to restore patients to the activities of everyday life, organ transplantation can put unbearable pressure on vital familial relations and weaken religious ideals pertaining to the sacredness of *all* lives and the importance of fortitude during God's trials.

MEDICAL MISMANAGEMENT, IATROGENIC RISK, AND PATIENT MISTRUST

Patients often told me that they suffered not only from disease but also from inferior medical treatment. Amin, a patient in his midforties who had both end-stage kidney failure and advanced liver disease, explained to me that the constant worry about his treatment was even worse than the disease itself. Whether the dialysis machines were actually working, whether his medicines were being administered properly, whether he would contract a disease through his treatment and blood transfusions were constant sources of worry. He said, "I heard that in the United States and Europe dialysis patients go [to dialysis units] as if they are going to a salon. They just drive there, and it is a nice pleasant room, and they are done and go on with their lives. If it were like that, it wouldn't be so bad. But here I have to worry all the time."

Only those patients who felt empowered to demand better treatment worried about the potential negative effects of their treatment. For them, worry about the treatment they were receiving seemed to supplant the more positive notion of "hope" of recovery. Fathallah, an agricultural laborer in his fifties, remained vigilant during dialysis, watchful at the insertion of the needle, shouting at the nurses if they did not use the proper amount of solvents in his machine, protesting if the physician did not stop at his bed on his weekly rounds. Others, particularly older patients, seemed utterly resigned to remaining ill and on dialysis for the rest of their lives and had given up worrying. They lay in their beds, their bodies heavy and still, periodically invoking God to foster within them steadfastness *(al-sabr)* and strong faith.

As medical anthropologists have noted, there are no patient support groups in the Egyptian medical sphere (Inhorn 1994, 2003), and efforts at group therapy in Arab countries have generally resulted in failure of improvement and even in adverse outcomes, because patients express strong preference for sharing the burden of care within the extended family and not with "strangers" (Al-Mutlaq and Chaleby 1995; Hamdy and Nasir 2007). Yet, by virtue of having to spend "half their lives," as the patients I spoke with put it, in a dialysis unit with other patients undergoing the same treatment, they supported one another. There were generally no partitions between the beds, which were arranged around the room, with the patients receiving dialysis as they lay side by side.[3] Many patients told me that having to go through the treatment alongside others somehow lessened the psychological burden of having to face their illness alone.

Moreover, the patients provided one another with information about managing and living with the disease. Their circle of exchange constituted a network that operated alongside the one connecting their bodies to the machines and to the hospital power supply, one that enabled alternative etiologies and practices of self-care in the clinic. Like chronic patients elsewhere, they had become familiar with medical terms related to their illness, often responding to the question "How are you?" with numbers indicating their most recent creatinine levels.[4] While being weighed, having their blood pressure checked, settling into their beds, and being hooked up to their tubes, patients greeted one another and exchanged news. Most significantly, in this makeshift community, patients identified with one another as the country's vulnerable, and now ill, poor *(il-ghalaba)*.[5]

The patients were keenly aware that the clinic's dialysis machines could never completely substitute for a pair of working kidneys.[6] "Good" solvents were too expensive to use in these second-rate machines, generations older than their counterparts in other countries. The patients, unable to afford expensive pharmaceuticals that increase blood protein, relied for this purpose on blood transfusions, which they feared were contaminated. Stories in the Egyptian press have revealed scandalous mismanagement of blood storage and processing. In June 2007, the Egyptian parliamentary member Hani Sorour was referred to criminal court after being accused of fraud and profiteering in 2006 in marketing three hundred thousand blood transfusion bags that violated Egyptian and international standards. Forensic studies reported that the bags caused bacterial poisoning and that they leaked anticoagulant liquid (Leila 2007).[7]

Regardless of whether they receive blood transfusions, dialysis patients are susceptible to infections, many cases of which have been reported in the press. In 1990, medical practitioners recorded eighty-two HIV infections at three dialysis centers in Egypt (Hassan, El-Ghorab, et al. 1994; El-Sayed, Gomatos, et al. 2000). The Egyptian Society of Nephrology's 2008 report states that 52 percent of dialysis patients tested positive for hepatitis C, and in the clinics that I visited, 70–80 percent of dialysis patients had contracted the virus through infection from dialysis machines.[8] Contracting hepatitis C made them vulnerable to liver failure, in which case they became medically ineligible for kidney transplantation, if they had not already been economically disqualified from eligibility. Dr. Charles, a British nephrologist who spent time working in an Egyptian dialysis unit through work with his church, once told me that patients should not think that transplantation will be the "be-all and end-all of the kidney disease. It should instead be thought of as a vacation from dialysis. The graft might last just five or six years, at which time the patient might be eligible for another graft." Of course, in England, patients are covered by the national health system and do not have to liquidate all their assets in order to afford a single kidney. In the context of poor Egyptians, the promise that transplantation can return a person to "normalcy" is particularly problematic, given the costs. Knowing that a graft would not last forever, some patients I interviewed wondered if it was more cruel to wager the gamble to earn them some time off dialysis if chances were that they would ultimately end up back on dialysis. Meanwhile, life on dialysis was depressing when there was no hope or end point in sight. As one Egyptian nephrologist cynically put it, "Dialysis is not a cure—it is like being in an ambulance. It can either take you to a transplant operation or take you to the grave."

University and other public hospitals in Egypt have been known to be bastions of mistreatment of the poor, who can receive services there free of charge or at very low cost in exchange for serving as teaching examples for attending physicians, residents, and medical students. The attending physicians receive very little financial compensation for their work at the public teaching hospitals and have little financial incentive to invest time in their patients there. Thus, many patients, even among the poor, have preferred to scrape together whatever savings they have to pay out-of-pocket expenses at private clinics, where the same physicians who teach in the public university hospitals during the day also treat patients in the evening for fees.

These private clinics are often not well networked with one another, allowing patients to fall through the cracks between specialties. Therefore, patients use common sense to match their symptoms with the appropriate specialist—preferably one who holds private clinic hours in the evening after his or her work as a faculty attending physician in the public hospitals. In Egyptian colloquial Arabic, medical jargon is rendered into unspecialized, everyday language. As we have seen, hemodialysis is referred to as "wash;" organ transplantation is referred to as "plant" (*zara'*, the same word one might use for planting a tree). Nephrology is referred to as "kidney," cardiology as "heart," and obstetrics as "birth." Rather than considering diagnosis to be solely in the realm of inaccessible, specialized expertise, patients tend to diagnose themselves and then turn to the physician for (belated) treatment. Patients are more likely to trust their own assessment of their bodily symptoms to select the appropriate specialist than to trust the referral of a primary care physician.[9] This is particularly the case when they see that the physician has a clear financial incentive to diagnose the patient's symptoms such that they correspond to the physician's particular specialty.[10]

However problematic this situation has been for the delivery of medical care in general, it has been particularly problematic in the case of kidney failure, which is characterized by wide variation in etiology and experience. Patients with kidney failure often simultaneously suffer from other illnesses, such as diabetes, lupus, hypertension, and heart disease, all of which affect kidney function, thus "conflicting against the notion of a diagnostic category as a bounded entity" (Kierans 2005: 345). Many of the Egyptian dialysis patients I met might have been able to prevent a terminal diagnosis and the remainder of their life on dialysis if they had had proper preventative care. Instead, they had suffered a broad array of symptoms before finally being diagnosed with kidney failure. In their profound mistrust of physicians, patients discounted medical knowledge that might have helped them come to earlier diagnoses of kidney malfunction. Or, put another way, poor patients did not receive reliable care that effectively intervened at early and, thus, more treatable stages of disease. [11] Although they were eminently grateful for their survival and for the treatment they received, they were also frustrated with greedy physicians, negligent nurses, and uncaring bureaucrats. Many of the patients had been misdiagnosed and mistreated prior to complete loss of kidney function. Some patients were prescribed the wrong medication, leading to acute kidney failure; others lost kidney function after botched operations to remove kidney stones.[12] Unable to afford expensive, five-star hospital treatment in Cairo or treatment abroad, poor dialysis patients in Tanta clinics knew that they were both critically reliant on and subject to local medical (mis)treatment. They formed communities out of a shared sense of vulnerability to a "failed state" and to corrupt and inadequate medical practice. These experiences of the medical risks in seeking treatment factored into patients' and family members' decisions about which level of medical intervention to pursue.

POLITICAL ETIOLOGIES AND ENVIRONMENTAL RISKS

The poor patients I spoke with were wary of more than medical institutions. They feared the very air they breathed, the water they drank, and the food they ate. "Do you see all of these sick people?" one patient in a dialysis-ward waiting room gesticulated at me in frustration. Imagining that I had come to Egypt to study kidney failure because it does not exist in "Amrika," he continued, "Did you see the filthy water in [Tanta's] irrigation canal? This is the water we drink from! And you want to know why there is so much kidney failure in Egypt? We get the bad genetically engineered food from other countries. They dump food on us, food that they would never let their own citizens eat. Our food is covered with pesticides, the water is bad, and now we are ill."

These patients linked their diseases and suffering to toxic air, dangerous pesticides and food, unsafe labor conditions, and medical mismanagement. The ways that patients linked the reasons for their poor health to broader social, environmental, and global economic forces, what I term their "political etiologies," served as a criticism of the medical reductionism they faced in the clinic. These understandings of disease were informed by medical studies, their physicians' views, newspaper and television reports, and their own firsthand experiences of toxic waste and poor medical care.

Mahdi, a fifty-eight-year-old man who received dialysis at a public hospital in Tanta, was accompanied by one of his six sons. Mahdi nodded and let his son do the talking while he secured the painful bandages around the tube that linked his flesh to the machine. His son explained,

> Kidney failure has really spread in the last few years. This could be because we are getting everything now from the outside—hormones in the food, pesticides in the fruits. These things are not natural; they are all poisons.
>
> They talk about advances in science, but [transplantation] is really not a solution to the problem, because there aren't kidneys available for all these people affected, and there are patients who have other problems. Like my father, he also has liver disease. [*Gestures to his father.*] And it could be that all his liver medicines are what caused his kidney failure. We are from the countryside. This [liver and kidney diseases] is all from bilharzias [schistosomiasis] too; it gets into the organs and into the liver and affects the whole body. So getting a new kidney is not going to lengthen your life.

Like Mahdi's son, other family members of dialysis patients and the patients themselves often appealed to a notion of a "local biology" (Lock 1993a, 1993b), in which their specific vulnerability—to poisonous food, a contaminated environment, parasitic infections, poverty, pharmaceuticals, and medical mistreatment—rendered organ transplantation inefficacious. Most of the dialysis patients' charts recorded the cause of kidney failure as "idiopathic," and the Egyptian Society of Nephrology from 1996 to 2008 reported that at least one-third of kidney-failure cases nationwide were due to hypertension, and another 10 to 20% of "unknown" etiology. This lack of a clear etiological explanation from medical experts was ripe cause for patients to develop their own ideas about their diseased bodies.[13] In the majority of cases in which kidney failure was diagnosed as secondary to hypertension or diabetes, these diseases, also ominously on the rise, were understood by patients to originate from the consumption of low-quality food and water. They dismissed the biological reductionism in medical diagnoses that indicated the disease was specific to the individual patient and located discretely in the kidneys. The patients in the dialysis ward, their families, and even their doctors linked their suffering to much wider political, social, and environmental causes. Kidney-failure patients all struggle with the stress (*al-daght*) of living in Egypt's cities today, caused by crowding, cramped living quarters, pollution, noise, rising costs, and falling salaries (Tabishat 2000). *Al-daght* is the term also used to describe the medical condition of hypertension, which is both a cause of kidney failure and an outcome of kidney failure and dialysis (Tabishat 2000). One physician from Tanta University Hospital even suggested to me that, unlike nephrological ailments of the past, which involved primarily rural patients with schistosomiasis (parasitic) infections, kidney diseases today are more aggressive, more complicated, and more persistent. He attributed this to an increasingly "unnatural" environment and diet.[14]

News media, particularly letters to the editor of the state-owned newspaper *Al-Ahram* and articles in opposition-party newspapers, have often reported on broken sewage systems and contaminated food and water unfit for human consumption as resulting in high rates of kidney failure.[15] In the summer of 2007, residents of villages across Egypt staged protests over water shortages despite their high monthly water bills. The print news media quickly dubbed the crisis the "water wars" *(fitnat al-miyah)*. In the village of Bishbiysh in Mahalla, residents faced a complete lack of water and sent appeals to the prime minister asserting that five hundred villagers suffered from kidney failure as a consequence of poor water maintenance. The villagers staged protests, and, in response to government threats to detain them, they dared the government to arrest them, saying that perhaps they would find clean water to drink in prison ('Arafa 2007; 'Imad al-Shadhili and al-Kashif 2007; al-Yawm 2007; Ghada 'Abd al-Hafiz, Abu-Zayd, and Nafi' 2007; Durrah 2007).

One nephrologist told me sadly that one-third of the patients in his private dialysis center came from the same rural area and that in one family he treated, five of its members were in end-stage kidney failure. This confirmed to him that toxic mismanagement in that rural area was a major factor in causing the kidney disease: "This isn't something that I like to announce, and let's not get into all of the conspiracy theories. . . . But there is some truth to them. The load of pesticides in the human body lasts around seventy years; even when buried in the grave, it will affect the next generation. I won't be around to see what the next generation is going to suffer." Focusing on Kafr al-Zayat, which is both a village in Gharbiya and the name of Egypt's major pesticide and chemical company, located in that village, he shook his head gravely and told me, "Don't these Kafr al-Zayat workers know that the water they drink is the same as the toxic waste? And when everyone finally realized this, what did the Ministry of Health do? Nothing!"[16]

Another physician from Tanta explained to me the link between adulterated food and the increasing number of diseases that he saw in clinic. We were sitting at his family's home, eating lunch. Pointing to the food that he was eating, he told me that formaldehydes are being used to preserve milk, leading to childhood blindness, that imported wheat and corn are now genetically modified and not stored properly, that pesticides declared too dangerous for use in other countries are dumped on Egyptian agricultural land. The imported variety of "white chicken," unlike the Egyptian country *baladi* (local) chicken, is pumped with hormones, he said, and fed all kinds of "unnatural" foods.

Several doctors cautiously pointed out to me that one toxic vector is the consumption of bread made from imported wheat (Johnston 2009). Instead of being grown and milled locally, more than one-third of Egyptian wheat is bought from the United States. This wheat, some doctors explained, sits in large barges in the Alexandrian port in hot and humid weather, a perfect environment for the growth of aflatoxins and ochratoxins.[17] Aflatoxins and ochratoxins also grow rampantly in local storage facilities in poor areas. These toxins constitute one of the many factors that have led to a large increase in renal and liver toxicity and carcinomas throughout the Egyptian countryside. Concerned public health researchers have continued to labor over the toxic etiology of liver and renal carcinomas in Egypt, revealing the links to aflatoxins and ochratoxins;[18] opposition newspapers have periodically reported on the problem, and letters to the editor in state-aligned newspapers have decried the ubiquity of "cancerous wheat" *(al-qamh al-musartan)*. Carcinogenic wheat has become a political rallying cry for oppositional political parties. For example, in May 2007, the government, fearing political unrest, agreed to an investigation of six thousand tons of wheat in the province of Daqahliyya (in the eastern Nile Delta). The investigation determined that the wheat contained dangerous levels of toxin and pesticide residue and was unfit for human consumption.[19]

With extensive subsidies from the United States, Egypt has become the world's third biggest importer of grain.[20] The increase in imported wheat reflects the diversion of locally produced coarse grains from humans to animals, whose meat products are chiefly consumed by tourists and other non-Egyptians as well as by middle- and upper-class urban residents (Mitchell 2002). Egyptian farmland that once grew barley, sorghum, and corn to feed the rural population is now used to grow grains to fatten cows consumed by those who are better off. Patients with kidney failure, in their own self-representations and in much of the rhetoric around the new "unsafe food," epitomize the vulnerabilities of detrimental state policies.

The link between "bad food" and the dramatic shift in Egypt's foreign and domestic policies has remained vivid in the living memory of Egypt's poor. After the 1978 Camp David Accords, in which Anwar Sadat removed Egypt from the pan-Arab alliance against the Israeli occupation of Palestine, the United States rewarded Egypt with a steep increase in aid, including food aid. Egypt became the second largest recipient of U.S. military and

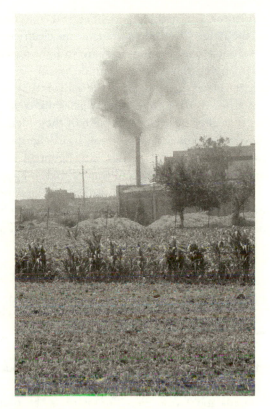

Figure 12.   A cement factory on agricultural land, in violation of the law, located along the road between Tanta and Cairo, June 2004. Photograph by the author.

economic aid after Israel. In 1982, under the pretext that Egypt had become a wealthier nation, U.S. food-assistance programs ended, and Egypt became the largest foreign market for U.S. wheat, with sales averaging $1 billion annually (*New York Times* 1981; Mitchell 2002).

The connection that patients have made between their illnesses and failed state policies is not merely abstract or cerebral; it is a connection that they experience in material and bodily forms as well. That is to say, these poor Egyptian patients suffering on dialysis are physically connected to machines that, in turn, connect them to the state infrastructure. These patients do not need to read science-in-practice theorists (Haraway 1985; Latour 1987, 2005) to appreciate the degree to which their cyborgian existence requires an extraordinary assemblage of human and nonhuman actors to link them to larger political structures. The machine-patient assemblage consists of bio-tech corporations, the state, nurses, doctors, engineers, electricity, machines, and the human body itself, each doing its share to fight against physical demise. Surgeons (many of whom, patients would say, are untrustworthy) rearrange the patients' blood vessels to allow the dialysis tubes easier access to their bodies. Attached to these tubes, their bodies are connected to the (erratic) machines that filter their blood in place of their "failed" kidneys. Dialysis patients are hooked to machines produced by foreign, profit-oriented corporations (suspected to have corrupt ties with Egyptian parliamentary members). The machines are imported and transported to Egyptian clinics (for use by those physicians with political connections). They are paid for by local government subsidies, and the patients using them must be approved for federal reimbursement by local parliamentary members (favoring, this time, patients with connections). The machines are inserted into (ailing) human bodies, and the resulting machine-patient hybrids are monitored by (negligent) nurses, supervised by (undependable) physicians, and tinkered with by (largely absent) engineers. Indeed, these assemblages are made evident every time a link in the chain becomes susceptible to breaking down. Patients experience their own vulnerability at every step, hitting the bumps of broken and missing links in the sequence.

Nowhere in the world has there been a holistic, organic, purely human dialysis patient unattached to the regimes of medical treatment and state infrastructure (Kierans 2005). And no nation-state has been autonomous within the global political economy. The Egyptian state, like the dialysis patients, is also hooked up to "tubes" and "machines" of U.S. liberal economic-development projects that have ultimately led to the exacerbation of socioeconomic inequalities (Mitchell 2002).

One columnist for the opposition-party paper *Al-Misri al-Yawm* encapsulated comments that I often heard among poor patients:

> The state does not pay a penny from its pocket to treat an Egyptian citizen. This is our money, the taxpayers' money. It is the right of the people, whose faith God Almighty is testing by thrusting on them a number of successive corrupt governments.
>
> More than half the population is afflicted with deadly diseases: 12 million are infected with liver and kidney related diseases, millions of others have suffered cancer, seven million are disabled, and, above all, there is the horrendous number of diabetic and hypertensive patients, as well as 40 million suffering from depression. These figures are based on statistics published in the daily newspapers, and not hearsay.
>
> Can anyone claim that God created these people sick, or deny that our corrupt government has neglected, ruined and even destroyed

people's health? Is it not the right of the citizen to be treated by the state? (Ramadan 2007)[21]

Following the lead of mass-media-hosted discussions of corruption, pollution, and medical mismanagement, kidney-failure patients have traced the etiology of their disease and their inadequate medical treatment to failures in state services and resources. Most dialysis patients are well versed in the toxic effects of pollutants that have been mismanaged throughout the Egyptian countryside. This informs their understanding of their illness as the outcome of a general weakening of the body attributable to a "toxic" *(musammam)* environment. They also feel weakened by what they describe as their "corrupt" *(fasid)* surroundings. The greed for profit and a lack of values, they often say, has led to the mismanagement of resources, pesticides, and toxic waste and to a situation in which medical care is substandard and the state's provision of services is detrimental. They do not completely accept the biomedical ontology of the body as an assemblage of parts, some of which function better than others. Rather, they conceive of their bodies as tired and weak, stricken by a toxicity to which everyone close to them is also vulnerable at all times.

Doctors who advocate transplantation constantly reiterate the biomedical claim that a person can live well with one-fourth of a kidney. In saying so, they mean to assure people that a living donor will not be harmed by having a kidney removed. Proponents of transplantation continually reiterate this statement of "medical expertise," which has also found its way into several fatwas that condone transplantation as an altruistic and commendable act. Many patients with whom I spoke could cite this "fact," yet they often cast it in a more cynical tone, because it seemed to have little to do with their lived realities. The generally detrimental environment makes patients reluctant to "take" organs from their healthy family members; they are disinclined to leave loved ones to fend for themselves in a polluted environment with only one kidney, half of what they themselves had when they got sick. As one hospital worker put it to me in response to the medical claim that a person can live with one-fourth of a kidney, "That is what they say. But where are they—all these people living well with one-fourth a kidney? All I see around me is people with *two* kidneys, and look at how sick they are getting!"

Understanding disease in terms of social inequality has particular salience in the realm of organ transplantation, a practice that presumes illness is located discretely in particular body parts that can be isolated, exchanged, and replaced. Anthropologists have demonstrated that biotechnological approaches to health more often exacerbate than erase social divisions, disproportionately intervening in diseases that are often themselves the end result of gross social inequalities (Farmer 1992, 1999; Kleinman, Das, et al. 1997; Scheper-Hughes 2000; Briggs 2003; Nguyen and Preschard 2003; Fassin 2007). This point is all too obvious for poor Egyptian dialysis patients and even for some of their doctors, whose political etiologies reject biomedical reductionism and form the basis of claims against the state for irresponsible care of its citizens. But they reject the extension of their suffering into the lives of healthy family members. Dismissing the notion that there can be such a thing as a "spare part"—for, surely, God created humans in perfect divine wisdom—many kidney-failure patients in Egypt cannot bear the idea of seeing their loved ones as bodily sources of medical intervention, even if a donated kidney might alleviate their own suffering.

SPIRITUAL RISK, EXPENDABLE BODIES

While in Tanta, aside from frequenting dialysis centers in major public hospitals, I also visited private outpatient dialysis centers. To my surprise, the patients at some of the private dialysis centers were facing even worse economic hardship than the patients in the public hospitals. The private centers accommodated patients who received government compensation for their dialysis treatments (*ʿala nafaq al-dawla*). Patients in these types of centers can be granted a space on a dialysis machine sooner than in the public teaching hospitals and can have the cost of their sessions paid directly by the Ministry of Health. I visited two such new private centers, one of which was an apartment in a dingy building in Tanta. The dialysis unit was on the third floor of this dark, depressing building, with a dilapidated stairwell and no elevators for the patients, some of whom could barely walk.

In the dark waiting room of this center, I spoke with Sabri, the husband of a dialysis patient. He stopped in the middle of our conversation to help carry an elderly lady, sitting in a heavy, rusted metal chair, from the dialysis center two flights down to street level. Down at the street, the family members wailed when they were forced to hail a cab—a great expense for them—to take them to the bus station, because the elderly lady could barely take a step. Sabri returned, out of breath, and resumed the conversation. While we were talking in the waiting room, loud shrieks permeated the entire building, originating from the dialysis center. I did not summon the courage to go inside the patients' room that day, remaining in the waiting area, where I spoke with patients and their family members before they went in or after they came out.

Sabri struggled to care for his wife, Khadra, and their child. Khadra had eclampsia (in Arabic, *tasammum haml*, literally, a "poisonous pregnancy"), and right after giving birth she was in pain and had swollen immensely. The obstetrician had told them the swelling was from the pregnancy, but after she delivered the baby it became even worse. Even after an arduous trial with the doctor from their town, then appointments with the Tanta city doctors, and finally a referral to the Mansoura Kidney Center, the symptoms continued to worsen, until years later she was diagnosed with acute renal failure. Sabri had been orphaned at the age of ten, and he told me that he had only his wife, Khadra, also an orphan, her mentally disabled brother, and their five-year-old son for family, and Sabri alone cared for them. Although he had a diploma as a technician, Sabri worked as a construction worker whenever he could. He said that the first five years of Khadra's treatment were enormously costly; before marriage he had saved up for a place to live, but by now they had spent all their savings on doctors' bills and prescriptions. On the days that he would try to find work and earn money, Khadra would plead with him, "Please, please stay with me. I feel sick, I feel like I might die." And so he would stay with her and would not go to work. "But she could do this, maybe twice a week," he told me in frustration.[22]

When Sabri heard about the possibility of a transplant, he considered donating his own kidney to Khadra but worried that he too would get sick after subjecting himself to the hospital. He said,

> If I get sick, well it's from God, but who will take care of her and her brother, who is sick, and our little son?
>
> People in our *balad* [town] said, "Take the kidney from her [mentally disabled] brother. You see he is not using it; he doesn't need his kidney for anything." But we felt that this was not right. How could I do this?
>
> So I sent a fax to Dar al-Ifta' [asking for a fatwa] to see if it is *haram* to do that. Of course they sent a rejection and said no to this. They said if he could understand what was happening and he agrees, then okay, but if he doesn't, then, no, it's not allowed, because you don't know what could happen to him. And this is *hurmaniyya* [sacred/forbidden]), it's *amana* [a trust from God]; you can't just take it. Like with someone's money, you can't just take it. So we rejected the idea. This was the first and only time we thought about a transplant.

People in Sabri's neighborhood placed less relative worth on the life and bodily integrity of his mentally disabled brother-in-law. They urged Sabri to see his brother-in-law as a repository of an "expendable" organ that could resolve the suffering of the larger family. The neighbors saw the brother-in-law's mental disability as the reason why his healthy kidney would be of better use in Khadra's body. Arguing that he was not "using his kidney for anything," they believed that his mental disability, his consequent inability to contribute economically to his household, and his inability to form his own family made him the most expendable family member. Organs should flow, in this logic, from the weak to the strong: to those who could "use" their bodies either productively, in financially supporting the family, or reproductively, in producing and raising family members.

But Sabri rejected this view. To him, his wife's brother was vulnerable kin who needed his protection. His brother-in-law's inability to comprehend what kidney donation entails was precisely what precluded him from being a donor in Sabri's eyes. According to the logic of the wider community, this inability was the very reason why he should be a donor. But Sabri had well-founded worries about the larger consequences of subjecting otherwise healthy family members to major medical intervention. While the townspeople, as Sabri described them, launched powerful moral reasoning based on the desperate allocation of scarce resources for sheer survival, Sabri appealed to authoritative religious discourse, now available to him in the context of the Islamic revival, to uphold his commitment to protect, rather than exploit, his vulnerable family member. Sabri exerted much effort in attaining what he considered to be the correct Islamic position on this question from the Dar al-Ifta' in Cairo. The mufti of the office ultimately confirmed Sabri's own position. He could not and would not take the spiritual risk of committing what was in his eyes a grave sin.

Sabri had sought a formal fatwa when his neighbors pressured him to do something that he intuitively felt was wrong. Worried that perhaps he *wasn't* doing everything possible to save his wife, that perhaps there *was* a way out, even if he felt there wasn't, he sought the counsel of religious scholars. Sabri appealed to religious scholars to confirm the fatwa that he had "received" from his own heart. By spending scarce resources and time on finding an office and sending a fax to Dar al-Ifta' in Cairo, he reassured himself that his actions were in conformity with authoritative religious reasoning. The majority of patients with whom I spoke in the dialysis centers did not formally ask for fatwas about whether or not they should seek a transplant. They were well aware of the debates through television and other media; they told me that they themselves knew their own situations more than any religious scholar could and that they did what they felt was right in their hearts.[23] Those who spoke of the importance of consulting their hearts struggled to avoid the spiritual and social risk of prioritizing their own needs at the expense of others'.

Had Sabri and Khadra gone along with the plan to "take" a kidney from Khadra's mentally disabled brother, they could likely have raised the funds to afford such an operation at a public teaching hospital in Cairo. But acting in conformity with what they understood to be morally correct took precedence over the impetus to reallocate their family's body parts to eliminate Khadra's suffering. For many, patterns in gifting kidneys reified hierarchical kin structures, such that resources—and organs—flowed to those seen as directly supporting the larger family unit. But others, like Sabri, appealed to Islamic discourses to act against this larger cultural logic, in a move they saw as protecting their marginalized family members and protecting their own moral integrity. Ultimately, the potential spiritual risk of "taking" what was not theirs was harder to bear than the significant medical, financial, and social suffering of their present situation.

WE COME FROM OUR PARENTS, WE BELONG TO GOD: MEDIATING SOCIAL RISK

Patients and their family members experience very little ethical quandary over parents donating kidneys to their children. While people generally have a hard time with the notion of "taking" a kidney from a living healthy family member, the antipathy is overcome when the kidney specifically moves from a parent to a child. This is considered the "natural" direction of how life should flow, as one patient put it, "as a branch grows from a tree." Parents often told me that they felt it was the most self-evident thing to do to help their children.

Parents have been the unquestionable source of kidneys for young patients when the blood type matches. Younger patients told me that they would accept an organ only if it came from a parent. Many patients and medical staff described mothers donating to their children as "natural," fitting with a mother's qualities of self-sacrifice for her children. Raghida, a young woman in her twenties, accepted a kidney from her mother, telling me that she would not have accepted a transplant from anyone other than her mother or father, not even her brothers or sisters. She said that she could not be sure that they would not have regretted this later, that they would not have been doing this only because of pressure from their mother

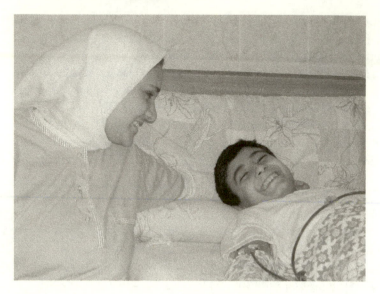

Figure 13.   A nurse bonds with her young patient who is on dialysis
preparing to receive his mother's kidney. Photograph by the author.

and father, or that their spouses would not have resented the operation.
"My mom and dad are the only ones that I could trust with this."

Both physicians and patients are less comfortable with the notion of
siblings as donors. Patients in need of the organ worry about interfering
with the more immediate rights that their siblings' spouses and children
have over them. One urologist at Tanta University Hospital explained to
me the problem of kidney transplants from siblings:

> I have seen many people who take a kidney from their mother or
> father—here there is no problem. But if he takes from his brother,
> every time he looks at his brother, he gets scared. If his brother devel-
> ops any small medical problem, he will blame himself. The wife and the
> children of the brother will always look at him as if he has stolen some-
> thing from their [husband and] father. Most of them [the recipients]
> develop psychological trouble. He blames himself a lot. If his brother
> gets the flu, he thinks, "I am the reason."

Khalid, age twenty-two when I spoke with him, agreed with this sentiment. When Khalid was serving mandatory time in the national army, he
suddenly developed vision so blurry that he could not see his hand in front
of his face. He could barely stand up, and every time he moved he vomited.
He was taken to the army hospital and started on dialysis. His parents
both immediately inquired about transplanting one of their kidneys to their

young son, but his mother was rejected as a donor because she had diabetes. Khalid had nine siblings altogether; three of them were half-siblings. He told me that although many of them offered to donate, he would never have felt comfortable with such an arrangement.

> From a sister, this is just *haram* to take from her, because she would be young and unmarried, so it wouldn't work. And even though your brother might really insist, a brother can't withstand such an ordeal. . . .
>
> With a brother or sister, they might offer and offer to donate, but then when the tests come back and there is no tissue match, they are so relieved and happy.
>
> A parent is a different story. With my father, it was the exact opposite. He was a little bit sick, and they told him it wouldn't work. His blood pressure was too high, and the whole reason it was high was that he was so upset [about my illness]. When they told him it wouldn't work for him [to donate], he started to cry. Then [after three years] he got his blood pressure regulated, and they said okay, he could do it. He was so happy that day.
>
> I would never take a kidney from a brother. He could come back to you after that and say to you, "I gave you my kidney." There would be—I don't know—I would feel guilty all the time. But not from my father. He's my father, and I came from his water.[24] What is his comes to me.

The specific kin relationship in this case, from father to son, was what established Khalid's ethical stance toward transplantation. There is less social risk involved when it is the parents gifting the organ. Receiving an organ, as many sociologists and anthropologists have demonstrated, often poses an intolerable burden, what Fox and Swazey memorably call "the tyranny of the gift" (Fox and Swazey 1974, 1992). The dominant cultural ideal for parenting in Egypt includes sacrifices that can never—and perhaps *should* never—be fully repaid by the child. It is thus acceptable that parents, who give life to their children, might also give pieces of their bodies, in the direction that life is understood to flow.

When I asked Khalid if he had sought the opinion of religious scholars, he answered,

> Yes, I asked a lot of *shuyukh*. They all said it was *haram*.[26] Some of the *shuyukh*—I would see them in the mosque that I prayed in, and I would ask. They even said that Sha'rawi had died taking a stance against this issue. But other people said that [it is *haram* only] if you are taking from the dead [without consent] or taking the organ for money or something. But a father or mother giving, this is okay.

They did put doubt into all of this. I was not convinced [that transplantation is okay] except for the fact that it was from my own father.
God made him good again; he returned to himself, and, glory to God,
it may be that God created two kidneys for this very reason. There are
people who can walk around with one-fourth a kidney, they say, and
they can go on functioning like that. . . .

The day we came out of the operation, I was wearing my surgical
mask, and I couldn't see anything, but there he [my father] was, and we
started crying when we saw each other, for happiness, knowing that it
had succeeded. Praise to God.

When I asked Khalid how he became convinced about proceeding with
the transplant if he had heard so many religious opinions against it, he
answered,

I don't see anything forbidden in it, because God created me, and I come
from my father. God created something in my father that came to me.
Praise to God, he [my father] has two kidneys that work well, so why
is it wrong if I take one? If it hadn't been my father, I would never have
done a transplant. But what convinced me was that it was my father,
and I come from him anyway.

So I made it *halal* [permissible] for myself because of this issue.
God created him with two kidneys, and I could take one. What could be
haram in it; if he is going to be well again, what will be the problem?
It is better than all of the dialysis and what it did to me. This is how we
reasoned then. This is how we saw it.

The implicit association of kidney transplantation with rebirth and
reproduction reinforces for people that it is "natural" for parents to
donate kidneys to their children (Crowley-Matoka 2005; Crowley-
Matoka and Lock 2006). Although Khalid had been told by local religious
leaders—those working outside official state positions—that transplantation is *haram*, he reasoned that it was permissible in his case because
the transplant came from his father. Khalid, assessing with the logic that
ethical positions operate through the contingencies of specific cases, saw
that the particularities of his situation rendered permissible what might
otherwise be forbidden. And because he was fortunate enough to have
a willing parent as a donor, less social risk was involved in bearing an
unpayable debt.

A year after receiving his father's kidney, Khalid and his young wife
had twins—a boy and a girl—completing their family in a way that had
seemed impossible in the days that Khalid was on dialysis. Indeed, there
was particular emphasis, among the patients and families whom I met, in
ensuring the reproductivity of their children; that is, mothers and fathers

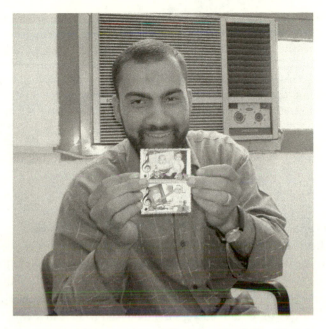

Figure 14. After receiving a kidney from his father, Khalid
fathered a twin boy and girl, whose pictures he holds up
proudly. Photograph by the author.

were eager to donate to young daughters and sons to ensure that they could
be married and have children of their own. The devastating diagnosis of a
terminal illness like acute kidney failure delivers the blow of the possibility
of not only a young death but also a death without marrying and having
children (see Smith and Mbakwem 2007: S40). Patients and their family
members understand attaining "normalcy" and "good health" in terms of
reproductivity and securing a family—the very point of life.[27] Among the
unmarried patients I spoke with and those who were in the early stages
of their reproductive years, there was great urgency for the larger family
unit to secure them a kidney to "restore" bodily function, often defined in
reproductive terms.

But even as a kidney graft offers the promise of fulfilling the important
"life projects" (Smith and Mbakwem 2007) of marriage and reproduction,
receiving a kidney can still be risky when the recipient feels responsible
for the sacrifice borne on his or her behalf. Khalid felt this burden acutely
and knew that it would have been insufferable had his donor been anyone
besides his father. When I asked him to talk about his life posttransplant,
he said,

When I was on dialysis I was better, because I could eat and drink what-ever I wanted, because I figured it would all come out in the dialysis anyway. . . . But having the transplant has changed my life a lot now. Now I'm afraid all the time, compared with before. I won't work all day. I can't be productive anymore. I'm so scared for the graft, scared about preserving it. I have, since the transplant, developed diabetes. So I'm very cautious now about what I do. Back when I was on dialysis, I did not hold myself back like this.

Although he continually thanked God for the "blessings" of the trans-plant, Khalid also felt burdened by a sense of responsibility not to "waste" this blessing given to him by his father. Khalid evoked the metaphorical understanding of dialysis (*al-ghasil*) as a process of "washing" the kidney; in this conception, any lapses from his strict dietary and medical regimen would be forgiven. On dialysis, the repletion of vitality and the slow dete-rioration of health were expected, not things for which he could be held accountable. But now posttransplant, Khalid had assumed an individual responsibility to "make the most" of his father's weighty bodily sacrifice. This pressure was significant enough to make him think things were "bet-ter" psychologically when he was on dialysis. Even though God had blessed him with the opportunity to accept his father's kidney, the remainder of his life would involve a struggle to protect this blessing from any harm.

GIFTING THE KIDNEY—RECIPROCITY, KINSHIP, AND REPRODUCTIVE RISK

Among the patients I interviewed, those without parents who could offer them kidneys, the decisions were much more difficult. Interviewing a sig-nificant number of kidney patients and kidney transplant physicians helped me uncover particular patterns in giving and receiving—patterns of which patients and physicians were not explicitly aware. Many patients simply did not have the right kin to "gift" them a kidney. Some were positioned as wives or mothers, adult married daughters, adult unmarried sons, or stepsons or stepdaughters—structural kin positions that decreased their likelihood of being offered the gift of a kidney. Others were in positions in which they actively refused to receive organs from their vulnerable fam-ily members, who were otherwise seen as the most expendable and, hence, the most likely organ donors. Most were without the means to buy a kid-ney, and some could potentially buy a kidney but were morally averse to the organ trade. Facing terminal illness on dialysis, many of these patients

actively worked to cultivate dispositions of steadfastness *(al-sabr)* in suffering as acceptance of God's will.

While the donations of parents to their children posed little ethical
quandary, in contrast, patients and physicians generally agreed that older
patients should not receive kidneys from adult children. The patterns in
the direction that organs moved within my informants' families reflected
larger cultural notions of the ways in which bodily resources should be
preserved and expended within a family unit. Because a kidney transplant
is such a costly procedure—in terms of financial, familial, moral, and bodily
costs—a place like the Mansoura Kidney Center, which relies on allocating
scarce resources, concentrates its efforts on its youngest patients. Adults
in their forties and fifties often consider themselves and are considered by
others to be "too old" to pursue transplantation. Ibrahim, a retired man in
his fifties, explained to me why he would not consider his son's incessant
offer to give him his kidney: "I am old—I am fifty-seven years old—so I
just depend on God. But my son, he still has his future ahead of him." A
prominent nephrologist at Egypt's top kidney center in Mansoura told me
that it is rare for patients to accept kidneys from their adult children. About
half of the patients he had overseen in his twenty years of experience had
come for transplantation with siblings as donors; the other half, with parents as donors.[28] Yet the preferences that patients and doctors held in terms
of cultural or kinship logics could not always be medically realized, given
other criteria for determining a good match.

Another longstanding nephrologist at Mansoura told me that as a physician he actively discouraged transplants from offspring to parent, which he
thought was immoral. Explaining his position to me, he stated,

> I have my personal opinion, and it is morally unacceptable for me at
> least, for offspring, let's say a twenty-five-year old, to give a kidney to
> his father who is fifty-five years old. I just can't morally digest it. What
> would the life expectancy for this graft be? Ten years? So you are giv-
> ing him an extra ten years? But on the other side, if this offspring lives
> the same length of time as his father, from twenty-five to sixty-five,
> that means for forty years you are putting him at a risk that is larger
> than the expected benefit [of ten years].[29]

The doctor continued, "When I see a couple like that [parent-offspring],
I try to find a way to reject this donor. I will ask the man to bring his
brother or sister who is [of comparable age]. But to take an offspring's
organ and put it in this man . . . Scientifically and legally it is okay, but
morally for me it is not." In any case, this doctor admitted that it was
not very common for patients to bring in their adult children as possible

organ donors; he estimated that he saw this in perhaps one out of every twenty patients.

In many cases, physicians thought of their medical advice and ethical advice as one and the same: they encouraged donation to occur within family patterns that resonated with "common sense." Yet some physicians saw their medical and ethical advice at odds; another nephrologist at the Mansoura Kidney Center told me that he agreed that parents donating to offspring is socially and ethically best but that medically, he encouraged sibling donation, so that the graft from the donor would be of comparable age to the recipient.

Among siblings the males are generally the ones to engage in transplants. That is, a brother is more likely to donate a kidney than a sister, and a brother is also more likely to be a recipient. A young woman in need of a kidney is most likely to receive one from a parent,[30] whereas young men receive kidneys from either parents or brothers. Female siblings do not generally donate organs because their "bodily resources" are to be channeled to their immediate families: their husbands and their children, through domestic labor, pregnancy, birth, and breastfeeding. Families worry about unmarried women more than men undergoing operations because of the great social emphasis on women's abilities to marry, conceive, carry potential pregnancies to term, and raise children. Women's fertility and reproductive abilities are closely safeguarded in Egypt (Inhorn 1994, 1996). This translates into many young women in the family being "protected" from donating kidneys to their brothers or sisters in need.

In the dialysis unit, Saʿid, a young man in his late twenties, was often accompanied by his mother. (His father was deceased.) She had undergone many tests to be able to donate a kidney to him, but she was rejected as a candidate because of her advanced age and her high blood pressure. Saʿid had an unmarried twin sister, who insistently offered to donate her kidney to her brother, but their mother adamantly refused. When the others in the dialysis room asked her why she would not allow her daughter to donate her kidney, she responded, "The girl is not like the boy. If he had a brother, I would allow him to donate, but not a sister." The women in the room all nodded in agreement. The unstated understanding was that such an operation might impinge upon Saʿid's sister's marriage prospects and reproductive viability. Also, because of the association of surgical "opening" with a loss of purity (Cohen 1999; Crowley-Matoka and Lock 2006), the general preference is for the male to donate. If a son is in need and the parents are medically excluded as donors, a brother is more likely to donate, even if the patient has sisters willing to donate. In all of the cases that I saw in which women did after all donate to brothers, the women were older, had finished raising their children, and were donating to younger brothers so that they might complete their families.

In general, a young couple who has not been able to bear children is considered to be in a "tenuous" marriage; often, women are blamed for the failure to reproduce and can be at risk of divorce (see Inhorn 1994, 1996). Women in kidney failure who have not yet borne children are thus in vulnerable social and economic situations. The primary concern about women's reproductivity means that women in kidney failure negotiate a delicate balance between their kidney function and their reproductive abilities. They know well that when creatinine levels indicate a stabilization in kidney function, their chances of bearing a child have increased, and yet at the same time they know that bearing a child will pose a significant and potentially very dangerous strain on their kidneys. Their hopes to recuperate kidney function *and* to have children are untenable if the patients do not have parents willing and medically eligible to gift them kidneys. In many cases, parents do everything they can to gift kidneys to their daughters or sons, to enable them to have children of their own—the very goal of a "good" and "normal" life. This is particularly urgent for a young wife, whose failure to reproduce puts her in a socially and economically vulnerable position, in which she may be divorced, because having children is what "ties" a husband to his wife (Inhorn 1994, 1996, 2003).

Yet even those young wives who are fortunate to have a mother or father gift them a kidney face significant problems, because a subsequent pregnancy can threaten the kidney graft. I witnessed several exchanges in which male nephrologists spoke harshly to women for "putting their lives in severe danger" by attempting to get pregnant posttransplantation or while in acute kidney failure and on dialysis. Young women often receive kidneys from parents in order for them to complete their life projects of marrying and bearing children. The nephrologists, in frustration, feel the women should "protect" their kidney grafts and resent that the kidney and surgery might be endangered by reproductive plans. But many women knowingly take this risk because they see marrying and reproducing as the very reason to be alive (Smith and Mbakwem 2007) and, in many cases, because of the tremendous amount of social pressure on them to do so (Inhorn 1994).

During one of my visits to the Mansoura Kidney Center, I accompanied the nephrologists as they made rounds in the hospital. One young woman, Samira, had received a kidney from her mother three years earlier and was readmitted because her kidney function was deteriorating. But rather than worrying about her kidney, she questioned the doctor only about her ability to get pregnant. The nephrologist's tone was uncompromising: "Listen. You cannot attempt to get pregnant. This will put both you and the baby at risk. You might lose your kidney." Samira looked dejected.

The nephrologist tried another tack: "You have a son. He will get married, God willing. So you just make sure he picks a good girl, and there you will have yourself a son and a daughter. And be content with that."

A young medical resident spoke up at this point: "But doctor, this is her second marriage."

Unable or unwilling to bear the expenses of Samira's illness and dialysis treatment, her first husband, and the father of her son, had divorced her, even though she and her natal family had made every attempt to find a new kidney for her so that she could resume her "normal" domestic duties in her married household. By the time Samira was able to get off Mansoura's waiting list for transplantation, with her parents at her side as potential donors, her husband had already divorced her. When she was finally admitted to Mansoura for an operation, her mother was able to donate her kidney to her. Then, a year after receiving the transplant, Samira remarried. But now she was afraid that she would lose her second husband if unable to bear him a child.

The nephrologist shook his head in exasperation, complaining to the residents in English, "She is afraid she will lose her marriage without a child, but she will definitely lose her marriage if she loses her kidney!" The medical residents and attending physician seemed to blame Samira for her ignorance and simplicity, even though she was in a structurally difficult situation in which women's bodies are expected to be reproductively viable in order to attain marital and financial security.

Among spouses, wives are much more likely to donate kidneys to their husbands than the other way around.[31] Because of the gendered division of labor, in which women within the domestic sphere play the role of nurturer and caregiver and men tend to work outside the home to provide for the family, wives contribute bodily to what is often a commonsense move to secure the family. Many patients I spoke with expressed cynicism when discussing transplants between spouses.[32] One woman, who was divorced during the course of her dialysis treatment, sullenly told me that some men think their lives are "worth more" because they are men. "If he had been the one sick," she told me, "I would have given him my kidney." Not only did he not do this, but tiring of all the treatment and expenses, he also divorced her, a fate not unfamiliar to other young women on dialysis. A fellow patient's husband, tending to his wife on dialysis nearby, heard the story of the woman after she had left and expressed extreme anger at her

situation: "What is wrong with people? What is wrong with
leaves his sick wife? Did she cause her own sickness? Didn't
young and beautiful and healthy? Does he not know God, t
from God?! Let's see who will care for *him* when he gets sick!
shaking his head, and later returned to the hospital carrying sandwiches for
his wife. He sat at her bedside and told me, "You see, I am lucky. My wife
became even more wonderful and beautiful since she started dialysis." His
wife smiled, bringing the hospital bedsheet to her face in embarrassment.

THE THREE BROTHERS: A CAUTIONARY TALE

It was not only patients or their family members who narrated to me how
cases of strained family relations, death, and morbidity shaped their ethical
predispositions toward transplantation. Doctors did this too. Dr. Yusuf, a
nephrologist in charge of a small private dialysis center in Tanta, was also
on the faculty at the Tanta University Department of Medicine. None of
the patients in his center had any hopes of having a transplant. Its cost was
far beyond anyone's reach, and many were not healthy enough to meet the
eligibility requirements at Mansoura for transplants.

Dr. Yusuf told me that among the young patients, all hoped for a transplant. But once they were in their forties or fifties, they gave up on the idea.
He said, "The young ones have the most hope and the best chances of benefiting, because they are less likely to have systemic diseases like diabetes
or collagen [systemic autoimmune] diseases. Other Muslim countries, like
Saudi Arabia, are more advanced in having developed transplant programs."
When I asked him why he thought Egypt has legislative problems with
instituting a national organ program, he first mentioned the black market
in organs. I asked him where he stood on the organ transplant debate. He
thought for a while and then said,

> Now before I answer your question, let me tell you a story. There were
> three brothers. The oldest one developed renal failure, and he died. The
> second brother—he was a doctor—he also got renal failure, and he
> took a kidney from his youngest brother. He did a transplant and then
> he died. So the third, the youngest one, was the only one left. He had
> given his kidney. And then he developed renal failure in the one kidney
> he had left. You see, God gave us two kidneys, and this young brother
> gave away one of his and had one left. So if he encountered any little
> problem, sooner or later, he would get renal failure. Well that's what
> happened. He got it, and he is now doing dialysis in the teaching hospi-
> tal to this day.

I was prepared for a generalized moralistic story (in the trope of "three brothers who . . ."), but I soon realized that Dr. Yusuf was speaking about an actual medical case history of a family. He ended by telling me that he had great reservations about transplantation from living donors: "The donor with one kidney, should he develop any little problem, would be threatened with renal failure and might have to end up on dialysis with all its problems. As for the recipient, it is true that he will be comfortable for about five years. He won't be stuck to a machine, but he'll still have to be on a regime of anti-rejection treatments. These have a lot of side effects. If you saw people after transplantation, with Cushing's syndrome, blood pressure problems—there are a lot of problems with it, and in the end, okay he left dialysis and doesn't have to depend on this machine, but he's not 100 percent cured."

Two weeks later when I saw Dr. Yusuf, this time at Tanta University Hospital, he stated his position in much stronger terms: "I'm against this coming from living donors," he said. "It's *haram*. How can someone 'give' something that doesn't belong to him? A person who does not own something cannot give it away [*man la yamluk la yu'ti*]." Dr. Yusuf's proposed solution was to establish a cadaveric transplant program. He explained, "If we could rely on dead donors, we would alleviate some of these problems." Yet when I asked him how to get around the question of determining if the brain-dead heartbeating donor is "really dead," he said that he did not know much about this but that the neurologists and Islamic scholars would have to define death and "solve this problem somehow."[33]

Dr. Yusuf urged me to speak with Sayyid 'Abduh, the "brother number three" of his story. The next day I went to the teaching hospital dialysis unit. With the help of the internist in charge, I found this brother. While he was receiving his dialysis treatment, his wife, who was a nurse, sat with him. There were actually *six* brothers altogether, with Sayyid being the youngest, but otherwise Dr. Yusuf's memory of the patient's family history was impressive. Sayyid narrated it to me, constantly interjecting questions to me and to the other medical residents who had assembled around me, curious about my "social science research" project:

> We had an officer [*zabit*] [among our brothers] who had kidney disease and died at the age of thirty-five. It was before anyone knew what this disease was. . . . He got it suddenly and shook; we said it was nerves. We took him to Cairo, to Ain Shams [Teaching Hospital], and they discovered it was kidney failure. But there was no dialysis back then. Is dialysis a new thing? This was back in the '70s. He stayed in the hospital, and he never came out of it; he lasted only about twenty days. I was

maybe twenty-three years old at the time—Is this in our genes, or what?

Then my brother who was a doctor, he got it when he was about forty. And he knew there was dialysis, but the machines were very bad back then. He said, "No, I can't do dialysis." He said, "I'll transplant," and he looked all over the family to find someone. I agreed. We did the analysis in Nasser Institute in Cairo. . . . [He consulted] a big doctor then; his name was Dr. Fu'ad something—I don't remember, but he did the surgery.

He [my brother] was thirty-eight years old. I was married. I was a teacher then. We had a sister who wanted to donate, but then I said, "I'll donate, for God and for my brother." They took the measurements [of the kidneys]. And they said the left one is better than the right, because the left is a little smaller. [*He laughs.*] But it turns out the right one got ruined too.[*He laughs.*] . . .

The one I gave—it lasted [in my brother] three years, then he got very sick. Some people last five years, but I never saw someone who transplanted last more than that.

This was nine years ago that I donated my kidney. Shouldn't this one I have left have lasted longer? Like twenty years? Why did it last nine years, and then I suddenly got sick? What is the reason? I don't know. Three got it in the family—that's a lot. The same disease! How can that be?

The internist and residents, five in total, had gathered around us, listening. The internist in charge, clearly affected by the story, shook her head and told me in English, "They did tests and took the better of the kidneys for the brother." She seemed dismayed to learn that the surgeons' drive to excel in new procedures had compromised the overall health of the donor.

The other residents around us started to ask questions, curious about Sayyid's history. Was his brother okay after the transplantation? "Not really." Are their parents related? "No."[34] If you could go back, would you still donate to your brother? He said, "Yes, yes, I would still donate to him. I did it for God and for my brother. He was a doctor, and he understood these things. So I said okay." By saying that he donated for God, Sayyid clarified that he had donated his kidney in order to do the right thing—that is, for his own spiritual reckoning with God—and not because he wanted anything from anyone else in return. When I asked him if he himself would ever consider getting a kidney transplant, he said,

No, I don't think about transplant. This needs a lot of resources that we don't have. And anyway, we experienced it and saw that it failed. Dialysis is better. Because having [a transplanted kidney] would be a third kidney to deal with.[35] Dialysis is more comfortable. The other one [transplantation]—it failed before my eyes.

I'm not so important that I need a transplant. *[He laughs.]* This is it, we are living, and this is it. We're surviving. This is God's will, what He intended for us. They say that if I stay on this and do everything right, I can last five years. These things [transplantation] are not guaranteed. They also have a time limit. So let's just live on dialysis. If I do everything right I can last five years, God willing.

Sayyid's story represents the actual reality of the fear of every would-be donor. The patients on dialysis next to him had all heard his story, and this of course worried them when they considered the consequences of "taking" the body part of a family member. As Sayyid's wife said, "He saw what happened to him, that he gave and then he got sick. So he will never take from anyone, because he would say that they would get sick too. Anyway, there is no way that we could ever afford it." Because she knew that Sayyid would never accept a kidney donation from a family member, his wife alluded to the expense of potentially buying a kidney. But for Sayyid, the sacrifice of a family member, the financial sacrifice of the cost of a kidney, and even the bodily sacrifice of an unrelated paid donor were all part of the same gamble that he had taken before and that he was unwilling to take again.

By calling himself unimportant in contrast to his brother—that is, not socially valuable enough to be a transplant recipient—Sayyid invokes Scheper-Hughes's (2000) observation that the flow of organs follows the flow of global capital, from the marginal to the more powerful. Within the microeconomy of this family, the better kidney of the brother who was a teacher (a low-paid job of little esteem in Egypt) went to the brother who was a doctor (a profession of high esteem).

But both Sayyid and his wife, Fatima, remained committed to the idea that God would reward Sayyid for his donation. Fatima said,

Maybe they didn't do the analysis properly; maybe they rushed to do the transplant. The brother lived for five years with it, but then it failed.[36] The body refused it after that. Of course Sayyid was very upset, but we all told him that he had done something very good for God but that God willed this to happen. We had wished that, well, as long as there was a new kidney—of course the lifespan is in the hands of God—but we had hoped this would help his brother, because of his children and all that, but it's all in the hands of God.

When I asked her what she thought of organ transplantation in general, Fatima told me, "I don't like it; I think it is *haram*, personally, because God gives us our body as *amana* [a trust] and because of our personal experience:

he [Sayyid] gave to his brother, and then he got sick. Only God knows if someone donates a part of his body what will happen to him; this is all from God."

Like Dr. Kotb and Shadya and other patients, Sayyid and Fatima phrased
their ethical reasoning in terms of religious permissibility, inseparably
bound up with assessments of medical efficacy, risk, and safety and also with
financial access and kinship relations. The administrative staff of the hospital, having heard the story of Sayyid ʿAbduh, who himself fell into kidney
failure after donating a kidney to his brother, pointed out that his case was
a moral lesson *(ʿibra)* sent by God to let people know that transplantation
is *haram*.[37] For many patients, it would not matter definitively if epidemiologists or physicians were to point out that the death and illness they had
witnessed were statistically unlikely. The doctors at the Mansoura Kidney
Center may have been mystified as to why Shadya suddenly took ill and
died immediately after the operation or why Sayyid ʿAbduh himself fell
into end-stage renal disease after having donated a kidney to his brother,
but the patients who did not have that much trust in medical operations
were not. Many perceived the people they encountered and the stories they
heard as divine signs meant to guide their own decisions.

SOCIAL LIABILITIES: NO LINEAGE AND NO GIFT

In the Tanta University Hospital dialysis center, I sat with a group of young
men in their twenties who were following a soccer match on a small grainy
television screen while they received their dialysis treatment. One of these
men, Muhammad, told me that he had been born with only one kidney and
suffered from hypertension. One day, he took the wrong pill for his high
blood pressure, precipitating acute renal failure. The physicians later told
him that if he had taken the full dosage—two pills—he would have died
immediately. But for some reason he took only one and ended up in a coma.

Muhammad was not particularly religious before his diagnosis, but since
that time, seeing his young life suddenly drastically changed, he said that
he would never miss any of the five obligatory daily prayers, nor would he
forget to thank God continually for still being alive. Before his illness, he
had worked in a small clothing store with a young woman and had recently
asked her family's permission to marry her. He said that she accepted the
proposal and that her mother also had accepted him into their home:

> This was last Ramadan. But it was her maternal uncle who opposed. He
> said to me, "Look son, this isn't because of the way you look or the fact
> that you are sick. It's just that I don't want my niece to be a widow in

a few months." He said it just like that, to my face. Just like that, he's telling me I'm going to die.

I told him, "But people live for years on dialysis." I was so upset. I kept thinking, if only God would let me get married and bless me with a son or daughter. But I've gotten used to my situation now. It's all over. Alhamdulillah, I come for dialysis, I pray, I know God, I have to bring myself above this kind of hurtful talk [*akabbar damaghi*] so that these things won't bother me and so that I can go on.

The doctors, too, told my family that it wouldn't work for someone like me to get married. I don't understand this. My family felt bad, saying that I was only twenty-eight and that I shouldn't hear things like that, so they didn't tell me. But I am not convinced by any of this. Look, there are people here who have been doing dialysis for years, and they are married. So why are they telling me that I cannot get married? Only God knows.

Muhammad had his whole life in front of him and suddenly saw it cut short. His difficulty in managing his disease was not merely in his physical pain and newly acquired disabilities. He told me that the most difficult change to endure was the ways that his illness had altered his social relationships: his inability to get married, to continue working, and to spend time with friends who fear his condition could be contagious. His physicians had stated that he could not get married, essentially issuing him a poor prognosis, which to him felt like a death sentence. Upon my questioning, the doctors later explained to me that, yes, they do indeed discourage patients such as Muhammad from getting married, because the physical and sexual side effects of kidney failure and dialysis would render such a marriage "not viable." As social gatekeepers, the Tanta hospital doctors felt responsible not only for the health of their patients but also for their patients' larger social networks. In this case, the doctor acted to protect the well-being of young women who might not understand the medical, social, and financial risks that they would face in agreeing to marry a terminally ill young man.

Being unmarried, still dependent on his natal family unit for support, and not directly responsible for the care of a wife or children made Muhammad less likely to be seen as urgently in need of a gifted organ. And because he was on dialysis, he was less able to be employed regularly and earn enough money to pay for a kidney. A final door was closed to him when his doctor declared him to be reproductively and maritally "unviable." Turning to the other young unmarried man beside him, Muhammad asked, "Does it make sense that they tell us not to get married? Aren't there men filling this [dialysis] ward who are married and having children?" His companion agreed, "Yeah, see those men there; they have young children, and some have even had more children after being on dialysis. So why do they tell us we cannot marry?" Muhammad shook his head and let out a chuckle, "We would take kidneys if we could. But there is no one giving them to us." Many of the young unmarried men in the dialysis ward were stuck in an awkward life stage; they were considered "too risky" to be married to, and because they were not yet married and supporting a family, their natal families felt less compelled to scrape together all resources in the hopes of what a transplant—another risky proposition—might bring. Muhammad told me that he now turned all his attention to God, trying as much as he could to interpret this "trial from God" as spiritually fortifying. God had chosen him, out of all people, to withstand a trial that forced him to remember God daily, eschewing the spiritual danger of heedlessness *(al-ghafla)*. If life on this earth was unviable, he would prepare, through prayer, for the next.

For those without parents healthy or young enough to donate or parents without the right blood type and matching tissue, the prospects of a kidney are wracked with problems. People at the margins of larger family structures struggle with their misgivings about not having the right kin to gift them kidneys. When I discussed these patterns with physicians who had long-term experience with transplantation, many expressed initial surprise that the ways in which organs are gifted within the family can be socially analyzed to reveal a consistent pattern. But upon reflection, these doctors affirmed that patients prefer kidneys to be gifted from particular family members and that certain members are deemed more or less urgently in need. These patterns make sense within the larger cultural logic that values biological reproduction as normative and as the major goal of life. Garnering resources toward the reproductivity of the family unit places those in particular kin roles (adult unmarried sons, wives, stepchildren, middle-aged people, adults with no children) in positions that decrease their chances of receiving gifted kidneys. In this sense, biotechnologies can reify hierarchies within family structures as much as they can disrupt them. At the same time, some appeal to an Islamic ethic of justice to protect their marginalized family members. And patients like Muhammad, who was deemed reproductively and socially unviable, seek to redefine their afflictions in terms of spiritual value. They argue for each person's intrinsic merits before God, independent of how that person fits within larger social and familial structures.

CONCLUSIONS

Inside and outside the dialysis clinic, people struggle with the ethics of transplantation by weighing the different types of risks involved in the context of scarce resources and vital kinship ties. Kidney transplantation requires enormous trust in medical institutions—trust enough to offer the healthy body of a living family member for invasive intervention. Most medical institutions have not earned that trust in Egypt, particularly among the poor. Many patients, and some doctors, do not accept that extracting a vital organ from a healthy family member is a tolerable medical risk. In a "poisonous" environment, in which the medical solutions offered do not appear beneficial, many patients resist the idea of turning to their family as a source of kidneys.

Aside from the significant medical risks, transplantation also poses social risks on the family networks on which it depends: the "gift" of a new kidney has to be sacrificed by a loved one or by a kidney seller who will henceforth live with only one kidney. And buying a kidney also relies on significant familial sacrifices—in financial rather than bodily terms—to forgo savings or to liquidate assets to be able to compensate the seller. Many are uncertain, in the end, about the price of this sacrifice. This uncertainty is most marked among poor disenfranchised patients, who are also the most vulnerable to medical mismanagement. Egypt's corruption and pollution, the subjects of much discussion in public discourse, have profoundly influenced patients' ethical dispositions toward their treatment options, particularly because they see themselves as the most damaged cases in a detrimental atmosphere in which all are vulnerable.

Aside from fear about whether the transplant will be successful, the "gift" of a donated kidney—even when it promises to restore health and enable reproductivity—also poses an unbearable burden on the recipient and fear of the donor's eventual resentment. The only direction in which kidneys are seen to flow without ethical quandary is from parents to their children, and then only when this is medically feasible and when resources are sufficient, bodily and economically, for this to happen. Patients' and physicians' narratives reveal their understanding of kin relations as ethical relations and demonstrate that arguments about belonging to God and the ethics of gifting and receiving kidneys are entangled with questions about medical mismanagement, environmental toxicity, and social position within family structures. Among my informants, many of those who might have been recipients of organs from marginalized family members exerted efforts to protect those relatives from an invasive extraction and to protect themselves from the intolerable burden of an unrepayable gift. The idea that the body belongs to God and that transplantation is, hence, not an appropriate medical solution was held by many patients and physicians alike, even among those who had directly participated in transplantation. Some asserted that the body is God's property as they took a stance against a kidney extraction from a vulnerable family member or against imposing an unbearable financial burden on the family. Others resignified the idea that the body belongs to God in ways that accommodated organ donation: patients argued that for a parent to gift a child a kidney is a sign of divine mercy and that God made life to flow from old to young. And many patients who were excluded from the promises of transplantation focused on belonging to God in cultivating the virtue of steadfastness *(al-sabr)* in the face of God's trials.

Of course, not all Egyptians are devout or conscientiously aim to bring their daily actions into alignment with Islamic ethics. Many patients I spoke with described the difficulties of living in an ethically bankrupt society overtaken by godlessness and greed. Some patients exploited their vulnerable family members or poor urban youth in order to survive; many physicians participated in unsavory but lucrative practices; many men abandoned their wives in response to staggering medical bills. Many patients spared themselves the tyranny of an unpayable familial debt by turning to a ready supply of seller-donors in Cairo. The next chapter examines more closely the so-called black market in kidneys and people's various engagements with it.

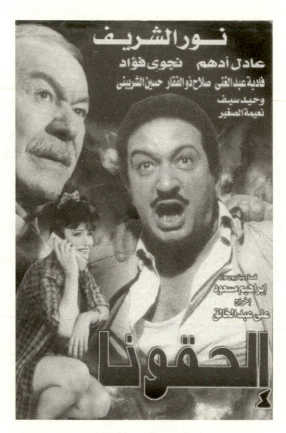

Figure 15.   Movie poster of the popular film
Ilhaquna! (Save Us!), in which the protagonist's
kidney is stolen by a wealthy businessman.

7. Principles We Can't Afford?

Ethics and Pragmatism in Kidney Sales

Although I interviewed many patients and doctors involved with kidney transplants from paid donors, I did not meet with those who sold their kidneys. The organ trade has been deemed a politically "sensitive" issue, and I already had difficulty attaining permission from the Egyptian Ministry of Security for my research. In any case, I had not originally set out to study "the organ trade" or to take up undercover reporting in Cairo; I was more interested in the ways in which people struggle with the ethics of their decisions surrounding organ transplantation in its legitimate and ordinary permutations. Through the course of my research, however, I came to realize how imbricated the selling of kidneys has been in all aspects of transplantation. No independent "black market" operates as a separate realm, as I previously imagined. Once I understood this, I became interested in how people come to decide, within the realm of monetary transactions, which transplants are legitimate or ethical and which are not. Islamic legal-ethical opinions, the voices of Coptic Christian leaders, global secular bioethics, and even the work of medical anthropologists (Scheper-Hughes 2000) have all converged in their unequivocal condemnation of buying and selling human organs. But even though the dominant discourse has been that all types of commodification are *haram*, for many patients and physicians, the dividing line between what is ethical and what is *haram* is not solely determined by whether or not money is exchanged for the kidney.

Indeed, there has been a curious disjunction in organ transplant practices in Egypt. On the one hand, it is common knowledge that the majority of kidney and liver lobe transplants have occurred through commercial live donors. By official accounts, commercial transactions have taken place in 50 percent—by unofficial accounts, closer to 90 percent—of all transplants in Egypt.[1] Although these individual monetary transactions have been accepted as a "necessary evil," physicians and patients often characterize them as a win-win situation, in which desperately ill patients can now survive and the desperately poor can now receive much-needed money (Cohen 1999, 2001). Paying for donors is a mundane practice that rapidly became routinized. On the other hand, press reports, often quite sensational, about the *trafficking* of human organs have been met by national outrage. The organized exploitation of the poor—by organ transplant brokers, "mafia" rings of doctors and middlemen, and transnational arrangements in which patients from the Arab Gulf have received organs from the Egyptian poor—has been portrayed as nothing short of a state of emergency (al-Irqsusi 1998).[2]

Different ethical distinctions *within* the realm of commercial transactions thus complicate the stark black-and-white division between "altruism" and "commodification" that pervades global bioethics and official religious discourse. There has been a seemingly broad tolerance for *some* local commercial transactions involving organ donations and a simultaneous disgust with its "excesses"—where and how is this line drawn? This chapter traces different ethical claims in the buying and selling of human organs in Egypt, demonstrating that for most physicians and patients involved in transplantation, much is at stake in separating tolerable financial transactions from those seen as excessive or exploitative. Many of Egypt's surgeons have adopted Euro-American transplant rhetoric that "decommodifies the commodity" by imagining organ donations to be "altruistic" and the ultimate form of selflessness that culminates in the "gift of life."[3] At the same time, Egyptian transplant doctors, particularly those in Cairo, have argued that the unavailability of cadaveric organs coupled with stark disparities in wealth make such proclamations impractical. The problem of organ sale indeed appears inevitable given the significant and growing gap between rich and poor in urban Egypt. The insertion of a biotechnology that cuts into one body for the sake of another has mirrored, and in some cases exacerbated, social stratification wherever it has been practiced.

ABOVEBOARD AND UNDERGROUND

All transplant physicians with whom I spoke stated that something has to be done for patients in organ failure who have no kin medically or socially eligible to give them kidneys. This was particularly critical in the absence of a national organ transplant system. Some of my informant physicians, like those in Mansoura, saw the turn to commercial live donors as a mere "safety net," with the clear preference that transplants be done though intrafamilial donations. But many physicians in Cairo saw commercial live donors as the primary source of organs. They reasoned that, with the exception of parents gifting kidneys to their children, transplantation from within the family is wracked with problems of guilt and compulsion that could be avoided with a one-time payment for a kidney, a payment from which a poor person might benefit.

As organ selling became further entrenched in the 1980s, in the following three decades, physicians increasingly placed the blame on the sellers themselves, many saying that it is *haram* to sell an organ but not to buy one. The "problem," as they saw it with organ selling, was that sellers cast their God-given bodies as profitable commodities. "God gave these people their bodies, and they choose to sell bits of them off," I heard many doctors and patients say, adding that the sellers exploit the desperation of patients in organ failure, by compelling them to pay for a kidney in order to survive.

As mentioned earlier, Dr. Mohamed Ghoneim's first kidney transplant operation in Mansoura, Egypt, in 1976 involved procuring a kidney from a mother and transplanting it into her ill daughter. Dr. Ghoneim's pioneering work took place in a provincial city that has not been characterized by the vast discrepancies in wealth that are commonplace in Cairo. But as Dr. Abdel Kotb's recollections revealed, the first Cairo kidney transplant in a prestigious teaching hospital involved a kidney donor who had made a financial arrangement with the recipient's family. In Cairo, the largest city in the Arab world, new treatment options were developed in a deeply stratified medical landscape. Cairo doctors then and now tend to take for granted the sharp discrepancies in treatment for patients of different socioeconomic standing.

No one questioned these doctors, for in the early years of transplantation they were the most elite physicians—on the faculty of prestigious teaching hospitals—and the only ones who were experimenting with the novel procedure. And they were generally above reproach. Many of them were trained in Europe and North America. They saw, in the absence of transplant facilities in Egypt, that transplantation was limited to only very wealthy patients who could travel abroad for treatment. Some of them traveled with relatives—oftentimes wives—who served as their donors. If they had no kin who were medically compatible, they were placed on indefinite waiting lists and given lower priority as noncitizens. Transplant surgeons reasoned that if these same wealthy patients had stayed in Egypt, they could simply have paid a poor person willing to part with his kidney for a sum of money.[4] This would have saved the ill patient the burden of travel, the high expense of treatment abroad, the difficulties in getting follow-up treatment from afar, and having to subject a loved one to a difficult and risky procedure while getting sicker on a waiting list. Physicians, of course, were interested parties: they wanted to establish opportunities within Egypt to practice new medical techniques. While they wittingly opened the door to the selling of kidneys for transplantation, the physicians saw themselves as saving the lives of very ill patients, particularly those who were without relatives to donate and who were facing certain death. Further, in adopting the logic that a second kidney was a "spare" part, they reasoned that they would be helping a young, healthy donor who needed the money and not inflicting undue harm. Many patients in need readily adopted this argument as well, as Nagla's story shows.

In a Tanta dialysis center, Nagla would fidget uncomfortably all throughout her dialysis sessions, telling me, "This dialysis is ruining me. Look at me. I'm ruined." On good days, she tried to cheer herself up by talking about the arrangements she was making for her older daughter's wedding. On bad days, she worried about whether she would survive long enough to see the wedding. She told me that she felt hurt that her husband would not donate his kidney to her. At the Mansoura Kidney Center, he had been rejected as a potential donor because he had hepatitis C. Nagla was not convinced that this was a good enough reason: "He's fine, really. He could donate to me if he wanted to. At Mansoura they want you to be 100 percent good, but anywhere else it would be okay. The truth is, he just wouldn't do it for me." While both her daughters, in their twenties, offered their kidneys to their mother, Nagla adamantly refused the idea. "My oldest is just about to get married, and the younger one, she's so weak and skinny. I could never take from them. I'd rather die."

Intent on seeing her daughter's wedding and refusing to accept the idea of spending the rest of her life on dialysis, Nagla began taking steps toward buying a kidney with her own savings from the days when she worked in petty business transactions. She had her bloodwork done at the laboratory of a public teaching hospital in Cairo and constantly inquired after a donor with compatible antigens who was willing to sell his kidney.

I met with Nagla over months, each time hearing about her progress and setbacks in finding a donor. Once she thought she had found a "young boy" who was a good match for her, but upon further screening, his bloodwork revealed that he had diabetes, which he had not even known about. A mere anecdote in Nagla's story, it nonetheless reveals the marginalization of potential organ sellers; this boy came to learn that he was diabetic not in the context of seeking treatment for himself but in the context of his disqualification as a donor. He was complicit not only in his own reduction to mere biomatter but also in coming to view this biomatter as of no value.

Responding to the look of dismay on my face, Nagla sighed and shook her head, saying, "Egyptians neglect themselves and their health."

Nagla described obtaining a kidney from "the outside," meaning outside the family, as an act of love, because she was sparing her daughters and making herself well enough for them. Lawrence Cohen describes these situations, in which patients "spare" family members the ordeal of donating by buying organs from strangers, in terms of Agamben's articulation of "bare life." As Cohen (2005) notes, prospective recipients see as ethical their refusal to let another (related) person make a sacrifice on their behalf, but they ignore the ways in which the seller, too, makes sacrifices, often to support loved ones, particularly in conditions of everyday or extraordinary debt.

"My daughters need me," Nagla would repeat over and over again. In the end, she finally made arrangements to buy a kidney from a poor woman who was the mother of five children. These children clearly needed their mother too. Nagla said that she connected instantly with her and liked the idea that she could help her and her children. They settled on a price of 8,000 £E.[5] Nagla remarked that after the transplant operation in a public teaching hospital in Cairo, her own donor recovered immediately and was discharged from the hospital eight days before Nagla could leave. When the donor was leaving, the hospital staff stopped her and offered her 7,000 £E more if she would now give up a lobe of her liver.[6]

"But she said no," Nagla continued. "She had had enough." Patients who bought kidneys often stressed the "perfect health" of the donors, as did Nagla, remarking on how they quickly recover. At the time of her discharge, in lieu of being offered care, medical advice, or follow-up instructions, this donor was offered the chance to sell another bit of her body. Not only did the hospital's offer efface the seller's sacrifice for her own family—that is, her motivations for selling her kidney—but it also effaced her right to bodily and psychological recovery from the major surgery. As part of their general disregard for seller-donors who sell their kidneys for money, many transplant physicians told stories of them fleeing the hospital hours before the operation but after having received the money, deserting both patient and surgeon. Doctors and family members spoke openly about the need to take precautions so that the paid donor could "not escape."

Nagla told me that she bought the kidney so that she could live, and she also tried to help this poor woman in need. She also claimed that she did not know that religious scholars have declared that paying for an organ is *haram*. It was only *after* she went through the operation, she said, that people in her neighborhood told her that buying a kidney is *haram*. Upon hearing this, she tried to make amends for what she had done and repeatedly asked God for forgiveness. "I did it so that I could live," Nagla told me over and over again. Not forgetting the dialysis patients that she left behind, she vowed to spend money on them for the sake of God. Shortly after her operation, she sent her sister to downtown Cairo to buy new linens for the dialysis ward.

Nagla told me that her "donor" periodically called her and visited her, and each time Nagla tried to give her money "to help her out" as much as she could. Nagla described a long-term relationship with the donor that did not end with a single transaction but rather entailed continual support. Some of the patients justified their purchase of kidneys through this very particular relationship of ongoing indebtedness to their poor donors. Some of the doctors I spoke with had a more negative view of this relationship of ongoing debt, describing their patients as being "guilt-ridden" and "terrorized" by organ seller-donors "for the rest of their lives."[7]

Another of the private clinic's patients, Ahmad, was a well-educated businessman who had also bought a kidney. He told me, "There was no other choice. There was no one in my family who could donate to me. And now we helped this poor man with his family. He was fine after the operation. And it saved my life." In speaking further, he said that the wealthy *always* benefit from bodily sacrifices of the poor: the clothes that we buy are made by poor people who work in factories for very small wages. "Do they have the chance to live lives that are as full and healthy as the life of someone who works in an office?" Ahmad in turn asked me rhetorically, "Don't the people who work on the pavements on highways risk their lives so that we can drive our cars there?" Ahmad pointed to the reality of social inequalities throughout the world and explained that buying an organ is the inevitable extension of these inequalities. As he saw it, when he bought a kidney, he saved his life, and a poor man's family could now eat. As for the arguments of the religious scholars that we should stay away from these things, Ahmad replied bitterly that *they* had never suffered kidney failure or life on dialysis. "It's all nice talk," he said, "but it's not realistic."

Ahmad legitimated his procurement of a kidney on the premise that his suffering from a chronic and incurable disease was intolerable and in need of correction, while the social suffering of the poor was simply a fact of life. This was generally the commonsense logic that abounded among the transplant physicians and financially secure patients I spoke with in Egypt who felt compelled to buy kidneys. The alternative to transplantation is slow death on dialysis. Survival and independence from dialysis machines come at the price of either subjecting a family member to a serious and risky operation or paying someone to spare her kidney.

NATIONAL HONOR AND SHAME IN TRANSNATIONAL ORGAN SALES

Estimating how many overall transplant operations have taken place is difficult, but it is clear that by the mid-1980s, the Egyptian Medical Syndicate had already lost, or abdicated, control over accounting for those occurring underground. In 2004, the syndicate recorded around 250 transplants yearly—that is, transplants that were performed in "legitimate" places by "legitimate" doctors. When the widespread trafficking in organs in Cairo began to draw international media attention in 2006, the general secretary of the Medical Syndicate at that time, Dr. Hamdi al-Sayyid, told reporters that the situation was not so drastic as compared with places like India, estimating that in Egypt only 120 to 130 such kidney transplants took place annually.[8] A World Health Organization report from 2008 put the estimate at four thousand.[9]

As more doctors in Egypt entered the field of transplantation in the 1980s, they expected that various legislative proposals outlining a national organ transplant program would soon be passed in the parliamentary People's Assembly. Legislators, however, continued to debate but not pass the proposals, while the press, including the newspapers of the opposition parties, took heed of Cairo's growing black market in organs. A large class of underemployed physicians, unable to get ahead in a medical profession with tight hierarchies and very few spots in the prestigious faculties of medicine, began practicing in small private clinics with little or no oversight.

Worries about the black market heightened the legislative debates, as lawmakers, physicians, and journalists debated whether or not organ sale is intrinsic to the practice of organ transplantation and whether and how the market can be controlled. But as legislation stalled, the uncontrolled black market grew more intransigent, more exploitative, and more complicated. Medical professionals expressed outrage against an "underclass" of profit-oriented physicians. Their condemnation fell in line with the elitism of the medical hierarchy, where those in established positions cast moral doubt on those on the margins of the profession. Moreover, medical professionals, characterized by nationalist sentiment, sought to protect the "national" honor, which, they claimed, was threatened by a predatory foreign demand for Egyptian organs. Transnational sales between foreigners and Egyptians provoked outrage throughout Egypt (al-Irqsusi 1998; Amin 2007a). There was broad tolerance, particularly in the first two decades of transplantation, toward transactions between Egyptian donor-sellers and other Egyptians. In contrast, reports about wealthier Arabs and other foreigners preying on Egyptians provided fodder for many columnists, journalists, and film-makers, who understood the movement of organs from Egyptians to other Arabs from the petro-rich Gulf countries in terms of national "shame" and "humiliation."

The idea that "Egyptian livers and kidneys" were for sale was, for these commentators, emblematic of the demise of the nation, of its inferior standing in comparison to richer Gulf countries, Europe, and North America. Other transnational flows certainly characterized this period. Laboring bodies of Egyptian men continued to migrate to the Gulf, with the hopes of earning enough money to return to build families and homes. The Egyptian intelligentsia, including the medical profession, likewise relied on migratory cycles to Gulf countries amid the unlivable wages of the Egyptian faculties. Many Egyptians reported feeling discrimination when working abroad. On the other end, Egypt, during the summer season, was on the receiving end of tourists from the Arab Gulf, who could enjoy entertainment, nightlife, and relative social freedom. Luxurious spaces in Cairo and Alexandria were increasingly cordoned off for tourists and marked inaccessible to local ordinary Egyptians, who experienced this deterritorialization as yet another way in which the "rich eat the poor," choking them off from their own resources (Singerman 1994; Kuppinger 2000).

Press reports, radio interviews, and popular films widely disseminated the notion that the poor were being exploited by profiteering transnational transplant brokers. In a popular 1989 feature film *Ilhaquna!* (Save Us!), the famous Egyptian actor Nur al-Sharif starred as a taxi driver named Qurashi, who chances upon a man severely injured in a car accident. Qurashi rushes to help the man and takes him to a hospital, where the doctors state that they need a blood transfusion. Qurashi turns out to be a perfect antigen match and donates his blood altruistically, nobly refusing to take payment from the man, who turns out to be a wealthy businessman and former politician. The rich man then offers Qurashi a job as his private driver and gives him a place to stay in his mansion, where Qurashi is well treated and well fed by the house staff. Meanwhile, the businessman requires further treatment. He has accumulated his wealth from a "touristic-hospital" business; one of his business partners, a doctor, artificially induces pain in Qurashi's abdomen and leads him to believe that he needs a major operation for it. Qurashi eventually discovers that his kidney was stolen during the operation and shipped off abroad, where the businessman received it in a transplant operation. The villains are transnational corporate profiteers, yet Qurashi blames the Egyptian government for failing to protect his body. The film's last scene is in a courtroom, and the camera moves from Qurashi to the judge and to the lawyers, and finally to a portrait of President Mubarak. Facing the president, Qurashi cries, "Are you happy? We have been robbed down to our flesh!"[10]

Throughout my fieldwork, patients alluded to this film—often replayed on Egyptian television—and spoke of untrustworthy doctors who had become "butchers and tradesmen." The dramatic film seems to encapsulate the vulnerability that poor Egyptians have felt to illness, disease, poor medical treatment, and transnational exploitation. The journalist 'Abd al-Hamid al-'Irqsusi wrote a book about the dangers of medical exploitation, organ theft, and the vulnerability of Egyptians, published by the state-aligned *Al-Ahram* newspaper and press and titled *Anqadhuna . . . fishash wa kalawi al-Misriyin lil-biy'!* (Rescue Us . . . Livers and Kidneys of Egyptians for Sale!). Like the film, it too is framed as a report addressed to the president of the republic, calling on him to act in the midst of a crisis in which "the Egyptian people were being sold off, piece by piece" (al-'Irqsusi 1998).

Organ sales continued and proliferated in clinics that were increasingly difficult to monitor; more complex rings of brokers and middlemen facilitated transnational transplants in private clinics. Brokers, notoriously, further exploited those selling their organs by usurping most of the payment. Commercial sellers often appeared at police stations with accusations that their kidneys had been "stolen." Indeed, claims of organ theft became a catchall for various forms of exploitation. That is, most of the time that people reported "kidney theft," their kidneys had not actually been extracted while they were unconscious, in the style presented in Egyptian films and television serials. Rather, their traffickers had taken most of the money that the seller-donors had been promised in their initial deals, or they had found themselves shoved into a cab in the middle of the night, only hours after the operation, some cash in their pockets, but without the appropriate time to heal or recover in the hospital. The seller-donors would realize they had been "tricked" into believing that the operation was simple and insignificant, that they would be well taken care of, and that they would receive more money than they did. Without a kidney, scarred and enfeebled, they had to face families and communities, who looked down on them for deciding to profit from their own bodies. Out of shame and humiliation at having been deceived, many commercial donors accused their brokers and the participating doctors of "stealing" their kidneys. Since the organ extraction had been performed outside any legal framework, they had little recourse to address their medical mistreatment. The term *organ theft* became the epitome of deception, exploitation, and dehumanization, and many commercial sellers seemed to feel that it aptly described their situation. For many, feelings of past deception or exploitation were what prompted them to sell their kidneys in the first place, because they had found themselves overwhelmed by extraordinary debt.

DONORS' HONOR AND SHAME IN ORGAN SALES

Emad, a father of three young girls, agreed to an interview with reporters from *Al-Misri al-Yawm* newspaper who wanted to know why he had hung advertisements reading "Kidney for Sale" all along Ramses Street in Cairo.[11] "Sometimes being sick is better than being in prison," he replied. The reporters wanted to know how he had gotten himself in this predicament. Emad told them that a year and a half earlier, at the age of thirty-five, he had decided to liquidate his assets in order to climb out of a life of rural poverty. He sold all of his cattle, and with the cash he received he made a down payment on a pickup truck, planning to pay off the balance in monthly installments. His plan was to work as a driver, taking workers from al-Khanka to all the different Egyptian governorates each day. At first it worked, Emad said, but then things took a turn for the worse: "Three months ago I had a terrible accident. My car turned upside down on the freeway and was totally destroyed. The accident left my right foot disabled, and I have no longer been able to work. Since then, I have been living a nightmare, as I have to pay the monthly installments and I have run out of all of my savings. Now I have a 29,000 £E debt, which I must pay as quickly as possible."

Emad received several phone calls after posting his ads; some were prank calls, and others serious. The highest sum offered was 25,000 £E. Focusing on family reputability, Emad was mainly concerned about his possible imprisonment for failure to pay his debts, which would destroy his daughters' chances at respectable marriages. Stating that he would "rather lie ill," Emad was cognizant of the physical risks entailed in donating a kidney, but he had reasoned that physical damages were more tolerable than social ostracism and shame.[12]

While Emad spoke of a prospective kidney sale as a way to maintain his honor, many kidney sellers spoke of their sale as a source of shame. Dr. Badr, whom we have already met and who worked only in private hospitals and his own private dialysis clinic, had asked donors upon whom he had operated about their feelings of shame. In this very interesting study that he conducted (in his possession), he found that twenty-three out of thirty (77 percent) answered that they felt ashamed to admit they had donated a kidney in exchange for money. About half of those who had donated a kidney to a relative (seven out of fifteen) reported feeling discomfort in facing the recipient, and seven out of fifteen of the donors reported that the recipients seemed to feel ashamed in their presence.[13]

Ayman Abdullah, an accountant in Upper Egypt, told *Los Angeles Times* reporters that he and his brother had taken their parents' savings and moved to Cairo to open a cell phone shop. They had teamed up with a man and trusted him more than they should have; their "partner" vanished with the money, and the brothers found themselves 75,000 £E in debt. Abdullah said, "I have two choices: pay my debts or go to jail. . . . I can't find any other solution. It's either the operation or I lose my freedom. . . . I started looking for ads where kidney patients look for doctors, but I realized that the maximum amount of money that I could get for a kidney is 20,000 pounds. Then in the same newspaper, I found an ad [posted] by a liver patient."

At the time of Abdullah's search, donor-sellers who subjected themselves to the much riskier, more complicated surgery of liver lobe extraction could expect to be paid as much as 40,000 £E. Abdullah's brother had already found a buyer whose blood type and tissue type matched his. Abdullah continued: "If God allows me to live after the operation, I won't stay in this country. I want to go work as a schoolteacher or salesman or do any kind of job in any Gulf country. After one undergoes this operation, he feels inferior to the rest of his people. I want to go somewhere with new people. I want people who don't know anything about me."[14] Many of these transactions, in which seller-donors sought out sick patients and negotiated deals, occurred in plain sight in Cairo's public teaching hospitals. Again, the dominant rhetoric about commercial donors has been that they are greedy or without dignity: if they do not respect their own bodies, then why should their willingness to part with an organ stand in the way of a terminally ill patient's chance at survival?

The bulk of commercial organ transplants have occurred in private clinics, some more or less beyond the scope of public scrutiny. The individual shame and humiliation of poverty, where better-off Egyptians benefit from the bodily "sacrifices" of the poor, has been easily naturalized and elided within the context of Cairo's deep social stratification. In a study of fifty donors, 78 percent reported deterioration in their health condition after their kidney donation (Budiani and Shibly 2006). Most reported financial decline as well, challenging the argument that organ sales generally help people in need. As many as 81 percent reported that they had spent the money within five months of their donation, and 73 percent reported a weakened ability to perform labor-intensive jobs, thus putting them in a less secure financial situation. Many said that they felt stigmatized afterward, and perhaps most striking, 94 percent reported feeling regret about their donation (Budiani 2006).[15]

Doctors in the "legitimate" public teaching hospitals have proceeded with their work in transplantation, seeing their own reliance on willing commercial living donors as wholly unrelated to that which has been practiced "underground." Their responsibility as physicians in teaching hospitals, as they see it, is to assure good surgical outcomes for donors and recipients.

Despite their national laws regulating organ transplantation from braindead anonymous donors and related living donors, countries like Saudi Arabia and Kuwait face a growing demand and a short supply of kidneys and livers. For those without kin eligible or willing to donate—or those who decide not to put their kin at risk—Egypt has provided a ready source of organ sellers and surgeons in private clinics willing to carry out these illegal operations.[16] As the transnational aspects of organ sales have gained more media attention, as well as the attention of legislators and established physicians, resentment has spurred people to call for a moratorium on the entire practice. Doctors in prestigious teaching hospitals initially felt immune to criticism, viewing themselves as entirely different from the "commercial" physicians who carry out hurried transplants in underregulated private clinics. But, in terms of public reaction, it hasn't been *where* or in which clinics the transplants are carried out that has been the problem. Rather, what has agitated a sharp public outcry is *who* is on the receiving end and *how;* the idea of Egyptian organs being exploited by the rest of the world by organized trafficking rings is simply intolerable (Jacob 2009).

As Egyptian physicians have faced unprecedented amounts of public criticism and suspicion in the official press, their image has also been tarnished in international circles by global media accounts of unregulated organ markets in third world capitals. Nephrologists in Egypt have been shocked to encounter colleagues from Western countries who scorn and dismiss them at international medical conferences for performing transplant operations from kidneys of "unrelated living donors." At home, not only has the lack of a national program to regulate organ transplantation left the poor vulnerable to exploitation and fears of organ theft, but also it has left medical practitioners open to false accusations of organ theft and to criminal investigation for participating in an organ trade. In response to the outcries about "mafia rings" of middlemen and surgeons, newspapers have reported cases of physicians and middlemen who have been criminally investigated and sent to prison for involvement in the "organ trade." These, predictably, have been physicians who work in the unregulated clinics, not those who hold positions in the high-status faculties of medicine. But it was only a matter of time, many physicians felt, before doctors as a whole would be criminalized for what many of them described as the failure of the state to legislate and regulate the practice. As the eye bank scandal described in chapter 3 indicated, what was normal practice for ophthalmologists one day—procuring eyes from the morgue—could become criminalized the next.

DOCUMENTATION AND MONITORING

Many critics, including Dr. Ghoneim of Mansoura, charge that the expansion of the black market in organs in Cairo cannot be attributed solely to the state's *inability* to regulate it; rather, the state has demonstrated a general unwillingness to get involved, given the wealth generated by the lucrative sales and operations.[17] In response to accusations about the involvement of more and more physicians in the organ trade, doctors and legislators have called for regulations. In the mid-1990s, realizing that a national program for transplantation was unlikely to materialize in Egypt anytime soon, the Egyptian Medical Syndicate, the professional organization that licenses doctors, took steps to regulate transplants itself.[18] Its first step was to limit transnational organ sales by precluding organ donation from citizens of different countries and by registering where (in which hospitals) transplants occurred. The syndicate produced a standardized bureaucratic procedure in 1996, adopting Euro-American models wholesale. On the surface, these guidelines seemed to prohibit the selling of organs.[19]

In the fall of 2002, I conducted fieldwork at the Egyptian Medical Syndicate headquarters in downtown Cairo, curious as to how the syndicate actually uses the paperwork to establish the line between "acceptable" and "unacceptable" transplant operations, when everyone knows that the reliance on commercial living donors has been the backbone of Egyptian transplant medicine. There I met Nasir, an administrator who occupied the office charged with monitoring "the ethical conduct of the profession" *(adab al-mihna)*, a phrase that was spelled out clearly on the sign over the door. A large percentage of his work was devoted to helping organ recipients and donors (mostly kidney and a few liver lobe) fill out their necessary paperwork prior to their operations. The documents would then remain on file at the Medical Syndicate regardless of the hospital in which the patients were treated.

I learned there that every organ recipient and donor pair in Egypt was required to appear physically at this office, to demonstrate that they were of the same nationality and to explain their blood relation. If no blood relation existed between them, then the potential recipient needed to explain why his or her family members were not candidates—that is, why they were medically excluded as donors. They were then to sign documents stating that no commercial exchange for the kidney had taken place. I spent some time in this office, watching encounters among doctors, would-be donors and recipients, and Nasir, the administrator.

Nasir was a jovial, deeply pious, and sympathetic man. He saw his job as important, because if the syndicate had not taken these measures, he told me, the market would be much worse. He listened to the patients' grievances and helped them fill out the paperwork. Many of them were compelled to produce the correct documentation in order for their physicians to agree to perform the transplant. At one of my visits to the office, a liver surgeon came in with two brothers who were to undergo a liver lobe transplant at a private hospital. The surgeon had brought the patients in himself to make sure they filed the paperwork, which would be on record in case any false claim was made about illicit financial transactions or organ theft. Both brothers looked ill to me—that is, to my medically untrained eye—the younger one yellowish and the older one greenish in complexion. As they filled out the paper work, Nasir asked them to mark the line testifying that there was no commercial exchange for the liver lobe. The older patient said, "He is my *brother*. Is there such a thing as a *brother* selling a liver?"

Nasir answered, "Well, actually, yes, we've seen cases like that—a brother who would say: I'll donate my kidney to you, but you will have to give up half your share of the inheritance."

The man was visibly distressed by this story. "A *brother* did that? A brother did that?" He kept repeating these phrases, shaking his head in disbelief.

He turned to me, after Nasir had stepped out of the room, saying, "But how could a brother do that?" The older brother explained that he could have gone abroad to do the operation. After having worked in the Gulf and saved money, he had the financial means to travel to another country, where the organ would have been from an anonymous brain-dead donor. But his younger brother insisted that he be the one to donate. The younger brother was completely silent while his older brother talked. They both seemed terrified. After they finished the paperwork, they left, accompanied by the doctor, and headed straight for the hospital to finish some more diagnostic tests.

The older brother, as a would-be recipient, had considered "donating family members" and "sellers of organs" to be mutually exclusive categories. Yet in Nasir's experience, according to several of the stories he told, this was not necessarily the case. Nasir—as a part of the Medical Syndicate's larger voice—contended that transplantation should be carried out "altruistically," free of the shadow of nefarious and greedy motivations, but actual patients continually came to him with stories that betrayed the "official line." Physicians and hospital administrators and staff narrated the story of the man who sold his kidney to his younger brother and the one about the young woman who donated her kidney to her father under pressure. Faced with such real dilemmas, doctors involved with transplantation had developed an ethical pragmatism in dealing with seller-donors. Too many terminally ill patients in organ failure had no kin to gift them kidneys. Many of them had families and young children to support. It made little sense to these doctors to police the boundaries between "altruistic" and "commercial" donations, especially when their experiences disproved the assumption that family donations are always altruistic and that commercial donations are necessarily more exploitative.

While Nasir worked on his papers, an older man came in to fill out the paperwork for his daughter, who was in need of a kidney. The old man explained that each of her brothers had a medical problem, that he was over sixty, that her mother had a heart condition, and that her sister lived in Saudi Arabia. The daughter's husband, tiring of her illness, the cost of its treatment, and her inability to tend to him and the home, had separated from her. Unwilling or unable to procure her own kidney, the woman had become resigned to her fate, but her father stepped in to provide for her, to care for her, in the only way he could. This father procured a kidney from an unrelated person and came to the Medical Syndicate to fill out paperwork, including the form on which he had to attest that he had not paid money for the kidney.

Nasir, the administrator, saw cases like this all the time. The old man leaned into him, his hands on Nasir's desk, asking him to read aloud all the information in the document—all the criteria and rules for a legitimate exchange. He hung on Nasir's every word. Nasir obliged, reading through the rules quickly: first all family members had to be medically excluded, including cousins, aunts, and uncles.

The old man drew a sharp breath: "Oh—my sisters and brothers! My nieces and nephews! But I could never ask this of them!"

Nasir nodded: "I know, I know." The Egyptian Medical Syndicate, as with its attempts at legislation, had imported the structure and content of organ transplant–related paperwork from the United States and European countries, without attempting to adapt the criteria to Egyptian practice. Family donations have rarely occurred outside the nuclear family in Egypt; the

Egyptians with whom I spoke considered first- and second-degree relatives unrealistic as natural candidates for organ donation. The idea of subjecting a healthy family member to a major medical operation is hard enough within the immediate family; it is much more so for a cousin, aunt, or nephew. Whereas "family" is generally a more extensive category in Egypt than in the United States, this has not been the case in regard to organ transplantation. Second-degree relatives generally do not count as potential family donors in the Egyptian context.[20]

The older man did not have to explain to Nasir why cousins were unthinkable as donors. Family members who donate generally do so because they endure physical and financial hardship when their children, siblings, or a spouse suffers. As demonstrated in previous chapters, quite unlike in Euro-American contexts, living organ donation in Egypt is not seen as a "medical miracle" to restore life. It is not considered a heroic or altruistic act born of a need to "make sense" out of suffering, to participate in medical triumphalism over death, or to see life regenerate and the dead "live on" (Fox and Swazey 1992; Joralemon 1995; Sharp 2001; Lock 2002b). Rather, in Egypt, people generally see organ donation as enormously risky, a last resort, a calculated measure for family survival (Scheper-Hughes 2007). Knowing this well, Nasir proceeded quickly through that section, dismissing it entirely as something that is clearly not applicable to the fates of the people whom he sees walking into his office every day. His practical knowledge functioned outside the traces of paperwork and documentation.

Nasir continued filling out the paper, checking the boxes for the old man, whose eyes were too tired to read the small print. Nasir also filled out the papers routinely for illiterate patients or patients not accustomed to the formality of official writing. The old man exclaimed gratefully, "May God be generous to your children!"

Nasir informed him that he needed to attach records of the kidney ultrasound and results of tissue-matching tests.

The old man sounded exasperated, "Just yesterday we made the trip to Mansoura to have the urine analysis completed."

Nasir assured him, "You still have time."

Nasir never made an issue of the organ recipient's father coming to fill out the paperwork rather than the patient herself. The forms presume that discrete, autonomous individuals represent their own wills when entering into these contracts of exchange. This same presumption underlies organ transplantation itself: the idea that discrete individuals might rationally choose to relinquish a body part in a transaction that will not alter either individual's sense of self. Yet, as we have seen, patients often spoke against these presumptions: they generally refused transplantation because they saw their healthy family members as materially and socially bound up with themselves; their parents, brothers, sisters, and spouses were also vulnerable to potential disease and suffering, and family members felt the need to protect one another. Here in the Medical Syndicate office, the father's life and self were bound up in his daughter's suffering, which he hoped to end by seeking and paying a donor.

The father had made many trips to Cairo's public hospitals in search of a blood and tissue donor who would be a good match for his daughter. The donor was one of untold numbers of people who had undergone diagnostic tests so that sick patients in need might contact him and offer money in exchange for his kidney. It was difficult for the older man to navigate Cairo's intimidating public hospitals and its hectic public transportation system, to interview donor after donor, while making sure his daughter underwent the proper diagnostic tests to remain medically eligible as a recipient. One can only imagine the difficulty if the dialysis patient herself had attempted these feats, particularly with her physical impediments and the risk of missing a dialysis session, compounded with the psychological challenge in accepting the idea that one's survival comes only at the high financial cost to her family and at the price of a stranger's subjection to the extraction of a vital organ. It seemed natural and perfectly unproblematic to Nasir that the father, who was "gifting" his daughter (another man's) kidney, could represent her in signed documents.

In my research, many of the patients who had paid donors for their kidneys were generally, like this absent daughter, passive in the process. Their well-meaning family members sought to "provide" for them by procuring a kidney that they were unable or unwilling to give themselves. Nasir, the administrator at the Medical Syndicate, encountered such people every day. In the case of the two brothers, Nasir had to ask if they were inserting trade into the family, for he had learned that sometimes a brother could sell to another brother. In the case of the old man and his daughter, Nasir recognized that family is often inserted into the organ trade: here, because the father himself could not donate his kidney to his daughter, he made this sacrifice through proxy by buying a kidney for her. Both situations seemed to indicate for Nasir the inextricability of family relations from the market in organs. His experience contradicted the popular notion that family is the one realm in transplantation that is safe from corrupting market forces.

As far as the administrator was concerned, the problem is far bigger than any regulations on paper could solve, and some leniency in enforcement is "more merciful" for everyone. He did not employ forgery or coercion to solicit signatures. When the old man came to the part of the form asking him to sign that he had not paid money for the kidney, he faltered. He looked up at Nasir helplessly as if to ask, "What should I do here?" Nasir nodded and told him it was all right, that he could sign it. Nasir implied, but never articulated outright, an understanding that this signature on a bureaucratic form was a necessary performance, that others in similar situations had come before him and had signed as well, that its primary purpose was to protect the doctors, and that there would be no negative repercussions against the man or the patient.

In creating their own regulations, the Egyptian Medical Syndicate wittingly shifted the burden of responsibility from physicians to patients to "regulate" the buying and selling of organs. The medical profession, backed by the syndicate, continues to perform transplants using seller-donors but only those who had signed that they had not received money. When Nasir told me that if it were not for him, the market would be much worse, he meant that the system could potentially filter out the "mafia rings" and lurid accounts of butchery that have been periodically reported in the state-aligned newspapers and the opposition-party press. The point of this bureaucratic system was to ensure that only those patients (of the same nationality as their donors) and physicians performing transplantation in legitimate hospitals would escape criminal investigation. The rest should presumably be vulnerable to prosecution, that seedy surplus of illegitimate transplant activity performed by unlicensed doctors in unlicensed clinics. The forms then, in this sense, have naturalized the selling and buying of organs by circumscribing the practice as "legitimate" when performed by the right doctors in the right places and when donor and buyer are of the same nationality.

The Medical Syndicate papers, the precursor to the law finally passed in 2010, claim to prevent the possibility of a commercial exchange in kidneys, whether within or outside the family. But in practice, the syndicate has aimed not at stopping the organ trade in Egypt but at protecting the (right) physicians from being held accountable for participating in it. The administrator told the old man to sign that there was no transaction, even though the man was undoubtedly buying a kidney from an unrelated donor. The bureaucratic performance was a practice in a cynical, yet still ethical pragmatism. Not all cases should be treated the same; a myopic focus on "financial transaction" and a comprehensive ban would, Nasir argued, lead to even more suffering. For Nasir, and for the doctors he represented, stopping a tired and desperate father from paying a man in debt to spare his kidney was pointless. The old man was doing all he could to save the life of his dying daughter; her illness had already led to the dissolution of her marriage and to the suffering of her natal family.

PAYING YOUR WAY OUT

The doctors and hospital administrators with whom I spoke in Cairo were resigned to the commercialization of organs as a "fact of life," but those in Mansoura were determined to curb organ sales. The majority of transplants in the Mansoura Kidney Center had occurred between family members. But here again, "the family" and "the market" were not entirely separable realms. As one Mansoura nephrologist told me, "Transplantation offers the best quality of life, so of course we try to encourage it, and because of the shariʿa problem of donation, we try to limit the [commodification/market] problem as much as we can. But of course, even living related donors sell, although they would never admit to it. For example, there was a daughter giving her kidney to her father so that he would give her a piece of land. This is a problem we can't really do much about."

Occasionally the doctors at Mansoura took on cases like that of Iman, a local Mansoura patient whom they had followed for years and for whom familial donation was impossible. Iman was a previously healthy married woman and mother of two young sons who became very ill during her third pregnancy. The doctors induced her labor in the seventh month of her pregnancy, but her baby died in the neonatal intensive care unit. Iman was diagnosed with acute kidney failure and put on dialysis. Her mother had died when she was younger, and she had only half-siblings with whom she was not close. Her husband offered Iman his own kidney to the outrage of his natal family, who protested against his undergoing such a risky operation for the sake of his wife. As Iman told her story:

> Back in the days that I was sick, my husband offered to donate his kidney to me. He would say to the doctors, "I will donate." But I would refuse. His relatives would call and say, "No! Don't donate your kidney! Don't do such a thing! You will hurt yourself."
> My husband was a very, very good man. He knew that I got sick from pregnancy. He said, "See the other patients who were with you in the hospital. They all got sick from pregnancy, so don't even think of getting pregnant again." So I never thought of having another child after the transplant.

In saying that he knew that Iman had fallen ill because of her pregnancy, her husband linked the onset of her disease with their attempt to make a mutually desired family. By telling her not to think of getting pregnant again, he was giving her assurance that their family was "complete," their marriage was already secure. Despite his family's protests, he went to Mansoura for tissue typing, but the doctors reported that his results were not a close enough match for them to proceed with the transplant.

After Iman's husband was disqualified as a donor, he traveled to Cairo to find her a better-matched kidney for sale. He now sought to provide for his wife through financial rather than bodily sacrifice. The analytic labs there, affiliated with public teaching hospitals, matched Iman's tissue test results with those of a young man of twenty-two years. He had come to Cairo's analytical laboratories to undergo tissue analysis, and since that time he had been waiting to be "matched" with a person willing to buy his kidney.

Analytic labs in Cairo's hospitals in many cases act as the "brokers" in organ deals (Budiani 2005, 2007). The hospital laboratories take in a large pool of "donors" and coordinate blood- and tissue-type matching with eager recipients. With enough people willing to sell their kidneys, the market has accommodated doctors' insistence on tissue-type compatibility. Here we find an interesting juxtaposition to the phenomenon that Lawrence Cohen (2001), an anthropologist who worked on organ transplants in India, described about tissue typing and the proliferation of an organ trade. Cohen argued that early on, transplant scientists had hoped that matching blood type and antigens (tissue typing) in donor and recipient, matches that were more likely to occur within families, would enhance graft survival. But, Cohen notes, it was the introduction of strong immunosuppressive drugs that has overridden the importance of tissue typing. Doctors around the world now rely less on tissue typing and count more on pharmaceuticals to prevent the recipient's immune system from rejecting the "foreign" kidney. Cohen (2001) described the change in goal—from "recognition" to "suppression"—as a key factor in materializing the organ trade, for now, with the knowledge that unrelated seller-donors' kidneys can fare just as well as "closer matches," there is less need to rely on families.

In Egypt, however, at the time of my field research, the prestigious medical centers and teaching hospitals did not rely on the idea of effective immunosuppressive drugs "trumping" tissue matching. Unlike in the situation that Cohen describes, an abandonment of tissue-type matching was not what drove the local organ trade. In fact, the opposite was true. In Mansoura, doctors insisted on an adequate tissue-type match between donor and recipient, which in many cases *precluded* intrafamilial donation. In cases like Iman's and that of 'Ali and his wife, described in chapter 5, transplant surgeons in other settings might have gone ahead with the operation, rely-ing on strong and highly toxic immunosuppressant drugs to override the lack of a complete antigen match between the spouses.[21] But because doc-tors on the faculties of medicine insisted on ameliorating the chances of graft survival without relying on high doses of toxic (and expensive) phar-maceuticals, the lack of adequate tissue typing within families drove people to look to paid organ sellers who might have a better antigen match.[22] Thus, adherence to full antigen matching does not necessarily equate with a pref-erence for intrafamilial donation; relaxing the criteria for antigen matching might have, in this case, encouraged intrafamilial donations—particularly interspousal donations—over the reliance on commercial live donors.

Paradoxically, even though this reliance on tissue typing in Egypt in many senses encourages patients to turn to commercial living donors, phy-sicians on the faculties of medicine understand their reliance on tissue typ-ing as another factor that separates them from the "unethical" practices of "organ-trade" doctors who work in unregulated clinics with brokers for transplant arrangements with foreigners. Those doctors, like those working in the Indian organ trade that Cohen described, allegedly have *not* bothered with careful tissue typing. From this juxtaposition, we can see that markets clearly work in different ways in different contexts. While technoscientific developments like tissue typing or immunosuppressive pharmaceuticals might lead to one outcome in a given context, they might lead to an entirely different outcome in another, even within the same local setting.

Moreover, Iman's story affirms that donations within the family, espe-cially in particular directions—such as husband to wife, brother to sister, or offspring to parent—can lead to never-ending cycles of guilt, accusations, and resentment:

> We paid him [the donor] 15,000 pounds. I used to wear a gold bracelet in those days; I gave it to him for his fiancée. I wore the surgical mask for four months after my operation. The doctors had to force it off me! I was just so scared that I would end up on dialysis again, I had to do everything to protect myself from losing the kidney. My sons were embarrassed about how strange I was acting, but I told them to mind their own business.
>
> Our arrangement with the donor happened right away. It cost 3,000 £E at the time for the lab to do the analysis and to get the donor. Now people say the price is 7,000 £E. The whole thing cost us over 25,000 £E. The boy wanted to have enough money to get married; he didn't tell his family that he was selling his kidney. He came several times after the operation to "borrow" money. We would give it to him, but we would never ask for it to be paid back.

Once he called and said that he wanted papers from the Mansoura Kidney Center here so that they could verify that he had his kidney taken out, to send to the military service. After that we never heard from him again; I don't even know if he got the papers.

My husband's sister, when she saw the donor that we paid, she said loudly so that I could hear, "Oh, the poor thing! Look at him! He is so young!"

Iman's mother—her most likely advocate—was dead, and her father and stepmother were either unwilling or uninterested in interceding on her behalf. She was thus completely at the whim of her husband's family, and as she told it, she was fortunate that her husband cared for her, against the wishes of his larger family unit. With no blood relatives as potential donors, her only "family" kin donor was her husband; as a nonbiological relative, he was less likely to have a full antigen match with his wife. Moreover, a husband's donation of a kidney to his wife was not an acceptable direction for bodily resources to flow; his family had made it clear that they would have made her life miserable had she received a kidney from him.

As it was, her husband's sister had already hurt her feelings by making the kidney that her husband obtained for her, from a seller-donor in the city, seem not only like a waste of resources but also sinful, given how young he was. After the transplant operation, Iman was hypervigilant about medical compliance, even adopting strange behaviors such as refusing to take off her surgical mask, out of fear that the resources spent on her might be "wasted" by a postoperative rejection of the kidney. If her husband's financial sacrifices on her behalf were already viewed by his natal family as "excessive," a bodily sacrifice, in the form of a kidney, would have been intolerable. She knew that relying on a paid donor rather than her husband for a new kidney, though still presenting problems, was more acceptable for her husband's family. But she could not have guessed how critical this wager was: "[After the transplant operation] my husband died two years later. He didn't have anything wrong with him. His heart just stopped beating. It was on a Friday, and he was watching a [soccer] match; he loved the Zamalek team. He watched the game, and then we had dinner. He said his chest hurt him. We read the Qur'an for him. Then he said he couldn't breathe, so we turned on the air-conditioning, thinking it was the stuffy, hot air. His brothers took him to the emergency room. When they came back, he was dead." Having unpredictably survived her husband, Iman's story in a sense exposes the faulty logic of the biomedical "urgency" that inspired scraping all savings together for one operation for one family member. How and why should all resources go toward one failed organ in a family of many intertwined bodies and organs, all of which are vulnerable to failure?

But at least money, as hard as it is to come by, is more replaceable than body parts. Iman continued: "Now I think: thank God we went with a paid donor, because everyone would have blamed me for my husband's death. God planned for me to have this donor so that I could be off dialysis and be able to care for my children." Among the patients and physicians I spoke with, the more complicated the family relations were, the less convincing it was to rule out paid donation, or to argue that paid donation was less ethical than familial donation. Why should monetary exchange necessarily change the way we view organ donation? It might be the case that commercial living donors are often exploited and ill-treated by physicians, but what if physicians screen these donors before hand? What if the physicians are assured of the donors' "informed consent" and commit to medically following both recipients *and* donors after the operation? Some physicians, like Iman's in Mansoura, directed only by their own conscience, have taken it upon themselves to follow what they viewed as the most ethical choice in a system of imperfect alternatives. From Iman's perspective, having paid for a kidney rather than accepting one donated by her husband, saved her and her children from an unbearable life of guilt and accusation. She would have been directly blamed for her husband's death had he lost an organ for her. Paying for a kidney was a shorter-term transaction, with presumably both parties in some way benefiting. After her husband's death, Iman continued to live in her married home, in an apartment flat in the same building as her husband's natal family. Receiving a kidney directly from her husband, who subsequently died, would have surely destroyed her already strained relations with her in-laws; now that she was widowed, she relied on them as kin and community, as she continued to raise her sons in their now father-less world.

CRACKDOWN: CAIRO AS "TRAFFICKING HOTSPOT" OF THE WORLD

In 2006, the World Health Organization began to call for greater transparency in the situation of organ trafficking in Egypt.[23] The Egyptian media had reported steadily on organ thefts and trafficking since the 1980s. Egyptian critics, journalists, physicians, and religious scholars had for decades decried the exploitation of the poor in organ donation, a practice that has been routinely ignored and denied.[24] Only when the international media began focusing on Egypt as a "trafficking hotspot" of the world, including reports issued from various United Nations agencies, did the Egyptian government feel pressured to act. The UN reports argue that poverty—not criminality or greed—and lack of governmental oversight fuel organ sales. Here again, state actors who ignored grievances of the local poor appeared responsive only when the injuries were to the "national image" and "national honor." In 2006, the Ministry of Health created a special unit to monitor medical centers and private hospitals in Egypt, where most of the unregulated organ transplants took place. In collaboration with the Egyptian Medical Syndicate, the Free Treatment Section of the ministry, which had the authority to arrest those suspected of organ trafficking, worked to track down organ brokers and donors and, in 2008, raided various private clinics found to be performing transplants on foreigners without certification.[25] But the private clinics have still remained difficult to identify and regulate.[26] As a Ministry of Health spokesperson told reporters of the television station Al-Arabiya, "Organ brokers have shifted their business away from certified hospitals and moved to shady areas in shantytowns and impoverished places in the outskirts of Cairo."[27]

The Medical Syndicate, lawmakers, and representatives in the Ministry of Health have spoken of the need to increase the supply of organs, given the overwhelming demand. Physicians have disagreed as to whether these bureaucratic measures put in place by the Egyptian Medical Syndicate have worked or whether the measure in fact has backfired, driving the practice further underground. In cases in which the donors or recipients have not been Egyptian, those involved will not even approach the syndicate for the required documentation.[28] Physicians' anecdotal evidence suggests unacceptably poor outcomes for transplant operations in "business-oriented clinics," as patients with botched operations have periodically appeared at more legitimate medical centers, and stories and rumors have circulated about organ rejection and death occurring in certain for-profit hospitals and clinics. Under *international* pressure to pass a law, lawmakers pushed for the legal permissibility of cadaveric procurement from brain-dead patients and were finally able to pass a law in 2010, which has yet to go into effect. In any case, given the significant increase in kidney failure, as well as Egypt's long history of experiencing the "overflow" of organ demand from neighboring countries with stricter regulations, the possibility of meeting the demand with cadaveric procurement from patients, those who die of major brain trauma with their bodies intact, is highly unlikely. Recognizing this conundrum in terms other than that of "organ shortage," Lesley Sharp has described organ transplantation as the "capitalist's dream," because the demand has been expansively increased—through earlier diagnoses of organ failure, more inclusive criteria of patients, and new transplant surgeries that can intervene in various diseases. Meanwhile, the supply will always be limited.[29] Whereas in the United States, this kind of capitalist entrepreneurship, which shapes the commodification of the body and its parts, has been medicalized, in Egypt it is simply "papered over."

There is some sad irony in the fact that as the global market in body parts has become more and more impossible to regulate, the more intransigent some of the stances against organ sales have become in much medical ethics discourse. This absolutism has ignored the vast range in exploitative practices in organ transplantation, whether "gifts" of organs occur within or from outside the family, for monetary exchange or not. The state-aligned Egyptian press's ridicule of Shaykh Sha'rawi for being tradition-bound and religiously archaic in his absolutist stance against organ transplantation is noteworthy given the press's own absolutist stance against organ sales, mirroring Euro-American stances articulated in the rhetoric of secular ethics. The topic of "organ sales," perhaps raising other specters—of slavery or sexual exploitation—has become so taboo that mere talk of regulating the market is regarded as crossing an ethical boundary.[30]

Moreover, much of the Euro-American condemnation of organ sales overshadows and, in some senses, shapes practices in Egypt that pragmatically seek to manage what has come to be seen as inevitable. Most religious scholars have echoed the absolutist stance, officially condemning any sale of body parts, claiming that the body is the sole property of God the Creator. But at the same time, some religious scholars, observing the intricate details of case after case of families wracked by devastating illness have, like many physicians, quietly offered other suggestions. I heard of several cases in which a doctor, his patient, and a seller-donor appealed to a high-ranking mufti, making it clear that the donor was indeed voluntarily selling his kidney. The doctor told the mufti that he was confident that the seller would be medically unharmed by kidney extraction, that the recipient would fare well, and that he would personally follow both of them after the surgery. Convinced that more benefit than harm could come from this particular case, the mufti offered a way out: "Surely, we cannot 'sell' what does not belong to us, but the donor can make this 'donation' to save the life of this patient. And the patient can charitably give him some money." In another case involving a middle-class Egyptian woman, the woman told her seller-donor not to mention anything about how much money he wanted, so that it would not resemble, in her mind, a transaction. She simply gave him a tidy sum (20,000 pounds) as a "gift" in exchange for the one he had given her.

The Medical Syndicate has effectively adopted an absolutist stance against organ commercialization, echoing the official policy of developed Euro-American nations. The substance of the bureaucratic forms has focused on the singular evil of financial transaction, marking it as the only ethical problem that should be considered in organ transplantation. Organ transplantation in reality is embedded in much larger problems for the world's poor. The great disparities in living conditions in Egypt render the lives of the poor expendable, their suffering natural. Patients in kidney failure link their disease to poverty and the mismanagement of toxic waste; patients in liver failure suffer from hepatitis C as the result of a mass treatment campaign gone amok. Patients greatly mistrust medical institutions; they worry about the strain on family dynamics that could come with intrafamilial donation, the prohibitive cost and medical risks of the operation, and the life-long regime of highly toxic immunosuppressants that are required in posttransplant life. In addition, the poor face these problems in a larger context of unsafe labor conditions, falling salaries, rising costs, debt, and the stresses of daily living in rural poverty or in Egypt's crowded, congested, and polluted cities.

The Medical Syndicate paperwork, initially created in 1996 to protect doctors from accusations of organ theft and trafficking and since 2006 used to distinguish between criminal and legitimate activity, has served as the connector between two commodified spheres of exchange: that of organs and that of medical services. The fallout is that structural violence, the stresses of poverty, toxic mismanagement, medical negligence, and poor laboring conditions have continued to be ignored. The assumption that "advanced Western" nations do not have the problems of commodified flesh that proliferate in seedy third world capitals undergirds Euro-American media accounts and a universalizing bioethics discourse, in a sense Orientalizing the question of a market in human organs. As Lesley Sharp (2006) has documented, the globalized rhetoric of "altruism" has dominated organ transplantation, while any mention of the ways in which organs are *necessarily* commodified in this most lucrative of medical practices is strictly taboo. This assumption overlooks the various ways in which "shadow markets" lurk in the realm of organ transplantation in places such as prestigious U.S. medical centers and how these supposedly different markets are actually linked to a common global system of commodified medical practice (Fox and Swazey 1992; Scheper-Hughes 2000, 2007; Lock 2002a, 2002b; Sharp 2006). It also exoticizes the problem as one that takes place among foreign Others distant from us, perhaps resulting from local corruption, failed polities, or strange "cultural" beliefs, Others who have deviated from the proper, rational, sterile practice of medical transplantation. Notably, in this neoliberal global health economy, the violence of poverty has escalated in recent decades, with the gap between rich and poor widening across the globe. Poverty has had disastrous health consequences, which have largely been met by a culture of indifference, much like situations of extreme warfare and terror (Arendt 1951; Farmer 1992, 1997, 1999, 2003; Briggs 2003; Nguyen and Preschard 2003; Nguyen 2005; Fassin 2007).

CONCLUSIONS

Doctors, family members, and patients draw the lines between "ethical" and "unethical" transplantation within the entrenched practice of relying on commercial live donors, even while voicing the dominant discourse that only "altruistic" intrafamilial donations should be ethically acceptable. As transplant physicians were quick to tell me, more than just wealthy patients benefit from organs from the poor. In many cases, the families of working-class or poor patients, who are medically ineligible themselves to be donors, have scraped all their assets together to come up with a sum of money acceptable for someone to part with his kidney. Many of these transplant doctors seemed to think that allowing some leeway is more merciful than rigidly opposing all types of transaction. "That would just mean people would die," one urologist told me. When I pointed out the vulnerability of the poor donors, several doctors stated the same thing: "There are *many* poor people in Egypt. Only a small number sell their organs." They explained that these seller-donors are generally not the desperately poor people from the rural countryside, that I might imagine. The seller-donors have often been young, urban men who want to get ahead: to put together some money to buy a kiosk or a minibus or to get married. Or they have been in extraordinary debt because some business deal went awry. The physicians I spoke with thus sympathized more with the patient-recipients, and less, if at all, with the commercial donors. Furthermore, these doctors did not consider the donors to be "patients," even though they must undergo major invasive surgery. Dire poverty is not what causes sellers to offer their kidneys for cash, they implied, but a clear disregard for themselves, perhaps a lack of dignity, which leaves them deserving little if any compassion.[31]

Many patients I spoke with struggled with what they saw as two evils. On the one hand, they could accept an organ from a family member and forever after live with an unpayable debt. Or they could pay someone to spare a kidney with some semblance of a legitimate contractual exchange. For most patients, the option of a family donation was not even a possibility. For them, the two options were to face death or pay someone else in order to survive. In practice, allowing for paid organs is sometimes the most ethical course of action. The "official line" for those promoting organ transplantation is that once a national system is regulated, the commercialization of organs will come to an end. But most of those directly involved with transplantation have seen that the buying and selling of organs is an integral aspect of transplantation, because the supply of "altruistically donated" organs will never meet the increasing demand. Some have argued, on this basis, that the commercialization of organs is not ideal but necessary to save lives. Others have argued that because commercialization is unstoppable, shunning transplants altogether is better. But this is difficult advice to follow for those who are dying or watching their loved ones suffer: those who sense a moral responsibility to continue to survive to provide for their families or those who are parents and feel a moral responsibility to buy an organ for their dying child if they themselves are medically ineligible to serve as donors.

On paper or, more accurately, by means of paper, the Egyptian Medical Syndicate has "regulated" the transplants and prohibited the buying and selling of organs. In the absence of a national law and amid increased scrutiny of physicians, the syndicate stepped in and shifted the onus onto the patients to make sure the transplants are "free of financial transactions" by having the donor and recipient enact a particular bureaucratic performance that elicits less than truthful declarations. The bureaucratic procedures at the Medical Syndicate have perpetuated a public secret that the syndicate simultaneously denies: the routine buying and selling of organs. I read this not as an instance of particular Egyptian duplicity but rather as a signal of a larger structural and philosophical problem involving our assumptions about the production of facts—about the body and about people's lives—that can be captured, isolated, and manipulated in discrete material cells, organs, texts, and institutions (Latour 2005; IRIN 2006).

It is public knowledge—outside the traces of documentation—that many of these transactions have indeed been commercial. Yet they are understood to have achieved an "ethical" standard, because they have been carried out in legitimate hospitals with reputable physicians. The implication, which to some extent echoes elitist hierarchies within the profession, is that prestigious and established doctors will ensure that the donors are there voluntarily, are in good health, and will be given proper medical treatment. But a more valid argument is that increased transparency, rather than criminalization, would better ensure that all donors—whether paid or not—are thoroughly medically screened, can be ensured proper surgical care, and receive follow-up medical treatment.

In saying this, I am not recommending that we justify organ sales or perpetuate the practice, which has clearly had adverse effects on paid donors (Scheper-Hughes 2000, 2005; Goyal, Mehta, et al. 2002; Budiani and Shibly 2008; Budiani-Saberi 2010). Rather, after having witnessed firsthand the struggles of organ recipients and donors, I suggest that the most practical interim step is to make all organ donation transactions transparent rather than turning a blind eye to or criminalizing them. This way donors can be given full information about the risks of surgery, the physicians can be held accountable for good surgical and medical outcomes, brokers can be eliminated, and donors might be more empowered, better treated medically, and decently compensated. The absolutist moralizing discourse adopted by Nancy Scheper-Hughes and others who outright condemn all aspects of paid organ donation has seized upon the commodification of the body as the ultimate insult and the logical consequence of neoliberalism and free global capital. Paid donors then have become the emblem for larger political arguments, but these arguments do not seem helpful in offering practical steps to alleviate the situation in which we are now mired. I agree with Scheper-Hughes that appealing to "individual rights" and "contractual exchange" is suspect within larger structures of extreme poverty and political repression. But I am also convinced that condemning all paid organ donation, or further criminalizing it, would be counterproductive to the aims of guaranteeing safe medical practice.

Criminalization, absolutist stances, and driving the practice further underground do nothing to address underlying social inequalities that have brought us to this situation. And as long as social inequalities persist, any organ transplant program will reflect them. Like Adriana Petryna (2009), who has studied globalizing clinical trials, I too have come to see "radical transparency" as a more ethical practice than increasing criminalization, a process that would require the creation of "criminals" and "victims," categories that do not accurately capture all the different exchanges that can go on between donors and recipients. (See also Warren 2010.) Sensationalized global media accounts about black markets in organs have overshadowed more subtle negotiations involving the ethics and pragmatics of the entrenched practice of buying and selling organs. It has become too easy to exoticize the problem of "organ selling" as one of third world nations, presumably impoverished in both ethics and medical authority. The sensationalism of "black markets in organs" has often obscured the structural violence of everyday stresses, toxicity, difficult labor conditions, and financial insecurity that have predisposed people to organ failure in the first place.

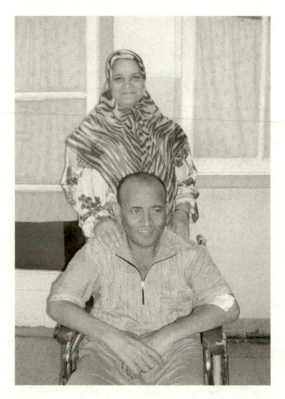

Figure 16.   Ola and her husband, Mahmud, who
refuses to take a kidney from her because, as they
both explain, "the body belongs to God." After
Mahmud had been on dialysis for eight years, this
was the first day that he could no longer walk, and
he entered the ward in a wheelchair. Other patients
tried to hide their distress at seeing him in this condition, and all put on a brave face. Photograph by
the author.

Conclusions

Where Cyborgs Meet God

While poor patients in organ failure were utterly vulnerable to medical mistreatment and state negligence throughout Egypt, the Mansoura Kidney Center had established a decidedly different model of care. Closing itself off from the problems emanating from Cairo, the center boasted impressive treatment outcomes and the enforcement of strict regulations, which included limiting the attending physicians to working solely in the hospital and not in private clinics. Hospital staff members were also proud to report that their poor rural patients received first-class treatment, including follow-up care and even their prescription medications at no cost to them. And although the physicians could not always rely entirely on familial kidney donation, they felt assured that they did not see patterns of exploitation of the poor by the rich. In response to Cairo professionals' seeming defeatism—and their justification of a world in which the rich "eat" the poor—Mansoura's transplant physicians insisted that it was their duty to play some part in delivering equitable treatment and social justice in medical care.

Contra Shaykh Sha'rawi's fears that transplantation might signal a person's wavering belief in God's ultimate power, devout rural patients in Mansoura exclaimed that their faith in and gratitude to God were *strengthened* by medical intervention. Within the walls of the Mansoura Kidney Center, the physicians generally saw their work of treating and healing the poor as pleasing to God. The patients expressed little doubt that they were doing the right thing in taking care of their bodies by receiving organs. And their family members felt virtuous in the sacrifices that they had made through kidney donation. In the Mansoura Kidney Center, the physicians, particularly since the last decade, exhibited both outward and inward

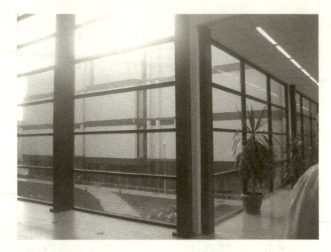

Figure 17. The interior of the Mansoura Kidney Center.
Photo by the author.

expressions of piety and religiosity; many of them were sympathetic to or were themselves official members of the Muslim Brotherhood, which holds a strong presence in Mansoura. And Mansoura's patients—of the nine million in population who are the rural inhabitants of Daqahliyya Province—expressed strongly cherished beliefs about the religious duty to care properly for dead bodies, about maintaining strong extended kinship ties, and about their place in the divine plan. Those who were involved in organ transplantation did not question whether that practice is proper or ethical; the medical results were compelling, the access equitable, and the rural poor felt justly and well treated.

The cases of Mansoura patients in the preceding chapters, in which marriages failed, pregnancies ended badly, guilt mounted, and the ability to attain a "fully normal life" after transplantation has faltered, all show the limits of a transplant's ability to really "cure" organ failure (Crowley-Matoka 2005). Patients might now have a body part that could function to pass urine, but life was far from normal again. The effects of disease continued to be felt, and new physical, emotional, and social burdens were added. Yet people in Mansoura's center generally did not blame organ transplantation itself for these shortcomings but rather blamed the intransigence of illness. Poor rural patients at the Mansoura Kidney Center were all immensely appreciative of the high-quality care they received, the respect with which they were treated, and the affordability of the treatment.

ROOM FOR HOPE?

The accomplishments at the Mansoura Kidney Center show disenchanted Egyptians that they have the potential to build successful medical institutions at the local level, founded initially with external funds and sustained by their own inhabitants, particularly when isolated from the unwieldy demands of Cairo's profit-driven medical landscape. This is particularly important to younger idealistic medical students but also to Egyptian intellectuals more generally. During my fellowship at the Center for Arabic Studies Abroad (2001–2), I distinctly remember a fellow American graduate student remarking that all Egyptians seem to do is complain about Egypt's many problems—corruption, backwardness, inequalities, poverty, crowdedness, pollution. She exclaimed, "Isn't there *anything* positive in Egypt today?" Our Egyptian professor of Arabic literature responded with an elaborate story about Dr. Mohamed Ghoneim from Mansoura and his accomplishments, both medical and ethical. Indeed, the first several times that I visited Mansoura, traveling along the *corniche* of the Nile, the inhabitants happily pointed me to the internationally renowned center, where they saw foreign students and residents come to study and train each year, the place they fondly refer to as "the center of Dr. Mohamed Ghoneim."

Another example of the pride the center invokes in Egyptians appears in a letter to the editor written to the newspaper *Al-Misri al-Yawm*, on March 24, 2009, in which a Cairo resident who suffered from kidney and bladder stones describes how he came to learn of an amazing center for treatment in Mansoura. After having visited a dilapidated and depressing theater hall in Mansoura, he went to the Mansoura Kidney Center, about which he writes, "And what a difference—the building was erected with the most modern marble tiles, surrounded by a garden filled with red flowers that welcomed visitors . . . leafy trees and the palm trees, and the peace of it, and the elevators, and the lounge chairs and the color of the furniture, and the neatly dressed nurses . . . ! My mind was overwhelmed by the level of cleanliness and precision of the place, as if I were in a hospital in Switzerland!" After his operation, the letter writer describes a surgery gone well and his great surprise to find that the services were free of charge to patients who could not afford the expense; he remarks, "I returned to Cairo full of praise and gratitude and prayers to those exemplary Egyptian scientists who achieved this miracle that restores self-confidence. . . . Ghoneim's international center is the pinnacle of modern achievement . . . !"[1]

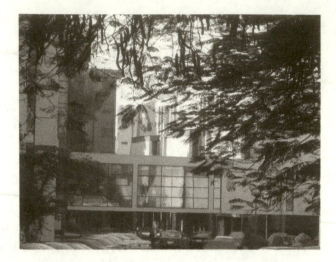

Figure 18.   Exterior of the Mansoura Kidney Center, built
on the grounds of a famous botanical garden. Photograph by
the author.

In April 2010, amid mass speculation as to whether Mohamed ElBaradei could successfully garner a meaningful democratic movement in Egypt
to counter decades of authoritarian rule, ElBaradei, the former director
general of the International Atomic Energy Agency and Nobel Peace laureate also visited the Mansoura Kidney Center during his campaign for
Egypt's presidency. In response to a personal invitation from Dr. Mohamed
Ghoneim, ElBaradei prayed with the doctor on a Friday during the Egyptian holiday weekend of *sham al-nasim* at al-Nour Mosque in Mansoura,
and later spoke to the local inhabitants. ElBaradei told them, "We must
move from a pharaonic regime to democracy. Egypt, with all its resources,
deserves better. It does not make sense that 40 per cent of the people are
still below the poverty line and 30 per cent are illiterate."[2] ElBaradei had
aligned himself with hope for a better Egypt by aligning himself with the
well-loved persona of Dr. Ghoneim.

But the question remains as to whether the Mansoura Kidney Center will be sustainable beyond the leadership of this charismatic doctor
of confidence. Did Dr. Ghoneim create a system that can maintain itself
beyond his direction, or is the center itself too much tied to a cult of an
authoritarian personality, all too familiar in Egyptian society? Many disaf-
fected professionals in Egypt complained to me about Egypt's syndrome
of the "one-man-show." A great organization, school, program, or center
might develop from the vision, leadership, and charisma of the founder,

only to fall apart as soon as the leader steps down. At one time, observers noted to me, the dietary requirements of all the patients at the Mansoura Kidney Center, based on their individual fluid and electrolyte statuses on a given day, were coordinated with the content of their individual hospital meals. So complete and seamless was the communication and organization of the center, from the physicians through the nurses to the cafeteria staff, that calorie, potassium, sodium, and protein levels were all adjusted daily to each patient. But since 2002, when Dr. Ghoneim stepped down from the directorship, according to some, the quality of patient services has already started to slip. Medical students, residents, and colleagues wonder what will happen when he retires completely. No one stepped beyond the bounds of his high standards out of love and fear under his authoritarian rule. How can this then be the "beacon of hope" in a country in which authoritarian rule is one of its many problems? When I spoke at length with a young heart surgeon working in Cairo in 2009, he told me excitedly about plans in Egypt to build a tertiary center for heart surgery, like the one Dr. Ghoneim had built for kidney and urological surgery in Mansoura, under the leadership of the world-famous heart transplant surgeon Dr. Magdi Yacoub. But a year later, this heart surgeon's excitement had diminished. He had grown disillusioned with what he called "yet another one-man-show" that seemed to offer few opportunities to build from the ground up or to train young aspiring doctors. Now looking to immigrate to Canada or the United States, this heart surgeon was joining a stream of medical professionals moving on elsewhere, leaving a deeper brain-drain in his wake.

The Mansoura Kidney Center should certainly inspire hope when one thinks of what has been accomplished by physicians adhering to high standards and social justice by blocking out medical corruption that was rampant in Cairo. In a provincial capital they have successfully built an alternative model in which the poor and the marginalized are treated with dignity and respect. Yet the question of whether this institution can continue as a counterexample to Egypt's broader medical landscape is a difficult one to answer. And it further raises the question of how one can begin to make a difference within Cairo itself. Young medical professionals doubt whether Mansoura has in fact changed the system at all, if, in order to exist as an alternative model, it has had to be tied so closely to an authoritarian and charismatic persona and has had to be so divorced from Cairo, Egypt's medical, political, and financial center. It seems to me, at the time of writing this, that only time and further research can fully answer these questions.

WAS THIS EVEN A RELIGIOUS DEBATE?

During the years that I conducted my research and worked on this book, friends and colleagues often asked me what my work was about. When I began to explain the issue of Egyptians' reluctance to accept organ transplantation, people looked disconcerted about what they assumed to be religious constraints to medical treatment. When I spoke of the black market in organs, uncertain surgical outcomes, or the high levels of toxicity and pollution, many would immediately appear relieved, more understanding, and more empathetic to my informants. It seemed reasonable, indeed rational, to them that people would consider medical efficacy in their treatment decisions. Yet they were disturbed by the mere thought of religion fostering antipathy to medical care.

I have tried, often unsuccessfully, to explain that these realms and logics are not mutually exclusive. People might come to *religious* positions by considering medical risk, safety, and efficacy, and these rubrics are further complicated by kinship and market logics. In frustration, I have realized that with our existing categories and analytical frameworks, the rift occurs not only because we tend to interpret "religious" practices in opposition to science but also because we have difficulty recognizing their hybrid nature at all.

Throughout the course of my fieldwork, I came across several transplant surgeons like Dr. Kotb, who admitted to me that they themselves would never undergo a transplant operation, because they believed that only God owns the body. In grappling with a way to make sense of this in my analysis, I found that our analytical toolbox in the social sciences leads us to view these discrepancies as ironic at best and hypocritical at worst. This has largely to do with our tendency to think of religious ethics as a set of codified rules that map onto or constrain practice, rather than viewing religious ethics as an embodied aspect of the self that is contingent on dynamic social processes (Asad 1993, 2003; Mahmood 2005; Hirschkind 2006; Agrama 2010). As Shaykh al-Marsafawy, an Azhar-educated religious scholar, once said to me about why he thought organ transplantation was *haram*, "Show me the day when organs travel from the rich to the poor. Then I might change my mind!"

In the Euro-American media, Muslim articulations against organ transplantation—assumed to be formulaically "religious"—are even deemed signals of "dangerous politics."[3] One popular book on contemporary Islam, written by Milton Viorst (1998), a self-proclaimed "Middle East expert," suggests that views on organ transplantation are indicative of the "liberal" or "conservative" leanings of particular muftis, which are essential to discern, because, as the back cover of Viorst's book describes, "without an opening-up of Islam, the Middle East will continue to lag far behind the West and even emerging Third World nations." Invoking the need to separate "good Muslim" from "bad Muslim" from the perspective of Western political interests (Mamdani 2004), Viorst specifically commends Shaykh Tantawi for permitting organ transplantation and for "challenging orthodoxy's contention that the body belongs to God" (1998: 44).

Shaykh Tantawi certainly never opposed the notion that the body belongs to God; to do so would be conceived of as meaningless. And it is unclear to whom Viorst refers when he describes this statement as "orthodoxy's contention." Yet the formulation that Islam is a constraint on scientific advancement and that this constraint condemns Muslims to lag behind on a linear march toward progress is certainly a pervasive sentiment. And it is not just the Euro-American media that rely on such assumptions when depicting Muslims or Islam. Even the Egyptian and other Arab media also, if describing a mainstream religious belief or practice that runs contrary to a nationalist ideal, often depict it as a gross distortion of religion, emblematic of dangerous or backward extremism (Abu-Lughod 2005; Hirschkind 2006). Journalists and physicians who consider themselves "progressive" have stated unabashedly that the views of the majority of Egypt's population are hindrances to "the advancement of science."

These commentators, in their pro-modern technology stance, seem not to have considered the stark differences in Egyptians' class positions in their assessments of organ transplantation's benefits and costs. The "transplant proponents" have failed to adequately address the vulnerabilities of the poor and the specific problems that arise when transplantation is practiced in a sharply stratified society. Of course, as Atul Gawande (2003, 2007) reminds us, all new medical skills and procedures, and even the routine training of new medical professionals every year, require risky experimentation on patients for the eventual improvement of medical technique. While organ transplantation had a rocky beginning in its early years in *every* place that it was practiced, in countries like Egypt the poor overwhelmingly and disproportionately suffered and continue to bear the brunt of the risks and uncertain outcomes of high-technological medical interventions. With the entrenchment of a black market in kidneys, exposés about the political etiologies of kidney and liver disease, and widely circulated reports of organ theft, it is more important than ever for everyone to acknowledge the vulnerabilities of the poor to exploitation and the results of state negligence.

Even Shaykh Sha'rawi, who argued in theologically abstract terms, still identified with the marginalized and criticized transplantation from the angle of inequality. His critics dismissed his arguments as a backward opposition to a potentially life-saving procedure. Yet the vast majority of dialysis patients who have been diagnosed as "in need of" a kidney and who informed this study explained their reluctance to pursue transplantation by affirming that their bodies, indeed, belong to God. They believed that God's creation should be protected from practices that promote social inequalities. Such beliefs did not prevent them from seeking treatment that would otherwise have solved their problems. Quite the contrary, their experiences made clear to them that this "treatment" could bring a host of problems of its own.

This brings us to a pressing question that remains unanswered: Was antipathy to organ transplantation in Egypt due to religion, or was it the result of the sociomedical problems it engendered? Related to this, we should ask: Are the problems of corruption, commodification, and theft intrinsic to the practice of organ transplantation in Egypt, or can they be separated from it? Disagreements over this question, that is, over the nature of organ transplantation itself and its potential for benefits and harms to Egyptian society, have fueled the organ transplant controversy. This question is what has led to disagreements among scholars—not one over scriptural interpretation or traditionalism. It illuminates little to ask who is a "liberal" or "progressive" or who is "traditional" or "conservative." Rather, we should interrogate who is really benefiting and who is not, what factors are calculated into assessments of "benefit," and how much benefit legitimates the undeniable suffering that has accompanied organ transplantation in Egypt.

In other words, to ask if antipathy toward organ transplantation derives from "Islam" or if it actually derives from an examination of social inequalities or medical efficacy misses the ways in which these interrelated factors *inform* Muslim ethical positions. When parents gift their organs to their children, they are doing what they can to correct the misfortune of seeing their children weaker than they, because they believe that life should flow from old to young. Ideas of gender and family role also inform decision making. Those without the "right" kin to gift them kidneys work to cultivate religious fortitude in themselves to foster the strength and steadfastness required to live with terminal illness and without the hope of life-saving treatment.

Thus, religion is not an a priori aspect of people's identities, nor is it merely an object external to people, something that they grab hold of to manipulate. When we ask whether the opposition to organ transplants in Egypt is due to Islam or actually due to issues such as social inequalities and geopolitical realities, we are analytically putting explanatory categories in opposition to each other, even though they are necessarily intertwined.

That is, social realities and religious experiences are mutually constitutive. Religious ethics, like bioethics, can be reasoned only in the context of particular social conditions (e.g., family relations, medical access and efficacy) and is necessarily informed by these conditions.

Indeed, the patients in this study themselves understood ethical formulations to be contingent upon the specificities of their social circumstances. Thus, they did not see themselves as "moral pioneers," as did the pregnant American women whom Rayna Rapp interviewed who, when they received a test result indicating that their fetuses bore the risk for genetic disease, were put in the position of choosing which lives were worth living and which should be ethically terminated before birth. Rapp captured a situation in which body-altering and life-prolonging biotechnologies shifted the social terrain so fast that ethical and legal norms could not keep pace (see also Fischer 2003). But my informants in Egypt did not perceive themselves to be in such a situation, because they understood the ethical and the social terrain as mutually constitutive. They would often maintain that Islam, as the ultimate ethical source, could address questions of "every time and place" *(li kulli makan wa zaman).* This is because they did not view religious ethics as an abstract realm to be mapped onto the social world. When they claimed that the body belongs to God, they were not merely invoking the words attributed to Shaykh Shaʿrawi as a memorized formula of Islamic "orthodoxy." Rather, patients, physicians, and religious scholars reiterated that the body belongs to God in the context of their larger grievances against state mismanagement of resources, exploitation of the bodies of the poor, questionable outcomes of transplantation, and underground trafficking rings, as well as within the context of cultural and social values that idealize dispositions of steadfastness and fortitude in the face of unavoidable suffering. Religious beliefs and timeless theological truths about God's purpose in creating human life gain new meanings when they are uttered in social and political-economic contexts that constrain, define, and enable possibilities of how that human life is lived.

UNBINDING AND REBINDING

The argument that ethical formulations are socially contingent should be an obvious one to muftis and other experts of Islamic legal-ethics, for whom study of the social sphere has long been recognized as an important factor in the formulation of jurisprudence (Kamali 1991; Messick 1993, 1996; Masud, Messick, et al. 1996; Hallaq 1997, 2001; Skovgaard-Petersen 1997;

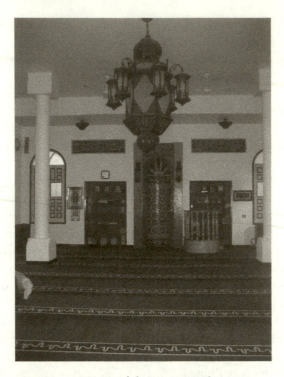

Figure 19.   Interior of the mosque at the
Mansoura Kidney Center, where physicians and
staff congregate for the five daily prayers.
Photograph by the author.

Jackson 1999; Johansen 1999; Haykel 2003; Murad, n.d.). Yet the increasing
demand for codified "religious opinions" to speak to the entire nation in
absolutist terms undercuts the ways in which people can engage meaning-
fully with Islamic legal-ethics to guide their lived experiences. Further, processes of modern state formation have resulted in the continual narrowing
of the wide terrain of Muslim ethics to the circumscribed field of legal jurisprudence (Moosa 2005). Egyptians are continually navigating, on the one
hand, between the fast-moving currents that dynamically shape religious
ethics and, on the other, the rock-solid hyperessentializing of Islam that
has come to the fore in domestic and international discourses (Salvatore
1997; Salvatore and Eickelman 2004). When legislators seek "the Islamic"
position on treatments such as organ transplantation, they often summon
"Islam" as a static set of rules that impose themselves on daily practice.
When they demand that medical practice abide by "Islamic law," they risk

codifying and essentializing forms of daily practice—medical encounters and religious ethics—that are necessarily contingent and ever evolving. The friction between codification on the one hand and the dynamism of social practice on the other is part of widespread perceptions that both medical and Islamic authority are in a continual state of crisis.

But when we trouble the notion that medical practice or religious ethics needs to be viewed in static, reified codes of law, then we can start to see crisis as less inevitable. Why should religious sentiment's meaningful adaptation to its context be rendered a crisis? Why is it a crisis that people with vastly different experiences, opportunities, resources, health statuses, and family relations approach biotechnologies differently? Commentators in Egypt often pointed to Saudi Arabia and Iran—countries that presumably operate under Islamic law—as evidence that Egypt's reluctance to pass a law can't possibly be because of Islam. But why should countries with vastly different resources, demographic distributions, and medical programs arrive at the same Islamic position?

Deliberating over multiple perspectives seems only reasonable when the stakes are as high, for example, as redefining the moment of death. Given that the demise of different bodily processes occurs at different times, it is understandable that not everyone will agree on the same particular moment as the one that constitutes death, especially since death is an emotionally fraught and biologically complicated process. What, then, lies behind the assumption that medical practice—or, for that matter, religion—should be unified and universal in its response to ethical debates? And why has the authority to determine the "Islamic" answer been left to the sole purview of muftis or other experts in classical legal texts? Surely the increasing complexity and fragmentation of today's society require input from specialists in other disciplines, including social scientists. As we have seen, it takes much rigorous study and the input of many disciplines and perspectives to begin to tackle questions about benefit, risk, cost, and other bases upon which people decide what is ethical.

Throughout this book, I have attempted to give a faithful account of people's ethical reasoning without losing sight of the tensions between the social contingency and dynamism of the Islamic ethical tradition, on the one hand, and the political and legal attempts to codify that tradition, on the other. The narrower the space given to Islamic discourse—despite the potential richness of its debates, methodologies, theories of reasoning, and its wide range of legitimate opinions—the more likely that the *necessarily* contextual and plural voices will be read negatively, as a "crisis" of authority. And the more that religious authority is described as in a state of crisis, the more likely it is that rigid and myopic views will vie for *the* final, normative, legitimate position to settle all debate. The force by which nationalist discourses have insisted on the singularization of modernity and the ways in which Islamist movements have mirrored this singularization with their own hyperessentialized Islamist platform have had a dramatic effect on the ways in which Egyptians themselves tend to understand plurality and divergence of opinion through the rubric of "crisis" (see Salvatore 1997). Meanwhile, the continual production and performance of crisis has long been in the interest of an authoritarian state and of protecting U.S. geopolitical stakes in the region, so that the suspension of the rule of law—Egypt's near-permanent emergency-law status—enables virtually unchecked power with little accountability.[4]

My research exposed to me the contradictions and complexities that high-tech biomedicine can entail, as well as to the contradictions and complexity of religious ethics. Each can offer salvation on the one hand and gross manipulation of power on the other. In this middle space between religious ethics and medical science, a delicate balance is always to be found between the imperatives to improve human conditions and to accept processes beyond our control. Often processes both within and beyond our control are understood to be the workings of nature or what many around the world conceive of, in one way or another, as divine will. Throughout the world, each introduction of modern technology—from the telegraph and the radio to contraception and prenatal genetic testing—provokes a rehearsal of this debate. The grand narrative of progress that technoscience tells of itself tends to elide questions about access, justice, and overall benefit. Thus, questions persist: If we can control nature's course, should we, or should it be considered God's will? If we should attempt that control, how best can we do so? The answers depend on a host of factors, foremost of which is how overall benefit, efficacy, and potential harm are defined and determined and by whom.

At the intersections between science studies and critical approaches to religion, we can rebind bioethics as a lived experience that is articulated in patients' discussions in their dialysis wards, in their care of their families, in their resignification of bureaucratic norms, at the knife's edge in a surgical theater, in the fatwas of Muslim scholars, and in the troubled hearts of those seeking to uphold values of social justice and self-care. By recalling the kidney failure patients as "cyborgs" (Haraway 1985)—both enmeshed in the tubes and networks of capital, economic development, electricity, substandard solvents, and human blood—we remember that there is never a "pure" body outside its social environment, there is no recuperable "pure" precolonial past, and there is no "pure" pristine Egyptian landscape to which we can return. The hybridity, enmeshment, and messiness in which we live should not seem problematic or crisis ridden. Medicine is less efficacious when it disregards the lived experiences of its patients, and religious claims are less meaningful when they do not correspond to believers' lived realities. An abstract religious argument like Sha'rawi's, which sought a blanket condemnation based on the "body belonging to God," misses the multiple ways in which people trace their belonging to God through their lived experiences. Sha'rawi was wrong to think that a wholesale rejection of a particular biotechnology was necessary for people to remember divine omnipotence. And secularists across the world are wrong to think that efficacious life-altering biotechnologies will soon make religion obsolete. Many contemporary Muslims have proven that technoscientific possibilities can, under particular circumstances, strengthen their connection to the divine Creator. Sha'rawi underestimated the potential of people to understand their lives on dialysis, their potential for recovery, and even test results that dash their hopes for a transplant all as the workings of a merciful God. As the dialysis patients remind us, a wholesale rejection of technoscience or the state—pulling out the dialysis tubing or the electrical cord—is neither practical nor desirable for those who care about social justice. It is in the engagement, negotiation, and appreciation of multiple voices and perspectives that we can get closer to representing and better manipulating the world in which we live.

Epilogue

The Ongoing Struggle for Human Dignity

On January, 25, 2011, a day meant to celebrate the Egyptian police force, protestors gathered at Tahrir Square in the middle of Cairo to call for justice and human dignity. Egyptians throughout the country were in no mood to honor the police. One of the calls for the demonstrations came from a Facebook group called *We are all Khalid Saʿid*, in reference to a twenty-eight year old Egyptian from Alexandria, who had uploaded onto the internet a video of police sharing the spoils of a drug bust. In retaliation, members of the police and security apparatus dragged him out of an internet cafe near his home and beat him to death. The Egyptian security forces tied to the interior ministry, together with the police were known for protecting a corrupt regime with utter disregard for the people. Images of Khalid's savagely disfigured corpse circulated on the internet. When his family asked for his body at the morgue, the medical report following the autopsy denied the violence done to his body.

More than eight hundred peaceful protestors were killed in the eighteen days that followed. The surviving protestors stood more resolute than ever after deadly violence was unleashed upon them by the police and armed thugs hired by the ruling party, corrupt business-owners and security forces. In the end, the protestors for revolutionary change prevailed, and Mubarak resigned from the presidency on February 11, 2011.

On May 28, 2011, I was back in Cairo, and I went to Tahrir Square to join the demonstrations that were organized to protect the initial aims of what is now called the January 25 revolution. Afterward, I went straight from the square to Agouza to see my uncle Ali, who, in his youth, was held without trial as a political prisoner for four years. This injustice was what led my father, Ali's younger brother, to leave Egypt. When Uncle Ali saw me, he cried tears of joy and told me that the victory of the popular revolt

253

could be understood in no other way than as a *miracle* from God. It is true that now, four months after the protests began, most people are cautiously optimistic, realizing that the regime has been decapitated while its roots are desperately clinging to power. But even in considering the formidable obstacles to change, there is a general realization that much has been accomplished. Finding a way to bring people together to demand basic decency and respect, finding a way to express words for the humiliation and pain of injustice—these achievements should not be underestimated.

I finished writing this book months before anyone dreamed of such an astonishing number of peaceful protestors precipitating the end of Mubarak's rule. Looking back at the years that I spent researching and writing, I feel as if I had spent a decade trying to make sense of the cacophony of a debate by trying to distill its elements and untangle its rhetoric, all so that I could tune in and make audible an underlying muted language. I struggled to decipher the meanings of pauses, the import of sighs, grimaces, and gestures. Amidst the vociferous assertions and argumentation, there was so much that went unspoken. But now there are words, audible and clear. *We have been denied our dignity.* Dignity! *Karama!* It was a word that I had been grasping at, as I tried to figure out what this book was about, and why I had intuited that these stories—about bodies in life and death, about injustice, suffering, and forbearance—revealed something even larger than the lives of the people who told them. After the protestors' exhilaration at Mubarak's resignation, another slogan emerged, asserting that dignity would be restored even in the face of atrocity: Hold your head up high, you are an Egyptian! (*irfaʿ rasak inta masri!*)

When the violence was at its highest, the protestors were not deterred; only more came out of their homes in solidarity. Neither did the regime's forces succeed in provoking the protestors to return the violence. The amazement of what could be accomplished with determination was coupled with sorrow that the regime had brutally repressed this great repository of strength and willpower that might otherwise have brought the country forward. The inspiring and multifaceted solidarity that was forged and displayed in the initial eighteen days of resistance at Tahrir square—across religious, class, and gender differences—symbolized to many the ideal enactment of what Egyptians *could be*. But outside of that circumscribed space and time, people were also awakened to the depths of desperation and despair, of the numbers of Egyptians who, having been deprived of basic human dignity and respect, may not have the same moral repository from which to act. If the days of Tahrir Square summoned Egyptians to enact their highest ideals—patience, steadfastness, wit, humor, solidarity, generosity, peacefulness—the pressures against them still threaten to rob them even of these.

As we celebrated the victory, we knew all too well that it was still too early. While amazed at the moral superiority enacted in those days at Tahrir, many in Egypt fear that the large-scale destruction of human health, vitality, and the social fabric that sustains these morals will be insurmountable. As I write, the regime is still in power, justice has not been served, the thieves have not been tried, the money stolen has not been returned, and those who murdered the demonstrators have yet to be held accountable. But a beginning has been forged—fear and silence have been broken, and ordinary citizens are now actively redefining what it is to be Egyptian.

This book poses questions about how people formulate ethical positions that make life meaningful, even or especially as that life is threatened. It is about what it means to call for ethics, or even the ethical "best" option within the context of rampant inequalities and a corrupt and brutally repressive regime. At the heart was a simple matter, even if the answer to how to attain it is not. *Karama.*

Notes

PREFACE

1. This phrase comes from Bronislaw Malinowski, who wrote that the goal of the cultural anthropologist or ethnographer is "to grasp the native's point of view, his relation to life, to realize his vision of his world" (1961: 25). Of course, anthropologists have since critically revealed the limitations of the term *native* and have also since broadened the goals of anthropology.

2. See Sholkamy 1999 for a discussion of the difficulties of doing social science research in Egypt and Kaufman 2000 about the delicacies of social science research in difficult medical situations.

INTRODUCTION

The opening epigraphs are headlines from, respectively, *Al-Liwa' al-Islami*, September 14, 1988; *Al-Liwa' al-Islami*, October 31, 1991; *Akhir Sa'a*, September 30, 1992; and *Al-Akhbar*, October 21, 1990.

1. The idea of organ transplantation as "life-saving but death-ridden" comes from Renée Fox, as cited by Scheper-Hughes (2002: 74).

2. *Al-Ahram*, November 24, 2008.

3. A law was passed in 1962 for the establishment of a national eye bank. However, as I detail in chapter 3, the conditions for extracting eyes from the dead were not legally enforced, leading to a national scandal and the shutdown of the eye banks in the mid-1990s.

4. The *infitah* ("opening") under President Sadat in the 1970s entailed the partial relaxation of state control over transnational flows of labor, capital, and goods and a series of legislative changes to attract foreign investment, to stimulate the domestic private sector, and to liberalize foreign trade (Wickham 2002: 37).

5. See, for example, the column by Sana' al-Bisi in *Al-Ahram*, January 26, 2006. She laments the current state of stagnancy and degradation and complains,

in exaggeration, that Egypt is the only country in the world without a national organ transplant law.

6. See Armbrust 1996 and Abu-Lughod 2005 for descriptions of the Egyptian state media's depictions of the "ignorant masses."

7. See Fox and Swazey 2008 for an analysis of the different narratives of the "birth" or "creation" of bioethics.

8. See Gregg and Saha 2006; Kleinman and Benson 2006; and Lock 2001 for the ways that "culturalist" analyses obscure an array of social, political, and economic processes that shape the clinical encounter.

9. See Agrama 2010 for a discussion of how the practice of requesting and receiving fatwas has long gone unrecognized in anthropology as an ethical practice.

10. The model of four principles is elaborated in the influential text *Principles of Biomedical Ethics*, the first edition of which was written in the 1970s by Georgetown University philosophers Tom Beachamp and James Childress, as the basis for a common morality to guide biomedical research and practice and was instrumental to the institutionalization of bioethics in the United States as well as other countries (Beauchamp and Childress 2001). See Fox and Swazey 2008 and Moazam 2006 for a discussion of this model and for a fascinating research study of how it was exported and adopted by the medical community in Pakistan.

11. From June 2001 to June 2002 I was a fellow at the Center for Arab Studies Abroad, an intensive Arabic program, during which time I followed press reports about the organ transplant debate and conducted some interviews with doctors and medical students. After this I devoted my full attention to research among doctors, medical students, journalists, religious scholars, and patients.

12. See Rapp 1999 for an analysis of the ways in which the "experts" of genetic screening failed to anticipate the complex reception of amniocentesis among women.

13. In 2001, the Egyptian Society of Nephrology estimated that 25,518 Egyptians were on dialysis and since this time has not updated the data (Afifi 2001).

14. At the Faculty of Medicine in Tanta University, urologists, nephrologists, and surgeons had once started a transplant program as an "experiment" in the late 1980s, but they reportedly "did not have success" with the patients. This, I soon learned, was a euphemistic way of saying that recipients, and in some cases even donors, died during or immediately after the operations. The doctors soon stopped the program. The physicians I spoke with in Tanta claimed that they still had the skills and experience to reinitiate their own transplant program but that it had been thwarted for a host of bureaucratic and inner-administrative reasons.

15. See Skovgaard-Petersen 1997 for a detailed account of the social transformations of the Dar al-Ifta' in Egypt.

16. The archives of many of the fatwas of Dar al-Ifta' are now accessible online.

17. For this I relied on the archives at the Al Ahram Information Center in Cairo.

18. For example, 'Amr al-Laythi is one such investigative reporter on the popular television news program *Wahid min al-nas,* which is broadcast on the Dream satellite channel. On a show aired on December 18, 2009, al-Laythi took his camera crew to a poor neighborhood in the October 6th district of Cairo called al-Rawahi. Following his interviews with people with alarming rates of kidney and liver failure in this newly built neighborhood, he investigated the water purification station, which was hidden from public sight by tall fences. He found that the facility had been built just above the sewage system and that a private water company was pumping water contaminated with sewage into the neighborhood water supply. The show had the water analyzed in a laboratory and found that it contained high levels of iron and that a large percentage of the thirty thousand neighborhood residents had kidney and liver diseases. In a heartbreaking scene, an elderly man openly wept, exclaiming that all he asked for from the government was clean water that he and his family could drink without getting sick.

19. Egypt's dreams of emancipation through greater control of its resources (with massive development projects like the Aswan High Dam) have resulted in adverse health effects not only for its own population but also for the populations of African countries upstream from it, who still face droughts and unstable food security. This has not gone unnoticed by government leaders in Rwanda, Ethiopia, Uganda, and Tanzania. See Hassan 2010.

20. Medical anthropologists have long criticized the tendency to blame the patient for his or her own condition, as well as the general focus on individual risk reduction in contemporary society. See also Beck 1992 and Sontag 2001 for further discussion of risk.

21. See Fassin's (2001) discussion regarding the problematic use of "cultural difference" as an explanation for patient noncompliance. See also Rapp 1997: 33.

22. I did not systematically include views of Coptic Christians in Egypt, who constitute an estimated 10 percent of the population. During the course of fieldwork in the hospital settings, I came across enough Coptic patients to offer some preliminary analysis; briefly, I found that Coptic patients had similar misgivings about organ transplantation, in terms of worries about harm to the donor, organ theft, and the black market in human body parts. The Coptic patients whom I interviewed discussed the same political etiologies, linking renal failure to pollution and the directionality of organs in the same kinship patterns described by Muslims. However, Egyptian Copts did not tend to speak of their misgivings in terms of the body belonging to God. Sociological, historical, and anthropological research on Copts in Egypt and on their relations with fields of medical expertise and with the increasing dominance of Islamic rhetoric in biomedical and other public settings is clearly needed.

23. This is in contrast to much work in the anthropology of bioethics that seeks to point out the differences among various cultural and ethical approaches to medicine across societies.

24. Lock reports that even after the first one hundred heart transplants in the United States, public opinion regarding transplantation was negative (2002b: 86). However, in a 1995 article she indicates a shift in public opinion such that transplantation was talked about in terms of the "gift of life," despite unfavorable survival rates for grafts and patients (391).

25. Layla al Marmush, from the *Hilal al Tibbi*, covered these stories; this information is based on personal communication with her and with liver transplant surgeons. However, quantifying the number of donor deaths accurately is difficult if not impossible, because they often go unreported. Liver transplant surgeons who do report their results in international medical journals report that *only* 10 percent of donors have serious complications after surgery, a percentage they consider to be evidence that liver lobe transplantation is a safe procedure. See, for example, Esmat, Yosry, et al. 2005; and Trotter, Adam, et al.2006.

26. As Talal Asad writes: "The term local peoples—now increasingly used by ethnographers instead of the older primitive, tribal, simple, preliterate, and so on—can be misleading in an interesting way and calls for some unpacking. Saudi theologians who invoke the authority of medieval Islamic texts are taken to be local; Western writers who invoke the authority of modern secular literature claim they are universal. Yet both are located in universes that have rules for inclusion and exclusion" (1993: 8).

27. Propaganda at the time of the Free Officers' Coup of 1952 claimed that, under King Farouk, one-third of the rural population was blind. While it was in the interest of the propagandists to exaggerate numbers, by all accounts blindness was widely prevalent (Hamdy 2005).

28. For the ways in which contingent social categories become naturalized as "types" of people, see Hacking 1999.

CHAPTER ONE

1. Those interested in Islamic reform may or may not be part of Islamist political groups, and in any case there is wide variation within this term. As Wickham writes, "The Islamic movement in Egypt in the 1980s and early 1990s encompassed a multitude of groups and organizations working in different ways to promote Islamic change. No single agenda united them, as their understandings of how Islam should be applied to contemporary social and political life and how Islamic change could best be achieved varied widely. Moreover, many of those in the Islamic movement did not openly identify with an Islamic *political* group or organization" (2002: 112).

2. This doctor has published prolifically in English medical journals under the spelling Mohamed Ghoneim. Muhammad Ghunaym is the academic transliteration of the Arabic spelling, based on the modified *International Journal of Middle East Studies (IJMES)*.

3. Nephrology and hemodialysis treatment are subspecialties of internal medicine, whereas urology is a subspecialty of surgery.

4. This was in Mansoura University Hospital, before the Mansoura Kidney Center was established, and what the center's staff refers to as the "mother hospital."

5. Transplant operations were conducted experimentally in the United States in the 1950s and 1960s, and the failure and death rates (when donor and recipient were not identical twins) were high until the late 1970s, when powerful immunosuppressive drugs were developed to control the rate of the rejection of donated organs (Fox and Swazey 1974).

6. Zamalek is the standard English spelling. In Arabic, the neighborhood is known as al-Zamalik.

7. Schistosomiasis is also known as "bilharzias," named after the German pathologist Theodor Bilharz, who identified the snail-transmitted parasite responsible for the disease in 1851. Egyptologists have found the eggs of schistosome parasites in preserved mummies, suggesting that this has been an endemic problem for millennia (see Lambert-Zazulak, Rutherford, et al. 2003), although its incidence has increased and decreased according to many factors, including climate change, water treatment and access, damming and irrigation practices, malnutrition and other forms of immunilogical stress, and access to efficatious health care. Dr. Ghoneim exclaimed that Egypt was the center of the battlefield, in an interview that I conducted with him in January 2008. His commitment to Mansoura and his challenge to the Cairo-centrism of Egyptian medicine are pervasive in his writings, work, and his reputation throughout Egypt. The information from this chapter about Mansoura is based on participant-observation there, previous interviews with Dr. Mohamed Sobh, senior nephrologist at Mansoura Kidney Center, the center's many publications, and interviews that I conducted between 2002 and 2004 with many other residents, fellows, and attendants there. I should also note that, according to many physicians with whom I spoke, creating an internationally renowned tertiary care center accessible to the poor would have been much more difficult (if not impossible) to accomplish in Cairo, given its complex and politically charged medical landscape.

8. The official name is Mansoura Urology and Nephrology Center. However, I refer to it throughout the text as the "Mansoura Kidney Center," to come closer to the Arabic phrase generally used for it (*markaz al-kila*).

9. The center is impeccably clean, patients are well fed and well cared for, and follow-up treatments are meticulously organized. Seventeen units within the center provide hemodialysis for two thousand patients with kidney disease (Ghoneim, Bakr, et al. 2001). One of the keys to its success lies in requiring all its physicians to work at the center full-time, thus preventing them from running private clinics on the side. The physicians at the center are paid salaries large enough to live comfortably, and unlike the physicians in any teaching university hospital in Cairo, they spend the bulk of their time treating patients, conducting both clinical and basic science research, and publishing in international medical journals. Mansoura residents are exceptionally proud

of the accomplishments of Ghoneim and his colleagues, as well as the medical fame that their small provincial capital has achieved. Some particularly important contributions that the Mansoura Kidney Center has made to the international medical research on transplantation have resulted from (1) its ability to follow patients in this single center with a uniform treatment regimen (as opposed to much U.S. research, which combines results of patients from various transplant centers) and (2) the "racial" homogeneity of its patient population, which can hold particular variables constant (in contrast to U.S. research, which has noted discrepancies in graft survival among different racial groups in its population) (Ghoneim, Bakr, et al. 2001; El-Husseini, El-Basuony, et al. 2004; El-Husseini, El-Basuony, et al. 2005; Sabry, El-Agoudy, et al. 2005; El-Husseini, Foda, et al. 2006).

10. Mansoura's records indicate that 43 kidney transplants took place from 1976 to 1983 (an average of 6 transplants per year), compared with the 1,458 performed between 1983 and 2002 (an average of 77 per year).

11. See Rutherford for a discussion of the ways in which the Muslim Brotherhood has called for increased governmental accountability and "regularly challenges and delegitimizes abuses of power by invoking Islamic principles of law and governance" (2008: 2).

12. Egyptian society is diglossic; that is, formal and written communications are rendered in modern standard Arabic, whereas spontaneous verbal communication is in Egyptian colloquial Arabic. The Egyptian medical sphere might be described as triglossic, with the third dominant language being English. All medical schools in Egypt provide instruction in English (lectures, notes, exams, and all text materials are in English), yet the clinical encounter takes place in Egyptian colloquial Arabic. Egyptian physicians are largely unfamiliar with medical terminology in standard or classical Arabic.

13. *Ghasil*, or "washing," refers to the kidney doing the washing (or, in the case of dialysis, the machine doing kidney-like washing), but it is the blood that is washed.

14. Note that patients distinguish this type of washing from washing the body or ritual ablutions *(wudu')*. The painful washing of the dialysis sessions is understood as an internal wash, to purify the blood of toxins.

15. Vulnerability to blood contamination is especially high among patients whose insurance does not cover the expensive (imported) erythropoietin injections that help reduce the need for blood transfusions.

16. In Egyptian colloquial Arabic, people often say, "I shall give you my eyes," to mean "I would do anything for you." Ragia's husband evoked this expression in a more literal reference to Ragia's blindness, although they both knew that such a transplant was not possible and would not enable Ragia to see.

17. In chapters 5 and 6, we will hear more directly from dialysis patients who were forced to discontinue work and experienced emotional, financial, and family strains.

18. See Jain 2010 on how such hope is put to use in clinical trials to recruit study participants.

19. As will be discussed in chapters 5, 6, and 7, buying a kidney was generally considered "worse" than accepting one from a family member, especially when people invoked religious language. However, some argued that paying for a kidney is better, because it saves their family members from having to undergo this burden and simultaneously "helps" a poor person monetarily.

20. There were, however, questions as to the efficacy and ethics of dialysis upon its first introduction. Many patients recalled to me having seen the horrific effects of past generations of dialysis machines on kidney-failure patients, who would "get immensely swollen" before the machine would brutally extract kilos and kilos of water from them. In its early years, many patients shunned dialysis, which was, in any case, not as accessible as it is today.

21. A few dialysis units existed in Egypt in the 1980s, and these were limited to urban centers and teaching hospitals.

22. For example, the show *Wahid min al-nas (Wahed Men El Nas)*, hosted by 'Amr al-Laythi (Amr El-Lithy).

23. Sandra Lane (1993) argues that patients and medical practitioners have vastly different definitions of what entails blindness or visual disability. Many patients who would be considered blind by medical standards do not consider themselves blind or even visually handicapped but merely as having weak sight.

24. These were operations for cataracts (referred to as "white water"; *mayya bayda* in Egyptian Arabic) and glaucoma (referred to as "blue water"; *mayya zarqa*).

25. Maghraby's chain of hospitals, eye centers, and optometry clinics stretch throughout the Middle East, Africa, and South Asia. Through Maghraby's initiatives, the equipment and skills for eye banking were established in Egypt's major public hospitals in 1987. At the time of my fieldwork (2002–4), Maghraby was the only government-compensated facility that provided cornea transplants (from imported grafts) for the poor. Ophthalmologists working in the public teaching hospitals often voiced resentment that Maghraby recruited the best residents and had somehow secured government relations that accorded them privileges. Several ophthalmologists suggested to me that there was something "suspicious" about the government "keeping" the public eye banks closed. As I explain fully in chapter 3, public access to corneas in Egypt was closed in 1996 with a legal decree to shut down teaching hospitals' public eye banks, following several scandals of allegations of eye theft. When these public banks were open, using local sources for corneas, the cost was only 240 £E per cornea graft. Now the government compensates poor patients who receive internationally imported cornea grafts at Maghraby, which cost 11,000–15,000 £E per cornea graft.

26. As part of the ethical procedures for interviewing human subjects, I began by telling all patients that all information would be kept confidential and that their names would not appear in any publications. However, Muhammad responded defensively and insisted that his name be written, stating that his illness was not something of which to be ashamed.

27. Medical anthropologist Soheir Morsy (1988) notes that even so-called Islamic clinics in Egypt (those established by social groups that aim to further "Islamize" Egyptian civil society), which operate alongside clinics provided by the state, do not offer an alternative medical model but are another elaboration of what she calls "biomedical hegemony."

28. Weber uses "ideal type" as an etic category of analysis, referring to the "construction of certain elements of reality into a logically precise conception" (see Gerth and Mills 1965: 59). In this case it is an emic ideal type that emerges in contemporary fatwas and nationalist narratives. For a very similar account of medical practice around kidney transplantation in Pakistan, see the work of Dr. Farhat Moazam, a pediatric surgeon and bioethical researcher who discusses how doctors are seen as doing "God's work" in Pakistani society (Moazam 2006).

29. "*Arif rabbina*" is literally one who "knows God," which implies knowing (what God has commanded to be) right or wrong and acting accordingly.

30. By "national narrative" I mean that this is how Ghoneim is depicted in the media and how he is famously and popularly known throughout Egypt.

31. For a similar account of medical practice and kidney transplantation in Pakistan, see Moazam's discussion of how doctors are seen as doing "God's work," albeit within a broken and corrupt system (2006).

32. The medical syndicate and the faculties of medicine at Egyptian public universities were politicized arenas, in which members of the Muslim Brotherhood and other opposition political groups, known for criticizing Egypt's heavy economic reliance on the United States, were closely monitored and excluded from university faculty positions. Mubarak's regime continued to operate under a "state of emergency," routinely arresting and detaining political opponents without trial. Ever since the assassination of President Sadat in 1981, Egypt has been under a continuous state of emergency. See El-Ghobashy 2006 for a discussion of its effect on the Egyptian polity and potential for political change. Reform of the extended uses and abuses of the emergency law was one of the calls of the popular protests in Cairo that began on January 25, 2011. One of the accomplishments of the popular revolts was to garner the promise to lift the emergency law after the first elections are held in September 2011.

33. Medicine remains one of the most prestigious specialties in Egypt, and all specialties are determined by one's results in taking the standardized national high school exams *(al thanawiyya al 'amma)*. Much discussion in Egypt centers on the sorry state of national education, of how faculty members in both public and private schools, from elementary to postgraduate levels, are paid such low salaries that in order to make ends meet they depend on private lessons (see also Armbrust 1996; Haeri 2003; and Abu-Lughod 2005). Thus, it has been in their financial interest *not* to teach well in the schools but to make students dependent on private lessons in order to learn enough to pass exams, although the cost of these lessons is an extreme burden on the average family. The issue of private lessons has made a mockery of standardization and "equal opportunity" *(takaful al-furas)* in national education, because clearly

the wealthier children have been the ones who can afford the best private lessons that teach to the test. If the students are lucky enough to score in the top percentile of the country, they rank specializations according to their interest, and medicine has to be ranked first if they are to stand a chance of admission. Furthermore, all medical faculties in Egypt use English as the official language of instruction, putting those students who were schooled in "private language" schools in an advantageous position. Meanwhile, official tuition rates at public institutions have been merely token amounts. For a discussion of the legacy of British colonial rulers who decreed that Arabic was a language "unfit for the sciences," see Cromer 1908. See Wickham 2002: 30,36 for a discussion of the political implications of the Egyptian state exams.

34. University tuition was reduced in 1956 and 1961 and then virtually abolished, aside from nominal fees, in 1962. (See Wickham 2002: 26 for a discussion of this.)

35. See Alaa Shukrallah 2012 on the politics of health in Egypt.

36. The problem with obtaining corpses for the purposes of medical education is similar to the problem of obtaining cornea grafts from corpses for transplantation, as will be discussed in chapter 3. Few family members are willing to turn over the bodies of their deceased. Officially, the corpses are supposed to be obtained from accident victims who have no surviving family members to claim them (and who may already be disfigured). Satisfying both of these conditions is considered difficult if not impossible; as one ophthalmologist put it: "Who doesn't have family members?"

37. Furthermore, it has been difficult for medical graduates to open their own private clinics, and many medical graduates have remained unemployed (Morsy 1988). Many students feel slighted by a system of nepotism, pointing to the ease with which well-to-do daughters and sons of physicians can pass the exams (in many cases, oral) and open up clinics, inheriting the capital and the reputation and, therefore, a ready patient base. These questions of inequality have been exacerbated in recent years by the proliferation of private medical schools for the first time in Egypt. The question of their legitimacy has been widely disputed; initially, it was unclear whether the graduates of these new faculties would be granted licenses by the Medical Syndicate and be able to practice in Egypt. (They were, not surprisingly, granted these licenses in the end.) Meanwhile, many graduates of the state medical faculties in place have remained unemployed or underemployed in fields other than medicine (Morsy 1988).

38. This current group of young scholars had studied under Shaykh ʿAli Gumaʿa, who was appointed grand mufti of Egypt at the time of my fieldwork. Shaykh ʿAmr says that the pursuit of any curriculum must begin with three questions: Who am I? What knowledge do I want to gain? How do I reach this knowledge? He feels that the biggest problem facing Muslims, aside from having lost a sense of traditional Islamic scholarship, concerns the first question: "We as Muslims have lost a sense of who we are." The curriculum should be based on deep knowledge of four disciplines: Islamic jurisprudence *(usul*

al-fiqh), religious principles *(usul al-din),* logic *('ilm al-mantiq),* and philology *('ilm al-lugha).* According to Shaykh 'Amr, these four disciplines constitute the fundamentals of the tradition; the Muslim scholar should also be philosophically concerned with the transmission of such knowledge and religiously concerned with the question of how to apply this knowledge to his or her life.

39. Shaykh 'Amr taught Muslim students from various countries, many of whom were American and acquiring degrees in the United States. He told me that in Egypt the modern educational system was inflexible and discouraged interdisciplinary work, but because I was in a U.S. institution, I could simultaneously explore philosophy, Islamic studies, medicine, sociology, anthropology, history, and so forth. When I confirmed his impression of my work, he smiled broadly at this type of intellectual freedom, which I seemed to take for granted.

40. On several occasions, Muslims involved with Sufi practice have explained Sufism to me by drawing a circle with a dot in the center, with the *circumference* representing God's (exoteric) command, the *shari'a,* and the *radius* to the center representing the Sufi *tariqa,* or mystic order (the esoteric path to pleasing God). However, Shaykh 'Amr did not explain his circle and dot this way; he wanted merely to point out that all human action, will, and thought should be done with the Creator in mind.

41. *Maslaha* literally refers to benefit or public welfare and is a tool of Islamic jurisprudence used to secure a benefit or to prevent possible harm. The concept of *maslaha* in Islamic legal theory was tangibly defined and elaborated upon by al-Ghazali (d. 505/1111), among other scholars. Al-Ghazali and other Muslim scholars categorized the *maqasid* (aims toward benefit) of Islamic law into five groupings, listed here in order of relative importance: the preservation of life *(al-nafs),* religion *(al-din),* intellect *(al-'aql),* lineage or offspring *(al-nasl),* and property *(al-mal).* These were also known as *al-daruriyyat al-khamsa* (Opwis 2005). Tools such as *maslaha* or *istihsan* (legal preference) are generally used to avoid rigidity in Islamic law and to ascertain the securement of the five *maqasid* listed above. Al-Ghazali argued that God's purpose in revealing the divine law is to preserve for humankind these five essential elements of their well-being (Opwis 2005: 188).

42. This is in contrast to other situations that anthropologists have described. For example, Matthew Gutmann (2007) describes how the state of Oaxaca in Mexico has declared that indigenous healing practice is equal to biomedicine in its legitimacy as a form of medical knowledge. (See also Farquhar 1994 and Langford 2002 on Ayurvedic medicine in India.) While Gutmann criticizes the state for making this rhetorical claim without providing practical support for indigenous health systems, even the rhetoric is unimaginable in the Egyptian context, where any healing practice other than that based on biomedical knowledge is unselfconsciously derided as "ignorance."

43. Religion in Egypt, at the national level, is framed in terms of either Islam or Coptic Christianity.

44. I thank my student Mark Caine for the term *(com)modification.*

CHAPTER TWO

1. Tantawi's answer to the question about brain death, that it was the same answer that he gave to other questions about medical ethics, including those about organ grafting and sex-change surgery (see Skovgaard-Petersen 1997).

2. Christian Barnard, the surgeon who carried out the first heart transplant in South Africa in 1967, boldly made the case that the donor was "dead" when he extracted her heart and transplanted it into the recipient (Lock 2002b: 82).

3. Of course, the extent to which someone can be a "native anthropologist" has been debated. See Spivak 1988; Narayan 1993; and Rosaldo 1993.

4. Many doctors in Egypt work combining nephrology and urology.

5. Linda Hogle (1999) explains German physicians' reluctance to take part in tissue procurement in terms of "national memory." They are haunted, she argues, by memories of state violence and its links to biomedical practice.

6. This is supported by Margaret Lock's (2002a, 2002b) anthropological fieldwork and interviews with thirty-two intensive care specialists in North America.

7. That is, transplantation using organs from various sources, such as: (1) a dead person with prior consent (2) a dead person with the consent of surviving relatives, (3) a dead person without either form of consent, (4) a living person who donates altruistically (5) a living person motivated by financial compensation.

8. Egypt's legal system is derived from French and English codes, a legacy of colonial occupation. The personal status courts and family law technically function under the shari'a as a consequence of secular governments' belief that "religion" should reside in the private domain. Many scholars have noted that the result of drawing on the European code has been "in some cases a much more rigid interpretation of Islamic law than had previously been customary" (Ernst 2003: 128; see also Tucker 2000). As for more recent Islamist movements, Skovgaard-Petersen (1997) explains that *shari'a* (literally meaning the "path" to follow God's command) has been a keyword of the Muslim Brotherhood and other Islamist organizations, but what they mean by this word is the rules of *fiqh* [human understanding and discernment about how best to follow God's command]. See also Lombardi 2006.

9. Skovgaard-Petersen notes that several decades ago the state mufti could display opposition to particular cases of the state apparatus, because then the legitimacy of the state was not at stake. But they can do so no longer, because, since the 1970s, the rise of Islamist groups has meant that others are posing as the representatives of Islam in Egypt: "The State Mufti and the 'ulama of al-Azhar can no longer claim neutrality or stand aloof: they are forced into the government's camp by both government and Islamists" (Skovgaard-Petersen 1997: 225).

10. Anyone can submit a question to Dar al-Ifta', and it can be as ordinary as asking for the correct way to pray during travel. New questions that have been

previously unaddressed are reserved for the grand mufti of the state, usually after an entire committee researches the question, and the formal fatwa that is issued is often published in newspapers.

11. The organ donation fatwa was issued just a few months before Mufti Gad al-Haqq was compelled to defend Law 44 on Family Status (the "Jihan" law), which was designed to improve the condition of women and children in family law and was attacked as being un-Islamic. See Skovgaard-Petersen 1997: 232.

12. In 1966, the Pakistani mufti Muhammad Shafi'i (d. 1976) ruled that organ transplantation (in all forms) was unacceptable in Islam. (See Moosa 1998 for a discussion of this fatwa in contrast to that issued by Gad al-Haqq in 1979.) In 1972, the fatwa committee of the Islamic Religious Council of Singapore also ruled that organ donation was unacceptable in Islam (the committee members modified their position in 1987.) In contrast, in the same year, the Algerian fatwa council ruled that donating an organ to another person was conditionally permissible, as did the fatwa council of Jordan in 1977. Fatwa councils in the following countries similarly issued fatwas conditionally permitting organ donation: Saudi Arabia in 1982, Kuwait in 1984, and the international Academy of Islamic Jurisprudence (Majma' al-Fiqh al-Islami) in 1988. In Saudi Arabia, an experimental phase of using brain-dead cadaveric kidneys began in 1983 and lasted until 1988, during which fifty-five kidneys that had been rejected by European centers were shipped to Saudi Arabia free of charge, an experiment which, in the words of the Saudi team, "emboldened" them to accept kidneys deemed unacceptable in Europe. Since this time Saudi Arabian hospitals have developed their own procurement programs from brain-dead persons, and ICUs are, in the words of the article's authors, "full of young highway accident victims" whose organs are deemed suitable for procurement. In 1997, 267 kidneys were transplanted. Beginning in 1994, other organs besides kidneys were also harvested (lungs, pancreases, livers, hearts, heart valves). The rate of consent among the surviving family members of potential donors has remained around 34 percent over these years (see Al-Khader 1999). In Iran, another country that purports to function under "Islamic law," the history of renal transplantation has occurred in three stages. From 1967 to 1988 all kidney transplants were from living related donors. In 1988, an ongoing program was initiated to regulate the financial compensation and transplantation of kidneys from living unrelated donors. In 2000, a law was passed to allow for procurement from brain-dead donors, but very few surviving family members have consented to this type of donation (see Ghods 2002).

13. Most official state fatwas on organ transplantation begin with the premise that the human body is outside the purview of financial transaction. This exemplifies the strength of the contemporary Islamic consensus (ijma') that human slavery is anathema to Islamic principles, in which all stand equal before God in divine judgment. Indeed, "slavery" in the nationalist imagination is not associated with Egyptian rulers' exploitation of slaves. (Nor is "colonialism" in the Egyptian nationalist imagination associated with the Anglo-Egyptian

colonization of the Sudan.) Rather, "slavery" has come to be associated with Egypt's colonized past, in which Egyptian workers were exploited in slavelike conditions for the glory of the British Empire. However, some more legal technical fatwas that draw on medieval sources use older language reflecting the existence of slavery in past Muslim societies; for example, Shaykh ʿAli Gumaʿa's research study in May 2007 discusses the bodily rights of the "free human." (For this report see Dar al-Ifta' al-Misriyya 2007; this report and other fatwas can be accessed online at www.dar-alifta.org.) Research studies from the Islamic Research Academy (Majmaʿ al-Buhuth al-Islamiyya) in Egypt also use the term *free human* when discussing the body as outside the purview of the market.

14. Popular views on the treatment of dead bodies are further elaborated upon in chapter 3.

15. The fatwa's paragraph on defining death was the eighteenth of a nineteen-paragraph answer to questions about the religious permissibility of organ transplantation in its various permutations.

16. The controversial Arabic terminology used in parallel to the English term *cadaveric* has often been *the recently dead*.

17. At this time, Shaykh Gad al-Haqq was the rector of al-Azhar (shaykh al-Azhar), the only official position more authoritative than that of grand mufti and perhaps the most authoritative position throughout the Sunni Muslim world in terms of religious rulings. Since 1895 shaykh al-Azhar has also been a position made by presidential appointment, which has somewhat lessened its authority, but al-Azhar still operates more independently from the government than does Dar al-Ifta' (Skovgaard-Petersen 1997). During and after the popular uprisings beginning in January 2011, discussion about the proper relationship between the religious scholars and the head of state has been re-ignited.

18. Lesley Sharp's work on U.S. transplantation calls into question whether the increasing demand for organs is a straightforward fact. She illustrates how even as the supply has increased, biomedical criteria for those in need of organs have also continued to broaden in recent years, creating a "shadow market in a gift economy," in which supply will never meet the demand of what is an especially lucrative biomedical practice (Sharp 2006). The recent study by Kaufman, Russ, et al. (2006) confirms Sharp's analysis by demonstrating that the expanding criteria for organ recipients have resulted in an increased pool of patients in need of kidneys, which now namely includes elderly patients, who turn to much younger relatives, such as grandchildren, to request kidney donations to sustain their lives a bit longer. In the early years of transplantation, candidates would be disqualified on the basis of advanced age.

19. Al-Mousawi does not, unfortunately, elaborate on what exactly he told the muftis in his "medical explanation" to them (Al-Mousawi and Al-Matouk 1997).

20. The following information comes from two interviews with Safwat Lotfy in 2002 (conducted with anthropologist Debra Budiani), his pamphlets and reading material, and my following of the press's coverage of him and his group.

21. Their phrase *"al-akhlaqiyyat al-tibiyya"*—a literal translation of *medical ethics*—was not generally used or recognized by patients or journalists in debates in the media. As I have mentioned, "ethics" is generally conceived of in terms of the correct thing to do from the perspective of Islamic jurisprudence *(fiqh)*.

22. Though rare, both Lock (2002b) and Egyptian physicians who worked in Saudi Arabia and Kuwait in the early years of Arab Gulf transplantation have reported cases of patients diagnosed as "brain-dead" coming "back to life." Also, several reports about such cases have been covered in the Egyptian media.

23. This call to more respectful treatment of the dying resonated among many Egyptians. See Hirschkind 2006 for how the medical (mis)treatment of the dying and the dead is taken up as a topic among contemporary Egyptian preachers who deliver sermons outside state officiated channels.

24. This hadith has been transmitted through the major compendia as follows: "On the authority of Abu Abdullah al-Nu'man ibn Bashir (may Allah be pleased with him), who said: I heard the Messenger of Allah (peace be upon him) say, 'That which is lawful is clear, and that which is unlawful is clear, and between the two of them are doubtful matters about which not many people are knowledgeable. Thus, he who avoids these doubtful matters certainly clears himself in regard to his religion and his honor. But he who falls into the doubtful matters falls into that which is unlawful, like the shepherd who pastures around a sanctuary, all but grazing therein. Verily, every king has a sanctuary, and Allah's sanctuary is His prohibitions. In the body there is a morsel of flesh that, if it be sound, all the body is sound, and that, if it be diseased, all of the body is diseased. This part of the body is the heart'" (recorded by both Bukhari and Muslim).

25. To be clear, I am using Moussawi's term *reeducate* ironically here to indicate the exact opposite meaning of what Moussawi intended.

26. For example, the late Muhammad Biltagi, a scholar of the shari'a at Dar al-'Ulum University, told me that he had originally considered this an issue to be decided by medical expertise, but it was Dr. Lotfy who made evident that brain death is not a "real" medical diagnosis but one invented to facilitate organ transplantation (personal interview with Dr. Biltagi, in Cairo, May 2002).

27. One prominent example is Dr. Maher Mahran, a former minister of health, who stood solidly against the idea that brain death is the death of the person. Although he himself was a medical physician, Dr. Mahran was unconvinced about the legitimacy of brain death and remained so until his own death.

28. This initiative was led by parliamentary member Muhammad Khalil Quwayta.

29. Lock (2002a) interviewed thirty-two intensive care specialists in North America.

30. Sharp goes on to say, however, "Donor kin frequently and vehemently reject themes reminiscent of rebirth or of a transmigrated soul, particularly after death is declared, organ removed, and they return home to grieve their losses" (2001: 114). Sharp also notes ironically that transplantation in the

United States has relied on the contradictory narrative that is offered to the transplant recipient: that the received organ will not alter his or her sense of self, that it is merely a part and nothing more.

31. Shbin al-Qum (commonly spelled Shbeen al-Kom) is the capital of Manufiyya and home to the first few liver operations in Egypt in the 1980s, all of which resulted in the death of the recipient and in some cases of the donor as well. Not much was publicized about them (as failures), and for a long time after doctors were reluctant to perform any more liver lobe transplantations. The procedure was restarted in the late 1990s in Cairo, with exchange programs with surgeons from Japan and France (see Budiani 2005; and Budiani and Shibly 2008) and became routine in the 2000s.

32. Marmush, it should be noted, only selectively associates Saudi Arabia with the "real religion" and finds much of Saudi practice to go against what she views as appropriate Muslim practice.

33. Marmush then told me a personal anecdote about having worked in Mansoura on a story about kidney transplants, where she met a physician who stopped her and asked her why she did not wear *hijab* (referring to the head covering). She grimaced as she told me this and made a gesture at her chin indicating that he had a long beard, which she associates with those who place exaggerated emphasis on outward religious symbols to signal their emulation of the Prophet. "This man," she said, "was a surgeon but wanted to spend his time preaching! I told him it was none of his business and that this was based on my own personal relationship with God, and wouldn't he be better off in the eyes of God to go spend his time in the hospital, treating people rather than trying to 'guide' them—and does this guy really think he is 'guiding' me?! . . . They want to focus on stupid little things, like whether a woman wears *hijab*. Is that really going to move society forward? Is that what we should be focusing on, when there are people who can't even afford to eat?!" (See Mahmood 2005 for an interesting discussion of different views of religious ethics in contemporary Egypt and their relationship to specific forms of ritual piety.)

34. By "tyranny of the gift," Fox and Swazey refer to that fact that "what is interchanged is so extraordinary that donor, recipient, and kin can become bound to one another, emotionally and morally, in ways that are as likely to be mutually fettering as to be self-transcending" (1974: 383).

35. Note also that while doctors dismissed the muftis as irrelevant when fatwas stood in the way of medical practice, the doctors were also willing to note that most of the religious scholars were in favor of it, thus simultaneously dismissing their authority and drawing upon it to add to their own.

36. Shaykh Guma'a had, in fact, studied in a Cairo business school.

37. Early in Shaykh 'Ali Guma'a's tenure as grand mufti, the Dar al-Ifta' released a detailed twenty-one-page study on organ transplantation and Islamic jurisprudence. See Dar al-Ifta' al-Misriyya 2007.

38. The Qur'an describes humans' divine duty on earth as *khalafa*, often translated as "viceregency." See Seyyed Hossein Nasr, who explains *khalafa*

thus: "The two primary features of being human are servanthood and vicere-gency: being passive toward Heaven in submission to God's Will, on the one hand, and being active as God's agent and doing His Will in the world, on the other" (2002: 13).

39. Hof and der Schmitten cited in Hogle 1999:1.

40. We can also see that this sense of a "unified" Western position is a racial-ized one as well, because it is often used to exclude and further marginalize racial, ethnic, and religious minorities. See Razack 2007. It is common practice in clinical encounters with minorities in the United States for clinicians to per-ceive their questioning of medical treatment or diagnosis in terms of "cultural difference" (if not pathology). See Fadiman 1998.

41. The report concluded that brain death should remain *the* sound defini-tion of death.

42. Note that my argument here is different from the assumption that "universal" principles can undergird bioethics that transcend place and time (Beauchamp and Childress 2001). How people approach bioethical dilemmas is everywhere rooted in historical and social contexts, and by expanding the object of analysis to include these contexts, we will be better placed to analyze how patients and their communities encounter biotechnologies. The more attentive we are to different forces, such as efficacy, cost, political-economic distribution, and access, the less likely we are to fall into the trap of "culturalist" explanations that assume more than they analyze.

CHAPTER THREE

1. By "the story" I mean the one commonly found in Egyptian newspapers as well as the one narrated to me by ophthalmologists, hospital workers, and lawyers to explain the closing of the eye banks. However, careful analysis of newspaper reports and my discussions with a Cairo prosecutor have revealed the occurrence of *numerous* complaints throughout the 1990s. In one interview I conducted with a public prosecutor in 2003, he related to me that in 1995 he had been ordered to file a report at the Kasr el Aini public morgue for the acci-dental death of a young girl, and there he incidentally discovered that the girl's eyeballs were missing. He marked this as the first time his office was aware of "eye theft for cornea transplantation" (personal interview, 2003). In other nar-ratives, the missing eyes were discovered when the families insisted on washing the bodies of their dead in their home villages.

2. Ain Shams Teaching Hospital, at Damerdash (in northern Cairo), is affili-ated with Ain Shams University. The older Kasr el Aini Teaching Hospital is affiliated with the Cairo University Faculty of Medicine. Kasr el Aini was forced to shut down in 1997 for one year, becoming semioperational again in February 1998, only to be shut down again in July 1999 (*Al-Ahram Weekly*, July 8–14, 1999, issue no. 437).

3. I have received varying reports from ophthalmologists and the press as to how many transplants were carried out before the shutdown, but they were

probably in the range of seventy per month at each hospital. Other public hospitals also performed transplants (Abu Rish Children's Hospital, Tanta University Hospital), but it appears (from my conversations with staff) that they too obtained corneas from Kasr el Aini or Ain Shams rather than from their own morgues. Although many press accounts railed against the sudden mushrooming of waiting lists for cornea transplants after the shutdown, a problem with cornea supply had existed long before the shutdown.

4. The Qur'an describes death as the transition to a second stage, and extrascriptural traditions have elaborated upon understandings of the dead as still sentient beings, as I elaborate further in this chapter.

5. In 1978, the eye surgeons at Ain Shams obtained microscopic instruments, making their earlier tools seem rough and rudimentary. And in 1989, a wealthy ophthalmologist and businessman, Dr. Akef Maghraby, the founder and chairman of the largest private specialized medical care network in the Middle East (El-Maghraby Eye and Ear Hospitals and Centers), in collaboration with Tissue Banks International of Baltimore, Maryland, donated eye banking equipment to Ain Shams Medical School, his alma mater. While Egyptian ophthalmologists had been making efforts to establish eye banks since the late 1950s and even had a law passed in 1962 for the establishment of a national eye bank, their plan had not come to fruition—for a host of bureaucratic and financial reasons—until Maghraby's intervention. See "For the First time in Cairo" *Al-Ahram*, December 27, 1983; "The First Eye Bank in the Middle East," *Al-Ahram*, April 18, 1989; "First Operation for Cornea Transplantation in Egypt," *Al-Akhbar*, July 3, 1989; and "Sidqi Inaugurates First Eye Bank in the Middle East," *Al-Ahram* June 25, 1989.

6. In fact, Shadi referred to the eye department as "the trachoma department" (*qism al-ramad*). Because trachoma has been such an important eye disease in Egypt, the specialty of ophthalmology has long been referred to as trachoma, and ophthalmologists are often referred to as "trachoma doctors" (*dakatra al-ramad*).

7. His reference to "the Arabs" is to the eminently successful ophthalmologist and businessman Dr. Akef Maghraby, who was born to an Egyptian mother and a Saudi father.

8. As Inhorn (1994) notes, a system of medical malpractice is comparatively underdeveloped in Egypt.

9. For example, in 2002, I spoke with a young pediatrician who had just graduated from Cairo's Medical Faculty and who was hired in a public hospital facility that paid her a salary of 250 £E (less than $50) per month.

10. See, for example, their discussion of the popular television serial *The White Flag* (Armbrust 1996; Abu-Lughod 2005).

11. Such narratives gained salience after the *infitah*, or Sadat's "Open Door Policy," which marked the decline of Nasser's socialist welfare state and the rise of the nouveaux riches (Armbrust 1996).

12. On social triage in medical anthropology, see, for example, Scheper-Hughes's (1992) discussion of "life-boat ethics" in the slums of Brazil or

Vinh-Kim Nguyen's (2010) discussions of the distribution of anti-retroviral medication in West Africa on the basis of people's relative contributions to AIDS communities.

13. Dr. Mustafa juxtaposes "truly dead" to those patients who are variously known as "clinically dead," brain-stem dead, or brain-dead. In contrast to the more dramatic examples of visceral organs, corneas in Egypt are procured from those whose hearts have stopped beating and who have stopped breathing. Most ophthalmologists with whom I spoke argued that cornea transplantation is "far removed from the controversy over brain death," but some argued that the need to remove corneas "immediately" can embroil this procedure in the problem of defining the moment of death.

14. For the ways in which the mass media have affected fatwa giving in the Muslim world, see Masud, Messick, et al. 1996; Messick 1993, 1996; Skovgaard-Petersen 1997; and Eickelman and Anderson 2003. For a more general account of religious discourse and television in Egypt, see Abu-Lughod 2005.

15. *Al-Wafd*, July 12, 1989.

16. In Margaret Lock's interviews with North American intensive care specialists who procure organs from brain-dead patients, the majority were not themselves signed on as organ donors (Lock 2002a).

17. As Lane (1994) and Rashad, Fiona, and Haith-Cooper (2004) have shown, patients are often poor, illiterate, and objects of research without adequate material or information about their decisions; whether their consent is ever truly informed in this context is in question.

18. The patients with whom I spoke could not understand why the imported corneas cost so much money if they were from nonprofit institutions and were supposedly donated "freely." But according to the international nonprofit eye banks, the high price reflects the costs of preserving, storing, processing, screening, and shipping the grafts.

19. I conducted this interview in January 2008 in Dr. Muhammad Ibrahim's private clinic in Cairo.

20. Dr. Mohamed Ibrahim received his general medical degree in 1954 and his specialty in ophthalmology in 1956. He was one of the main founders of the discipline of ocular ophthalmology in Egypt in 1964.

21. An important note here is that when medical students, residents, and physicians with faculty positions at university hospitals talk about patients (*al-marda*), they are often speaking specifically about the poor; physicians teach in public teaching hospitals and learn clinical skills on poor patients, who in turn receive care at minimal or no cost. Eye doctors often complained to me about "ignorant"—that is, poor—patients, whom they described as "too irrational" to approach about bequeathing eyes for cornea transplantation.

22. Thus, the doctors saw the excessive lamentations among Egyptians over the dead as "cultural" obstacles to science and did not recognize the "stoic" attitude among the English as an equally culturalized expression; they simply saw one as an obstacle to science, the other as "civilized."

23. The film was directed by the prolific Egyptian filmmaker Kamal 'Atiyya.

24. See Gordon 2002 and Abu-Lughod 2005 for a discussion of cinema and television in the context of Nasser's development plans.

25. The film *The Lamp of Umm Hashim* is but one example from Egypt's rich popular and literary culture that illustrates the extent to which blindness, especially blindness caused by trachoma, is linked with ideas about Egyptian ignorance. Indeed, the period of the *nahda*, known as the "Egyptian Enlightenment" or "Renaissance" of the late nineteenth and early twentieth centuries—a period of intellectual and literary modernization and reform—is saturated with metaphors of sight, vision, awakening, and light. Taha Hussein, one of the leading figures of the *nahda*, whose autobiography *The Days (al-Ayam)* has become one of the best-known works of modern Arabic literature, suffered from trachoma as a child in a poor Egyptian village. When the village barber was called in to heal Hussein, the "folk" treatment ended up permanently blinding the young boy. In his autobiography he expresses painful regret that his parents were not educated enough to have thought to call a modern doctor instead. Throughout his adult life, Taha Hussein would call for a struggle against ignorance, blindness, and the rote mimicry of backward tradition.

In the literary work on which the film *The Lamp of Umm Hashim* is based, the novelist Haqqi reverses this famous incident of Taha Hussein's life—an integral component of Egyptian national history. In Haqqi's novel it is biomedicine that can blind, and traditional healing that can help regain sight. Yet the filmmakers who translated the text into the cinematic medium in the late 1960s did not allow for Haqqi's unsettling of the dominant historical narrative that emphasizes modernity as the only avenue to progress. See Hamdy 2005.

26. This line of questioning is inspired by the work of Talal Asad (1986, 1993, 2003) and Saba Mahmood (2005).

27. A popular American bumper sticker to promote organ donation spells this idea out bluntly: "Don't take your organs with you to Heaven—Heaven knows we need them here!" Death *in the body* is cast as selfish and ungodly; the righteous path is to recycle body parts; the body's role is to serve life on earth; the spirit will accrue rewards for the afterlife. There are, of course, many competing discourses on death, the soul, and the importance of the material body in Euro-America that are drawn upon selectively toward different ends. In the case of organ transplantation, the material body is detached in meaning from the "person" or spirit. But this understanding of dead bodies is not mobilized consistently by the U.S. media, for example, when rescue teams, following a natural or political tragedy, work to restore the human remains to family members out of "respect and dignity."

28. This event took place six years after the eye bank had been shut down, and Tantawi was asked to address the issue of cornea transplantation, which doctors and journalists deemed a life-saving medical treatment impeded by "incorrect religious views." When Shaykh Tantawi walked in, there was a murmur and buzz in the audience. He walked briskly to the front, wearing his long flapping robe and turban, flanked by the other men, all physicians, in their contrasting black suits. A film crew from Egypt's national television station

ensured the forum would be accessible to the public on Channel 1. About two hundred people were present in the conference hall of the Royal Nile Hilton, one of Cairo's ritziest hotels. The conference was open to the public, and lavish leather portfolios and brochures were handed out as promotions by the Pfizer pharmaceutical company, which had donated samples of its antibiotic Zithromax to the developing world as part of the World Health Organization's program to eradicate preventable blindness.

29. Dr. Muhammad 'Awad, who sat at Tantawi's side on the panel, was the minister of health at the time.

30. Those who argue that organ transplantation is *haram* because it leads to other things that are clearly *haram* (theft of body parts, trade in human organs) are drawing on an Islamic legal tool (from the field of scholarship known as *usul al-fiqh*, the methodology of jurisprudence) called *sadd-al-dhara'i'a*, or "the blocking of means." See more on this in chapter 4.

31. I recorded this speech while attending the conference.

32. Sahih al-Muslim is a major hadith compendium that can be found in various forms and in many translations, texts, and online resources.

33. See Langford 2009 for an argument about the denigration of the materiality of the dead in biomedical and mortuary rituals in the United States, to the dismay of Southeast Asian refugees.

34. By "Islamic tradition," I am referring to the lived interpretations of the Qur'an and its exegesis, the hadith compendia and their exegesis, the *sunna* more generally (teachings from the life of the Prophet and his companions), and the dominant ethical, theological, and legal commentaries that emerged from them.

35. Performing these rites for the dead in *fiqh* is an example of *al-fard al-kifaya*, meaning that it is not incumbent upon each individual Muslim to learn how to perform these rites correctly as long as a sufficient number of community members have attained this knowledge. (The same applies to attaining specialized medical or Qur'anic knowledge.) This is in contrast to *al-fard al-'ayn*—which refers to a duty that is incumbent on every individual Muslim, such as learning how to correctly perform the daily prayers.

36. Similarly, as Hogle (1999) and Kaufman (2000) discuss, U.S. medical practice continues to exhibit its own ambivalence about the living and dead qualities of a brain-dead body from which donations are taken.

37. This Prophetic saying was recorded and transmitted by Ahmad, Abu Dawud, and Ibn Majah.

38. The charitable organization for the blind in question was Mu'asasat al-Nur 'Amal, or the Light and Hope Foundation, famous in Egypt for its musical performances.

39. The actual text of the fatwa continues, "As for the issuance of a law that would allow for taking the eyes of the dead, we qualify its permissibility under the condition that it is restricted only to the cases of dire necessity and that it does not extend beyond the dead with no surviving family members. As for those with surviving family members, then the case of taking the eyes of the dead should be only under the power of the family and with their consent;

if they consent then it is permissible, and if they do not consent then it is not allowed. And with this, the questioner knows the answer. And God knows best."

40. In contrast, other muftis, including the late Shaykh Gad al-Haqq, Shaykh Nasir Farid Wasil, and the current grand mufti, Shaykh 'Ali Guma'a, have made consent *(wasiyya)* an explicit condition, as well as stipulating that there be no profit or "trade" in corneas. Tantawi might argue that precedents exist in Islamic law that could justify overruling individual preference (for the deceased body to remain untouched) in the case of clear overriding benefit of society as a whole (a source of grafts to restore sight to the blind). Yet most Egyptian muftis do *not* argue on this logic, instead insisting on individual consent, which may demonstrate their reluctance to entrust contemporary medical institutions to distribute corneas justly and without class or geographical prejudice. Their insistence on the requirement of consent has been an attempt to preserve patients' autonomy as a counterpoint to the potential of state institutions' misuse of power.

41. An alternative explanation is that those who survive the dead can intend to make a *sadaqa jariyya* on behalf of the dead's spiritual accounting. But who would have the authority to intend a *sadaqa jariyya* for the dead? The family members? The hospital staff procuring the eyes? To imagine a member of the hospital procurement staff declaring his spiritual intention for the dead donor clashes with the popular image of the workers stealing body parts from the morgue.

42. For instance, in the United States, the perception among African Americans that most organs will go to wealthy white individuals provides little incentive for these individuals to become donors (Siminoff and Saunders 2000: 64–65).

CHAPTER FOUR

1. Several scholars with whom I spoke in Egypt and in Syria suggested that Sha'rawi had, in fact, formulated his position against organ transplantation through conversations with Shaykh 'Abdallah al-Ghumari. A Moroccan scholar of hadith and a great defender of Sufi discipline and practice, Ghumari (d. 1993) had studied at al-Azhar and made his home in Egypt for many years. Al-Ghumari's pamphlet, written on behalf of "the scholars of al-Azhar," is titled *Ta'rif ahl al-Islam bi-an naql al-'aduw haram* (Letting the followers of Islam know that transplanting an organ is *haram*) (1987), and it states that he came to his position on organ transplantation when asked about it by a group of medical students in Alexandria in 1983. He responded that this procedure is *haram* because the body belongs to God. Yet rather than suggest that his own position might have influenced Sha'rawi's, al-Ghumari (1987) writes that he was later pleased to read of Sha'rawi's position in *Al-Liwa' al-Islami*, which confirmed his own view. Thanks to Suheil Laher and Jonathan Brown for information on Ghumari.

2. During his exile, Sha'rawi worked in newly founded Islamic universities in Saudi Arabia and Algeria.

3. See Carrie Wickham's discussion of Nasser's and Sadat's different versions of presidential self-styling (2002: 95).

4. Sha'rawi's shows were given different names throughout the years, including *Nur 'ala Nur, Khawatir Imaniyya, Liqa' al-Imam,* and in reruns *Ma'a al-Sha'rawi.*

5. I have no interest here in making judgments about the personal character of Sha'rawi, who has long been the subject of much controversy among more "liberal" intellectuals in Egypt; I leave this task to historians and his biographers. Neither am I interested in evaluating Sha'rawi's particular religious and political positions. Rather, my interest is in the ways in which his statements about organ transplantation, medical technology, and the body have been taken up and made meaningful by those directly affected by the possibilities of organ transplantation as well as by those in the wider Egyptian society. During the course of my fieldwork, no other Islamic scholar's name was invoked as often as Sha'rawi's in discussions about organ transplantation.

6. Sha'rawi's "fatwas" refer to spontaneous answers to questions posed to him by his audience members, not to "official" fatwas authorized by the state institution Dar al-Ifta'. By referring to his responses as "fatwas," his followers work to decenter the authority of fatwa giving *(ifta')* from the state. In explicating the groundbreaking aspects of the mass media, Skovgaard-Petersen notes that these fatwa collections were suddenly sold in the hundreds of thousands and were found in the homes of many "first-generation literates" in the 1990s (1997: 12). Examples of compilations of Sha'rawi's fatwas include *Al-Fatawa al-Kubra* (see al-Sha'rawi 2002) and *Al-Fatawa: Kul ma yuhimm al-muslim fi hayatihi yawmihi wa ghadihi* (see al-Sha'rawi, 1999).

7. Wickham (2002) argues that Sadat and, initially, Mubarak in this sense underestimated the political relevance of the "Islamic trend" *(al-tiyar al-islami).* See also Mahmood 2005 and Hirschkind 2006 for a discussion of how seemingly unpolitical acts of piety counter many assumptions of secular liberalism.

8. Sha'rawi's biographers note that he grew up in the purity and beauty of the Egyptian countryside and that as a child he was one with nature, taking in the beauty of the full-moon nights and offering companionship to the birds in flight. Sha'rawi himself narrates that the rural environment in which he was raised was pure and God-fearing and free of the temptations that exist in the city (see Hasan 1990: 8).

9. See Skovgaard-Petersen 1997 for an overview of Egyptian state muftis of the twentieth century.

10. While Carrie Wickham (2002) suggests this group is composed mainly of "old guard elites," anthropologist Jessica Winegar's (2006) study of fine artists in Egypt demonstrates that not all "cultural producers" oriented toward cosmopolitanism come from elite backgrounds.

11. These fatwas/responsa are to be found in the compilation *Muhammad Mutwalli al-Sha'rawi: Al-Fatawa al-Kubra,* Cairo: Maktabat al-Turath al-Islami, 2nd ed. (Cairo: Maktabat al-turath al-islami, 2002).

12. *Min al-alif ila al-ya'*, presented by Tariq Habib, December 23, 1988. Thanks to Reem Saad, who first alerted me to the importance of this television episode.

13. It should be noted that Tariq Habib is a Coptic Egyptian Christian, and this influenced the way in which his exchange with this important Muslim leader has been interpreted. As a non-Muslim, Habib was not asking Sha'rawi for counsel, to guide him on what he might do if faced with such a bioethical dilemma. Rather, he was asking Sha'rawi to represent his religion's view, addressing him as a spokesperson for Islam writ large. This is partly why his fellow Muslim critics responded to Sha'rawi's answer with such discomfort and embarrassment.

14. Note that Hasan, the author of the quoted biography, is using the term *fatwa* in its looser, wider meaning, as the (nonbinding) opinion of a scholar in response to a question. Scholars who have insisted that Sha'rawi's view was "not a fatwa" are using *fatwa* in a narrower sense, as an opinion based on Islamic jurisprudential reasoning. Also the end of the sentence reads in full: "all because of his opinion on organ transplantation and terminal illness." Hasan's inclusion of "terminal illness" refers to patients in organ failure and in need of transplantation as well as to Sha'rawi's argument against what he sees as medical futility. See Hasan 1990: 84.

15. In a recent opinion piece by Sulayman Guda (2008) titled "The Shaykh's Approach," Guda writes, "When [Shaykh Sha'rawi] objected to blood transfusion and organ transplantation saying that they are forbidden in religion, he was wrong and he should have been challenged on this matter because such statements go against the interest of many patients. The shaykh himself needed blood transfer when he underwent surgery in London and had a cornea transplant at a Saudi Arabian hospital."

16. *Al-Ahram al-Riyadi*, August 22, 2001.

17. For insightful discussions about who gets to speak for the Egyptian nation, see Saad 1998 and Abu-Lughod 2005.

18. By issuing *Al-Liwa' al-Islami* newspaper, the Egyptian government has sought to counter the publications of the Muslim Brotherhood, whose monthly journal bears the similar name, *Liwa' al-Islam* (Wickham 2002: 135).

19. The argument that Muslims have a duty to take good (medical) care of their bodies because of the Qur'anic prohibition against suicide was echoed to me by many physicians. During an interview with Dr. Nuha, an internist in a dialysis ward in a public hospital, she explained people's reluctance to donate body parts thus: "The body is a sacred creation. We have always had this belief. A person is not free to do whatever he wants with his body. Our bodies are not our property. Like in times of war there were people who would mutilate the corpses of the enemy. Islam forbade all of this. So people don't want to give from the body, because this type of mutilation [tamthil] and disrespect [ihana] of the body is *haram*." Sha'rawi had also extended this argument to people engaged in "suicide operations" in the name of Islam.

20. *Al-Liwaʾ al-Islami,* February 26, 1987.

21. *Al-Liwaʾ al-Islami,* February 26, 1987.

22. *Al-Liwaʾ al-Islami,* February 26, 1987.

23 Shaʿrawi's insistence on God's infinite control over every infinitesimal process of human life echoes that of the great Ashʾari theologians. Egyptians who associated with Sufi *tariqa*s also claim Shaʿrawi as a great Sufi, their evidence being his tremendous amount of respect and devotion to *ahl al-bayt* (the family of the Prophet). An annual *mulid* now commemorates Shaʿrawi's birthday, in which many Egyptians who associate with *tariqa*s take part (Mittermaier, personal communication, 2006). I find it less interesting a question to ask whether Shaʿrawi himself was a Sufi or saw himself as one than to ask how he is perceived and taken up in wider Egyptian culture.

24. *Al-Liwaʾ al-Islami,* February 26, 1987.

25. *Al-Liwaʾ al-Islami,* February 26, 1987.

26. This interview was conducted in the office of the grand mufti at Dar al-Iftaʾ in Cairo in May 2004. *Madhhab* is more commonly used in reference to particular "schools" of Islamic jurisprudence.

27. Shaykh ʿAli Gumaʿa referred to Egyptian journalism as "not quite yellow journalism" *(al-sahafa al-safraʾ)* but, rather, as "pumpkin-seed journalism" *(sahafat-al-lib),* pumpkin seeds being the snack that Egyptians eat during shows and fairs (akin to popcorn eating at U.S. movie theaters).

28. Narrated by Imam Bayhaqi (994–1066) in *Al-Madkhal ila al sunan al-Kubra lil-Bayhaqi.*

29. Cited in Hasan 1990: 85. Again, Shaʿrawi did not coin new or modern *legal* terminology; rather, he asserted truisms of Islam in order to counter trends in modern society toward godlessness and heedlessness of the divine.

30. By "road of caution" (cited in Hasan 1990: 85), ʿImran is evoking the concept of *waraʿ,* which is the avoidance of something out of prudence, even if that thing is not clearly forbidden. For example, some people avoid eating at large gatherings out of fear of gluttony; some speak only reservedly out of fear of backbiting; some avoid contact with members of the opposite sex; et cetera.

31. When people in this context note that "healing comes from God, not from the doctor," this is *not* meant as a prohibition against seeking treatment from a doctor. The doctor's treatment is not exclusive from God's treatment; rather, God is the ultimate Healer no matter what forms this healing takes or from where it originates. Therefore, this statement *approves* medical treatment by saying that any legitimate healing is ultimately divine in nature. See Solomon 1997 for similar discussions of the role of medicine in Jewish ethical thought.

32. Cited in Hasan 1990: 85.

33. Shaʿrawi's responses, however, did little to abate the criticism against him, even after his death. Posthumous criticism of Shaʿrawi (such as Guda's above) continue, more than a decade after his death.

34. Umm Kulthum, Egypt's most famous singer and entertainer of the twentieth century, was placed on an artificial respirator at Badrawi Hospital before her demise.

35. Cited in Hasan 1990: 88–89. While such sentiments about not prolonging death through technical means may sound familiar and agreeable to European and American readers, in Egypt death, dying, and illness are much less dominated by biotechnology. Official discourse is focused more on increasing patients' access to medical treatment. That is why the idea of a shaykh saying "Let them die (mercifully)" caused so much anger among "progressive" journalists in the press, who see the main problems in Egyptian health care to be the ignorance and neglect that prevent uneducated poor Egyptians from seeking treatment.

36. Felicitas Opwis (2005) does an admirable job tracing the "rational objectivism" in Islamic jurisprudence throughout Islamic history. Shaykh Muhammad 'Abduh, known as the great Muslim reformer who served as grand mufti from 1899 to 1905, drew on several classical sources that asserted the importance of rationality in Islamic law. He wrote in his famous *al-Tawhid*, first published in 1897: "[Islam] is not a religion of conflicting principles but is built squarely on reason, while Divine revelation is its surest pillar" ('Abduh 1966: 39).

37. In explicating the difference between a mufti and a *qadi* (a judge), Skovgaard-Petersen notes that a judge is consulted by litigants and must endeavor to find the facts behind what they present and be skeptical toward what they say. In contrast, a mufti is consulted by only one party and does not investigate the truth of the information presented to him (1997: 7). However, if the fatwa is going to address as broad a topic as the permissibility of organ transplantation in the state of Egypt, a mufti in the position of state mufti now appears to have a conflation of roles between *qadi* and mufti: he cannot trust the information presented to him by only one party (e.g., a particular medical practitioner) if his fatwa is going to affect all parties (i.e., all medical institutions, patients, donors), although Tantawi appears to have done just that. Further, in the absence of Islamic courts managing such issues in contemporary Egypt, the role of the mufti, at least in the case of organ transplantation, is further conflated with that of the *qadi*, in that the fatwa issued has immediate practical effects (to bear upon legislation in Parliament), even if in theory fatwas are nonbinding. Furthermore, most state-issued fatwas use the main categories of permitted *(mubah)*, obligatory *(fard)*, and prohibited *(haram)* (as is the traditional case of the *qadi*), disregarding the additional, ethically oriented concepts of recommended *(mandub)* and disliked *(makruh)*, which may also be used in fatwas.

38. Cited in Hasan 1990: 89.

39. More than a decade later, Sha'rawi is quoted as saying that God had disgraced those who had permitted organ donation in the case of a patient mistakenly declared to be dead. *Ruz al-Yusuf,* May 18, 1998, 84.

40. The study begins with philological analyses of the word *ownership (milk)* of the body and humans' rights to "deal with it" *(al-tasarruf fih)* before it addresses the specific legal requirements and conditions of permissibility.

41. This legal tool is accepted in only some of the schools of jurisprudence *(madhahib)*. An example is a ruling in which the Prophet forbade a creditor to accept a gift from his debtor lest it become a means to usury. It is usury that is

explicitly forbidden in Islam, not accepting gifts from creditors, yet the latter is prevented to avoid leading to the former (see Kamali 1991). The theorist of Islamic law Felicitas Opwis describes *sadd al-dhara'i'* as "the principle of eliminating pretexts" and as a prime example of substantive rationality: "Whenever a formally legal transaction leads to something contrary to the purpose of the law, it is considered illegal and void, such as a deferred sale *(bay' al-ajal)* that results in charging illegal interest *(riba)*" (Opwis 2005: 192).

42. *Al-Liwa' al-Islami*, July 14, 1988.

43. In contrast, the fatwas of South Asian scholars, most prominently Mufti Shaf'i of Pakistan, suggest discomfort with blood transfusions because of the *najasa* (impurity) of blood once outside the body.

44. *Al-Liwa' al-Islami*, February 26, 1987.

45. Some of the Egyptians who are increasingly disenchanted by biomedicine, as well as those who seek to restore all traditions of the Prophet in daily life, seek to revive this medical practice (see also Sholkamy 2004). The prevailing viewpoint in Egypt and elsewhere in the Muslim world, however, has been that such practices of the Prophet were a reflection of the time and place in which he lived, and not a part of *wahy*, the divine (eternal) revelation.

46. Egyptian legal scholar Tariq al-Bishri also argues that blood, because it is a renewable resource of the body, is a matter to be considered separately from other body parts: "[Blood donation] has been practiced for decades, and we can still remember the long line of blood donors from among the youth and public citizenry during the days of war. This practice has not been opposed or debated from the arenas of religion, Islamic jurisprudence, the laws of the *shari'a*, or those of civic law" (2001: 4).

47. Here, Dr. Walid refers to the Qur'anic prohibition of wine and intoxicants. But one can read the Qur'an as going directly against his logic, for the Qur'an itself states that drinking wine has certain benefits but that the sin outweighs the benefit (Sura 2:219). That is, weighing good against bad always involves a calculation.

48. Rationalist objectivism is also sometimes referred to as *philosophical ethics* (humans can know what is right and wrong on the basis of their own reasoning), and theistic subjectivism as *religious ethics* (right and wrong is based on what God tells us). Rationalist objectivism is associated with the Mu'tazali theological school, and theistic subjectivism with the Ash'ari school, which is the dominant theology for Sunni Muslims today. Historical and sociological analyses reveal much messier interconnections and medial positions between and within these two approaches, however, than such a neat dichotomy would imply. As Carl Ernst points out, most religious ethical systems are based on both rationalist objectivism and theistic subjectivism (2003:110). Also, as Opwis notes for the case of Islam, "Neither of these two positions in unadulterated form was historically viable" (2005: 190). Rationalist objectivism would eventually lead to the diminishing of the role of revelation as social conditions change, and theistic subjectivism would be unable to answer new questions that arise that the revelation does not directly address. Opwis notes that indeed one

of the major reasons that the Ash'ari school has been able to gain the status of orthodoxy in Sunni Islam is through its rapprochement with rationalist objectivism (2005: 190). While recognizing their permeability, it is still helpful to consider these two broad tendencies within Islamic legal thought and theology in order to understand how Muslims today variously engage with new ethical dilemmas upon which they struggle to bring Islamic reasoning to bear. This is not to suggest that ordinary (unscholarly) Muslims are necessarily acquainted with the histories and genealogies of the various theological schools but rather to point to the way in which these scholarly categorizations can broadly help us to understand different ethical positions toward which people tend. While the state muftis clearly appeal to tenets of rationalist objectivism, Sha'rawi remained theologically subjective in his stated reasoning.

49. Recent scholarship has contended that the use of *maslaha* does not merely signal a "modern invented tradition" to authorize present practices through an authoritative appeal to the past (Dallal 2000; Opwis 2005). Opwis' (2005) reading of classical legal texts demonstrates that it was premodern jurists, and not modern secular visionaries, who expounded on the legal aims of *maslaha*, and that the premodern jurists' arguments were later taken up by Muslim reformers.

50. Muslehuddin cited in Krawietz 1997: 186.

51. Birgit Krawietz has written extensively on the use of Islamic legal theory in twentieth-century Egypt in cases of new medical procedures. About the specific case of organ transplantation, Krawietz writes, "I cannot imagine a comparable test case which offers such a scope of issues with regard to conceptions of *maslaha*" (1997: 187).

52. In several of his obituaries in the English-language press, his position on organ transplantation was stated. See, for example, the obituary by Salah Nasrawi in the Associated Press, June 17, 1998.

53. An oft-cited tradition of the Prophet Muhammad is: "For every illness there is a cure, so seek treatment (*li kulli da'in dawa'*)." Physicians in Egypt habitually recite this hadith to convince reluctant patients about a particular medical procedure.

54. See, for example, "Shaykh Mutwalli Sha'rawi in a frank conversation: 'If a mother saw her child dying she should leave him and not give him her kidney.' " *Ruz al-Yusuf* news magazine, May 18, 1998.

CHAPTER FIVE

1. On October 6, 1973, Egypt launched a successful surprise attack against Israel across the Suez Canal to regain control of the Suez and the Sinai, which were lost in the demoralizing defeat of the 1967 war. Negotiations toward a permanent ceasefire began in December 1973. On June 5, 1975, the Suez Canal was reopened.

2. The donor kidney is washed of its blood after being extracted. After the donor kidney is connected to the recipient's vessels, the surgeons must wait (in

this case five minutes) for the donor kidney to be reperfused (filled with the recipient's blood).

3. The casualties of this war included an approximate eight thousand Egyptian fatalities.

4. The great saphenous vein is the vessel in the leg that is most commonly used for coronary artery bypass grafts.

5. The Holy Qur'an, 95:4. The fatwas issued by state muftis *permitting* organ transplantation also reference this Qur'anic verse, for example, the 1993 fatwa issued by Muhammad Sayyid Tantawi, in his role as state mufti.

6. Kotb was convinced that "developed countries" around the world no longer perform operations on living donors, although I tried to tell him otherwise. He was under the impression that "only places like Egypt and India" rely heavily upon transplantation from living donors and, worse, from living unrelated donors. Hence, he described the practice as "uncivilized."

7. See Annemarie Mol's (2008) discussion of the logic of care as opposed to the logic of choice in health care.

8. Scientists in many different cultures have integrated religious conceptions into their scientific views and practice, even those who consider themselves adamantly unreligious (Haraway 1989; Keller 1992; Gusterson 1996; Helmreich 1998). In Dr. Kotb's arguments, like those of other Egyptian physicians, he seamlessly and conscientiously integrated a religious conception of the world—with God the all-knowing Creator at the center—into his understanding of human anatomy and physiology. In his *Science and Religion: Some Historical Perspectives*, John Hedley Brooke notes the difficulty in using "science" and "religion" as analytical categories; as a historian writing about western Europe, Brooke cautions, "Precisely because the boundaries have shifted with time, it would be artificial to ask about the relationship between 'science' and 'religion' as if modern definitions of their provenance had some timeless validity" (1991: 8). This same precaution should be taken with respect to different social and cultural contexts as well.

9. In 2005, the going rate for a kidney was 20,000–30,000 £E, approximately $3,500–$5,000.

10. In contrast, dialysis patients who are candidates for renal transplantation living in Europe and North America describe dialysis as time standing still, during which they wait in limbo for a kidney transplant, which they see as a new chance at life (Fox and Swazey 1974; Joralemon 1995; Gordon 2001; Gordon 2002; Kierans 2005; Russ, Shim, et al. 2005; Kaufman, Russ, et al. 2006). In the United States, the question often asked is *when* a transplant candidate will receive a kidney (how much time will be spent on the waiting list), not *whether* he or she will receive one. As of 2005, most candidates for kidney transplantation in the United States received a kidney within five years (Scientific Registry of Transplant Recipients 2005, www.ustransplant.org (last accessed 8/22/2011).

11. According to the Egyptian Society of Nephrology's annual regsitries, in 1996 the prevalence of end-stage renal disease was 225 per million. In 2004, the number had soared to 483 per million. The registries can be found on the

official website of the Egyptian Nephrology Society at www.esnonline.net. See also Bakr 2000 and Barsoum 2003. Less than one-fourth of the donated kidneys were from family members, as I explain more fully later on. The general assumption within the Egyptian medical community is that donors who are unrelated are paid for their organs. An exception to this is spouses, who are often labeled as "unrelated" (biologically) if not specifically labeled as "emotionally related."

12. The cost of a lifelong regimen of expensive immunosuppressants, however, is prohibitive for many patients.

13. This system for obtaining government-sponsored treatment is known as *nafaq al-dawla*.

14. Medical data show that recurrent lupus nephritis rarely reappears in the newly transplanted kidney of a lupus patient, but when it does appear, the patient is at increased risk of kidney graft rejection and death (Schiezer 2009).

15. *Nasib* literally means "portion," as in what is allotted to you in life.

16. The reasoning behind quick action is based on the biomedical assertion that the longer a patient is on dialysis, the worse the final outcome for kidney graft survival.

17. Dr. Badr designed a sociological study in the form of a questionnaire that he asked the donors to fill out, the results of which he shared with me. Between 1998 and 2001, he asked forty-five kidney donors (thirty had benefited commercially, and fifteen had donated to relatives), most of whom he personally saw for follow-up treatment, to fill out a confidential questionnaire about their feelings posttransplantation. He asked them: Is your life better now that you received money in exchange for your kidney? What did you do with the money? Has your financial situation improved? Do you feel ill after the transplant? Two-thirds (twenty out of thirty) of the commercial donors reported that their financial situation had worsened, but they reported that this was because they had not spent the money in the right place, or that they had received less money than anticipated from the buyer, or both. Only five of forty donors who answered this question (12.5 percent) reported worsened health conditions; thirty-seven of these forty underwent medical follow-up treatment. Out of the thirty who had sold their kidneys, twenty-six said that they felt they had sacrificed a lot for their families; thirteen of these (43 percent) said that they regretted their decision.

18. Armando Salvatore (1997) discusses what he calls the hyperobjectification of Islam among both Western observers and contemporary Muslims who draw on Islamic rhetoric for political ends. 'Ali, in his politicized form of Muslim identity, stands out from the other patients (many from rural backgrounds) stating things such as "Religion is the only thing stopping me." Most of his fellow patients do not articulate "religion" as an autonomous agent in this way. And while I argue further on that 'Ali does not experience "religion" as an object external to himself, he does, in instances such as in the above statement, participate in an increasingly dominant discourse that represents religion as an objectified agent.

19. The army and other state employers who provide insurance coverage that pays for treatments have calculated that the costs of transplantation end up being less than years on dialysis, and many encourage their employees (who continue to receive salaries although unable to work) to seek transplantation.

20. *Salat al-istikhara* is generally two prayer cycles *(raka'a)* long, after which the person asks God directly for guidance.

21. The more powerful current immunosuppressive drugs make complete tissue match less necessary, so many in 'Ali's position would have proceeded with the transplant anyway. In his case, refusal to proceed was a combination of reluctance both on his part and on the part of the physicians. Because the number of patients needing transplants at the time of my fieldwork far exceeded the facilities available, physicians in Egypt (in state hospitals) were disinclined to proceed with transplants without a full tissue match, to increase chances of graft survival.

22. This mystification is especially the case with organs procured from brain-dead patients. Yet living kidney donation is currently on the rise in the United States, exceeding cadaver donation for the first time in 2001. The greatest increase in live donors has been among individuals unrelated to the recipients. Whereas in 1988 the proportion of living and deceased donors was 32 and 68 percent, respectively, by 2000 it was 50–50. In 2003, 47 percent of kidneys transplanted were from deceased donors, and 53 percent were from living donors (out of 15,135 total kidneys transplanted) (Kaufman, Russ, et al. 2006: 82).

23. Hence my slight difference from Hania Sholkamy's important discussion of forbearance in Egyptian medical experiences, where she writes: "God, as the ultimate source, is a formula that helps *ex post facto* acceptance but is not one which precipitates an *a priori* fatalism. It is a tenet that leaves plenty of room for people to take initiative in defining, managing, and protecting their health and well-being" (Sholkamy 2004: 122). For 'Ali, what was important was a *continual* alignment of himself, and his own desires, with what he understood to be God's will.

24. This hadith is well known and oft cited among Egyptians. It can be found in the modern Islamic scholar Sayyid Sabiq's compendia of hadith traditions, *Fiqh al-sunna* (Sabiq 1994).

CHAPTER SIX

1. As Vinh-Kim Nguyen (2010) has demonstrated in his work on antiretroviral drugs among AIDS communities in West Africa, scarce drugs are allocated not to those most vulnerable (e.g., mothers and children) but to those who are able to support more community members (e.g., workers in the cause of securing access to therapy).

2. See Comaroff and Comaroff 2000 for a discussion of the ways in which "gambling" becomes a salient trope in our contemporary neoliberal era, as the expectation of a person having safety nets provided by social networks or the state has shifted to the expectation that each individual will either succeed financially or fall to his or her own ruin.

3. A few dialysis clinics, including those in military hospitals, attempted to provide separate spaces for women and men to ensure more privacy, but most dialysis wards did not do this, because the patient group continually changed and men generally far outnumbered women.

4. Creatinine, a waste product formed by muscle contractions, is passed through the kidneys. It is also found in protein foods, mostly muscle meats. When the kidneys do not get rid of creatinine, it remains in the bloodstream. Elevated levels of creatinine signal that the kidneys are not eliminating this waste from the body.

5. *Il-ghalaba* is a colloquial expression referring to those who are downtrodden. I render it in the colloquial transliteration because this term rarely appears in print media.

6. The dialysis machine performs three major functions: (1) it pumps blood and monitors blood flow; (2) it cleans wastes and toxins from the blood; and (3) it monitors blood pressure and fluid removal.

7. In an article in *Al-Misri al-Yawm*, Sabir Mashhur (2007) reveals the contents of a report done by the British Quality First Institute, which inspected Sorour's private company, the Hidelina Company, in 2002 to determine whether it should be granted an international standardization (ISO) certificate. The report found that the dialysis filters and solutions manufactured by the company were stored improperly such that they were exposed to the sun, which altered their effect and was dangerous for patients. The report also found that the water at the manufacturing plant was unclean, the water pipes were rusty, and there were cracks in the ceiling, making it a breeding ground for bacteria. The *Al-Misri al-Yawm* article goes on to say that Sorour's response to the report was to attempt to export his company's dialysis filters to China. A Chinese delegation inspected Sorour's factory, objected to the proportion of urea in the kidney dialysis filters, and noted that the company should have used a machine to run tests on the filters at zero degrees. Sorour then bought a machine from a company in a neighboring building; the machine's gauge did not read less than zero, so Sorour fabricated one with the right numbers and stuck it on the machine. The Chinese apparently discovered this attempted forgery and rejected claims that the company's technicians had made the necessary changes (Mashhur 2007).

8. The Egyptian Society of Nephrology and Transplantation reported that in 2004, 82% of dialysis patients tested positive for Hepatitus C. See www.esntonline.com, last accessed 8/22/2011.

9. A negative consequence is that patients often misdiagnose the nature of their illness and go to the wrong specialist, who also does not correctly identify the problem, as with Shadya's family misidentifying lupus as a skin condition and one of her initial doctors mistakenly treating her for rheumatism of the heart.

10. This is why many patients are initially reluctant to accept medical orders from profit-oriented dialysis clinics for immediate long-term dialysis treatment.

11. In Egypt's 2008 Demographic and Health Survey, information collected on 6, 578 women and 5,430 men revealed that 13% of women and 11% of men were hypertensive. In Egypt, hypertension (high blood pressure) is the

leading cause of kidney failure. The rate of hypertension was significantly higher among those who did not complete primary school. Thirty-two percent of women and 21% of men were aware that they had high blood pressure but were not being treated, and another 27% of women and 53% of men were unaware of their condition. Fourteen percent of hypertensive men were being treated but still had elevated blood pressure, measured at the time of the survey (El-Zanaty and Way 2009: 228–234).

12. The nephrologist in charge of the dialysis ward during the time of my research confirmed these particular patients' claims that botched operations and the misuse of pharmaceuticals had played a large part in precipitating their kidney failure.

13. In my ethnographic work, I found that patients put uncertainty to productive use, that is, as a space in which to formulate criticism of social inequalities and state irresponsibility. See also the challenges of Petryna (2002) and Whitmarsh, Davis, and colleagues (2007) to the standard claim in U.S. biomedicine that uncertainty acts only negatively, upsetting patients who need to know the diagnosis and its cause.

14. Medical researchers from the Cairo University Department of Nephrology studied etiologies of serious renal disease in Egypt by registering all patients ($n = 155$) who came to the nephrology service at the university during a period of sixty-two days in 1993. They reported, "The most common specific etiology for chronic end-stage renal failure was diabetes mellitus type II in the older patients; second most common was Schistosoma in the younger ones. Most diabetic patients came from the city. All but one Schistosoma patient came from rural Egypt. In the 22 patients who underwent renal biopsy the most common diagnosis was mesangio capillary glumerulonephritis. The prevalence of acute renal failure, particularly iatrogenic-toxic, is increasing" (Essamie, Soliman, et al. 1995). This last sentence about increasing acute nephrotoxicity corresponds to the suggestions of the nephrologists I interviewed that a change is occurring in the etiology of kidney disease.

15. Columnist 'Adil Ibrahim, of *Al-Ahram*, often writes of "economic dangers." See, for example, Ibrahim 2007.

16. The Kafr al-Zayat Pesticides and Chemicals Company (KZPC) was established in 1955 as a state-owned entity and held a monopoly over the pesticides market in Egypt until liberalization policies began in the early 1990s. The company was privatized in 1996. An alarming report on the health status in the impact zone of the Kafr al-Zayat chemical plant was published in March 2006 by a global NGO project called the International POPs Elimination Project (IPEN; "POPs" is the abbreviation for persistent organic pollutants) in partnership with the UN Industrial Development Organization (UNIDO) and the UN Environmental Program (IPEN 2006).

17. Aflatoxin is produced by fungal action during the production, harvest, storage, and processing of food. The U.S. Food and Drug Administration (FDA) considers aflatoxins to be unavoidable contaminants in foods, and its strategy

has been to minimize consumer risk by controlling their levels. In a comprehensive review article on aflatoxins in developing countries, Jonathan H. Williams, T. D. Phillips, and their colleagues argue that methods used by the FDA to manage the problem "cannot realistically be used in developing countries, because of the characteristics of the food systems and the technological infrastructure in those countries; therefore, aflatoxins are uncontrolled in these situations. The result is a 'divide' in the prevalence of aflatoxicosis exposure between people living in developed and developing countries" (2004: 1106). Williams, Phillips, and their colleagues advocate pharmacoprotection: use of a food additive that acts as a binding agent to prevent the digestive tract's absorption of toxins.

18. Most noteworthy in this regard is the overview by Dr. Rashad Barsum (2002), a leading Egyptian nephrologist. A recent study found that babies who were exclusively breastfed were vulnerable to renal toxicity because of elevated levels of ochratoxins that were passed via breast milk (see Hassan, Sheashaa, et al. 2005).

19. The issue of "cancerous wheat" has precipitated mass demonstrations and political movement among members of opposition parties, students, and youths, especially in Daqahliyya Province. Many reports have expressed surprise that members of Parliament acknowledged the situation and demanded action to correct it, including the government's guarantee that the toxic wheat would be destroyed and not sold for consumption. For print journal reports, see *Al-Ahali* 2007; *Al-Misri al-Yawm* 2007b; and *Al-'Arabi* 2007. Information has also been disseminated, organized, and historicized on Web sites of active political parties in the region. The Kifayya political party initiated demands for quick government and legal action during May 19–20, 2007. The Muslim Brotherhood followed suit, with online articles informing people about the wheat and demanding clean and safe food and water. These online sites continually change as government agents work to dismantle them.

20. See Mitchell's critiques of U.S. development reports that consistently attribute Egypt's need to import food to the country's desert geography and "population explosion" and, therefore, its "natural" inability to feed itself. Mitchell (2002) demonstrates how the restructuring policies of USAID and the IMF have increased inequalities by removing price subsidies and altering what Egyptian farmers grow.

21. Columnist Khayri Ramadan (2007) goes on to make a plea for the state to intervene in the treatment of the intellectual and academic scholar 'Abd al-Wahhab al-Massiri, who has been afflicted with leukemia since 2001 and has submitted requests to the presidency to be treated at the expense of the state. Ramadan argues that the state is quick to pay for treatment when a famous actor or movie star is ill.

22. Although patients widely perceive public hospitals as bastions of corruption and mistreatment, there is even less oversight and surveillance of private clinics by the Ministry of Health. Two years after I met Shadya and her

mother, I found out that prosecutorial authorities had shut down the make-shift private dialysis clinic where Shadya was being treated, after numerous complaints from patients and family members. The attending physician was arrested for fraud and malpractice. This action was taken under criminal law, not under regular surveillance by the Ministry of Health. In another dialysis unit, reporters from *Al-Misri al-Yawm* found dialysis patients neglected while doctors and nurses were engrossed in watching a television soccer match (*Al-Misri al-Yawm* 2007 a).

23. Interestingly, two of the Islamic legal scholars whom I interviewed also offered such a statement: "The person in question *[sahib al-amr]* knows his case better than anyone and is in the best position to make an ethical choice," deferring their own authority back to the questioner.

24. There are many references in the Qur'an to God's creation of humans from "water" (i.e., a liquid)—often interpreted as seminal fluid or as a mixture of male and female reproductive fluids. See Inhorn 1994 for a discussion of Egyptians' various understandings of reproduction and fluids.

25. While this may be a generally accepted phenomenon, in the example of the mother with two sons needing kidneys, the gift of the kidney to one of them did cause familial disruption.

26. While all the major religious authorities and all those in state-appointed positions opined that organ transplantation is conditionally permissible, I have shown that on a more popular level there is dissent on this question. Many shaykhs who work in local mosques, and especially in areas outside Cairo, are likely to follow the same logic as that of Shaykh Sha'rawi and say that organ transplantation is not allowed because the body belongs to God. Others would argue that it depends on whether the organ is given altruistically, with consent, and so forth.

27. Daniel J. Smith writes of Nigeria: "Having children is not only a means to individual personhood, but also a fulfillment of one's obligations to kin and community" (2001: 139). In the context of HIV/AIDS, the promise of antiret-roviral therapy makes possible again the crucial "life projects" of marriage and reproduction.

28. From 1976 to 2004, a total of 1,569 kidney transplants were recorded in Mansoura with data about the donor-recipient relationship. Of these, 26.4 percent were from parents to children, 47.9 percent from siblings, and 1.7 percent from offspring to parents. Thanks to Dr. 'Amr el-Husseini, a nephrologist at Mansoura, for providing me with this information.

29. This doctor's reasoning might seem questionable, because he is compar-ing having a life-threatening illness with the *risk* of illness. Yet as someone who works at the Mansoura Kidney Center, he must be extremely selective about which patients he operates on, because the demand continues to be so much higher than the number of transplants that can be practically performed.

30. I observed no preference for sons over daughters in parents donating kidneys to children.

31. From the years 1976 to 2004, data were collected on 1,548 of the kidney transplants carried out in Mansoura. Of these, 1,158 were for males and 390 for females. Unfortunately no good sociological data exist on specific family relationship between donors and recipients.

32. Nancy Scheper-Hughes writes that in general the circulation of kidneys follows established routes of capital, for example, from poor to more affluent bodies and from females to males. She also notes, "Women are rarely the recipients of purchased or purloined organs anywhere in the world" (2005: 150).

33. Also interesting to note is the scant discussion in Egypt of current practices in the United States and elsewhere in which kidneys are extracted from patients immediately after their hearts stop beating. These are orchestrated deaths, in which a patient who goes into cardiac arrest and has a "do not resuscitate" order is rushed into surgery for organ retrieval. For a very short time in Egypt, kidneys were extracted from executed prisoners after their hearts stopped beating, before the practice was exposed and ordered to stop. Extracting kidneys from hospital inpatients after cardiac arrest is unlikely to be feasible in Egypt anytime soon. No coordinated legal, bureaucratic, and technical infrastructure exists to support it, many families are unlikely to agree to it, and no concept parallel to a "do not resuscitate" order exists.

34. Physicians often ask if intermarriage is the cause of a high burden of disease within a single family; many tend to stigmatize patients for consanguineous marriage (usually between first or second cousins) and subsequent medical problems.

35. Indeed, in organ transplantation, the recipient's two failed kidneys are usually left in the body, so the transplanted kidney becomes a third kidney, though in Sayyid's case he only had one kidney left, so a transplanted kidney would be a second one.

36. In Sayyid's narrative, his kidney lasted three years in his brother, while in Fatima's narrative it lasted five years. It may be that after three years, the brother began to experience chronic (rather than acute) rejection and died after five years.

37. Other "moral lessons" were narrated to me throughout my years of research into Egyptian medical practice, such as women who suffer from infertility after having themselves opted for tubal ligation and later changing their minds (Hamdy 1998) or after having sought abortions and later being unable to get pregnant again (also described by Inhorn 1994, 2003).

CHAPTER SEVEN

1. Afifi (2003) reports 50 percent; Budiani (2010) reports 90 percent. After 2003, the Egyptian Society of Nephrology ceased to provide this information in their annual Egyptian Renal Registry.

2. As the work of Scheper-Hughes has shown, the nationality of the clientele and brokers quickly changes as organ routes adapt to a dynamic market; my reference to Gulf Arabs reflects the local discourse currently in the Egyptian press. Israeli military aggression against Palestinian bodies has also extended to the realm of organ transplantation with allegations of Israelis secretly harvesting organs from Palestinian (victim) bodies. See Weir 2009.

3. Tober cited in Sharp 2001.

4. I write "his kidney" because the vast majority of paid kidney donors in Egypt are male, although the number of female commercial donors has increased in the last few years.

5. People from the Delta provinces of Gharbiyya and Daqahliyya (where Iman and Nagla lived) reported paying much lower prices than people in Cairo, although all the donors were from poor areas in Cairo. For patients (recipients) in Cairo, the general range seemed to be from 10,000 to 30,000 £E, with most transactions around 20,000 to 25,000 £E.

6. The practice of transplanting pieces of the liver from living donors, less common in Europe and the United States because of the grave risk it poses to the donor, has taken off in countries like Japan and Egypt, where there is greater antipathy toward harvesting whole organs (such as livers) from brain-dead donors.

7. I heard three different organ recipients from Tanta who had received kidneys from commercial donors in Cairo describe this type of ongoing relationship. But according to the studies conducted by Dr. Badr and Dr. Budiani (described below), this is generally not the norm and certainly not the norm within Cairo.

8. Dr. Hamdi al-Sayyid is reported as saying, "The total number of transplants taking place every year ranges from 120 to 130. In comparison to India for example, the number isn't so high" (IRIN 2006).

9. WHO report cited in El Katatney 2009.

10. For more commentary on the film, see Tabishat 2003.

11. The following discussion of Emad comes from Zalat and al-Bahnasawi 2007.

12. Lawrence Cohen's words seem to characterize Emad's narrative aptly: "What is exceptional in these situations is less one's reduction to a zone of indistinction in which political life and bare life collapse together, but a more articulated zone in which one trades in one's bare life—kidneys, other biomatter—in order to remain a political subject of sacrifice and love" (2005: 82–83).

13. In the study by Dr. Badr (in his possession), his questionnaire asks similar questions phrased in different ways. For example, seventeen out of forty-five answered yes to the question "Do you feel an injustice was done to you after donating your kidney?" Sixteen out of forty-five answered yes to the question "If now, after donation, you could go back and undo what you did, would you?" And thirteen out of forty-five answered yes to the question "Since the donation, do you regret your decision?" See comparative information on paid

donors in Moazam, Zaman, et al. 2009, published in a recent *Hastings Center Report*. Also see Ghods 2002 for discussions of Iran's regulated program for unrelated living donors.

14. Cited in Fleishman and El-Hennawy 2008.

15. Debra Budiani, a medical anthropologist, began her own nonprofit organization to address the problem of commercial live donors and organ trafficking in Egypt and other countries. See also her film, *Organ SOS: A Plea from the Shadows* (2010).

16. Poor Egyptians, as well as refugee populations in Cairo, such as the Sudanese and Somali refugee communities, have felt particularly vulnerable to organ theft during operations and have avoided Egyptian doctors and health clinics (Budiani, personal communication, 2003). Whether these fears are founded or not, they profoundly influence poor and marginalized people's interactions with health care (Scheper-Hughes 2000; Tabishat 2003; Budiani and Shibly 2008). Barbara Harrell-Bond, who as a professor at the American University in Cairo teaches forced migration and refugee studies, said, "Many refugees in Cairo, particularly the Sudanese, express their self-marginalisation from Egyptian society in terms of their fear of Egyptian doctors and the threat of organ theft" (quoted in IRIN 2006).

17. Mohamed Ghoneim is quoted as saying, "No one wants to approach the issue of human organ trafficking in Egypt because trafficking is a huge source of wealth" (IRIN 2008).

18. See IRIN 2006.

19. The regulations have had to be updated continually as the organ trade itself has changed. They were initially designed to limit transplant operations to biological relatives or "emotional" relatives (i.e., spouses). But when several press reports exposed the trend of Gulf Arabs coming to Egypt, marrying a "seller-donor" for the purposes of the transplant, and then divorcing afterward, amendments were proposed, such as the requirement that the couple be married for five years (or three if they had children) before the operation. In my interviews in 2003, I found that many of the Egyptian medical professionals who claimed that a "crackdown" on the organ trade needed to occur wanted to place a moratorium on transplants outside the public teaching hospitals, where there was more transparency and oversight. In the first two decades of kidney transplantation in Egypt, doctors imagined a strict divide between operations performed by the faculties of medicine in teaching hospitals and those by doctors in unregulated clinics. But some doctors in public teaching hospitals grew more and more emboldened in their practices and in their disregard for sellers, and many doctors performed transplant operations in both public teaching hospitals and for-profit clinics. As Dr. Badr quickly pointed out, for doctors to limit transplant operations to the public teaching hospital clearly served these doctors' own interests by stamping out the (private sector) competition. In August 2008, the Egyptian Medical Syndicate provoked another controversy by giving this nationalism a religious-ethnic spin: in claiming that many poor Muslim Egyptians sold organs to wealthier Coptic Christians, they proposed

a limitation on organs transplanted from one religious group to another. Human rights groups quickly called foul, sensing that this move would do no more than inflame interreligious tensions and put the Coptic Christian minority at a disadvantage in receiving organs. The proposal was quickly withdrawn.

20. In Mansoura, a prominent nephrologist with whom I spoke extolled the family values of the close-knit *fellahin,* some of whom have considered cousins as donors. Yet the way in which he glorified this practice further confirmed that it was outside the norm.

21. The criteria for tissue matching differs from doctor to doctor and clinic to clinic, but most of the doctors with whom I spoke sought at least a three out of six or four out of six HLA match. See also Ghoneim, Bakr, et al. 2001.

22. My findings in Egypt also complicate the now standard narrative in the organ transplant literature that the introduction of cyclosporine (a specific immunosuppressive drug) drove the organ trade (e.g., Cohen 2001; Scheper-Hughes 2001) or even drastically changed the graft survival rates of kidney transplantation (e.g., Fox and Swazey 1992). Dr. Ghoneim and his team in Mansoura, in their study of graft survival and the nephrotoxicity of the new and old drugs, found that the results obtained through the use of cyclosporine did not warrant its prolonged use primarily because of its prohibitive cost (El-Agroudy, Sobh, et al. 2004).

23. This call for greater transparency was made in consultation with medical anthropologist Debra Budiani.

24. Even when captured on camera, the realities of organ trafficking tended to be denied by government officials. In a documentary film focusing on youths in slums of Istabl Antar (a slum within the wealthy Ma'adi suburb, home to many American and other foreign ex-patriot residents of Egypt), the director, Yasmine Abu-Youssef, portrays the "mafialike brokers" that entrap poor young men in organ trafficking. The film was met with denial by officials in the Cabinet and the Ministry of Health and Population. See Amin 2007a.

25. Salah 2009.

26. The Ministry of Health reported a slight decline in the number of transplants in 2007 but then a rise in 2008 (El-Katatney 2009). Given that part of the problem has been an inability to estimate actual figures of clandestine operations, these figures can be interpreted only as conjectures.

27. Abdel Rahman Shahin, the spokesperson for the Ministry of Health, cited in Awad 2008.

28. Nasir, the employee at the Medical Syndicate, agreed that this was the case, and Dr. Alaa Fayez, professor of children's surgery at Cairo's Ain Shams University, was also reported to have said, "It's very difficult to control the activities of small private clinics, which are very widespread in Egypt. . . . Often, donors will be from Sudan, for instance, while recipients may be from the wealthier Arabian Gulf." In this same report, journalist Ibrahim Othman said, "It's not unusual for secret agreements to be made with Saudi Arabian patients

willing to pay thousands of dollars for a transplant. Such operations totally circumvent stipulations laid down by the syndicate" (IRIN 2006).

29. In Egypt, the limited supply is particularly critical in light of endemic hepatitis C. As mentioned in the introduction, in the 1960s and '70s, a government campaign featuring tatar-emetic injections to treat schistosomiasis, before the availability of disposable needles (which were not available until the 1980s), inadvertently spread the hepatitis C virus among the population. Estimates vary widely: at least nine million Egyptians (between 10 and 30 percent of the population) test positive for hepatitis C. The impact of this virus—liver failure—is now clinically overloading the health system, and Egyptian medical experts say that liver disease has become the number one health care priority for the country. Approximately 70 percent of all liver deaths in Egypt are due to hepatitis C. The sobering reality is that liver transplantation is not a realistic solution to what has been dubbed Egypt's "viral bomb." See McGrath 2009b.

30. See Pharma and Healthcare Insight 2010.

31. People subjected to highly invasive and risky surgeries in the extraction of vital organs are always referred to as "donors" and never as "patients" in medical discourse, obscuring the suffering that is necessary to sustain organ transplantation, a point that anthropologists Lesley Sharp, Margaret Lock, and Nancy Scheper-Hughes have also made. These anthropologists have also pointed out that the "sacrificial violence" of living donation is further rendered invisible with the powerful metaphors of "saving" and "gifting" life. The language of "donation" also obviously obscures the financial transaction, when present (Fox and Swazey 1974, 1992; Lock 2002b; Ong and Collier 2005; Scheper-Hughes 2005, 2007; Sharp 2006, 2007).

CONCLUSIONS

1. *Al-Ahram* 2009. Not withstanding its positive associations, note that the Mansoura Kidney Center operates with the biomedical tendency to focus reductively on pathology without assessing wider social, economic, and political ills.

2. "Pharaonic regime" was an allusion to Murbarak's rule and the *sham al-nasim* holiday that Egyptians have celebrated to mark the coming of spring since the time of the pharaohs. See *Al-Misri al-Yawm* 2010a, 2010b.

3. As several feminist scholars working on the Middle East have demonstrated, violence against women as "cultural" or "religious" (such as in "honor killings") is received in the Euro-American media and academic scholarship with moral outrage, while the everyday violence against women throughout the world remains invisible. Didier Fassin (2003) has argued that "exotic" and supposedly traditional African beliefs—such as sex with a virgin will cure AIDS—do much to pathologize Africans and do little to shed light on the ordinariness of sexual violence and rape that have been exacerbated by historical patterns of colonial violence, geographical dispersion, migratory labor patterns,

and the dismemberment of families. And Talal Asad (2003) has recently questioned why it is that global media discourses judge violence committed in the name of religion so differently from violence and terror committed in the name of secular ideals. See also Hafez 2011.

4. See Agamben 1998; Khalidi 2009; Rutherford 2008; and El-Ghobashy 2006 for a nuanced discussion of the state of exception in the rule of law.

Glossary of Frequently Used Arabic Terms

al-Azhar:

The premier institution for the study of Islam in the Sunni Arab world. Founded in 970 in the heart of what would later become the center of the emerging city of Cairo, it was modernized in 1961 into a state-run university, which, while specializing in the training of Islamic scholars in the various fields of Islamic studies, now also offers a variety of academic disciplines, including medicine and clinical training. The rector of al-Azhar, or shaykh al-Azhar, and the grand mufti of the republic are the two most authoritative state-appointed positions of religious scholars. See studies by Chris Eccel (1984) and Malika Zeghal (1999) on al-Azhar and the changes it underwent through the modern period.

daʿiya:

An individual who attempts to spread the call to Islam through various missionizing efforts. While most who take on this role have attained a significant level of training in Islamic scholarship, their activities are geared toward the accessibility of the Islamic message and its relevance to daily practice and spirituality.

Dar al-Iftaʾ:

The Egyptian state bureaucratic office responsible for issuing official opinions (fatwas) according to Islamic legal precepts. This institution was created in 1895, to give the modern state more direct control over muftis' authority. Since that time, the head of the institution, the "grand mufti" or the "mufti of the republic" became a government employee appointed by the president of the republic. Since 2003 Shaykh ʿAli Gumaʿa has sought to reform its practices and raise its profile as the authoritative locus for issuing fatwas.

darura: Need, or necessity. As a technical term of Islamic juris-prudence, there are specific criteria for what constitutes *darura* such that an ordinary ruling can be relaxed, in order to uphold the major goals (*maqasid*) of the shariʿa. These are, in order of importance, the preser-vation of (1) life *(al-nafs)*, (2) religion (*al-din*), (3) the intellect (*al-ʿaql*), (4) lineage (*al-nasl*), (5) and prop-erty (*al-mal*). These were also known as *al-daruriyyat al-khamsa* (Opwis 2005). In conjunction with the legal tool of *maslaha,* the aim of employing these tools is to avoid rigidity in Islamic law in cases in which rigid-ity might restrict rather than uphold the major prin-ciples of Islam. This notion of "necessity," as it is often glossed in English, has become used with increasing frequency, fewer restrictions, and more overt political motivations of state interest, becoming a particularly contentious topic.

daʿwa: The efforts undertaken to summon both Muslims and non-Muslims to the call of Islam. The craft of *daʿwa* differs from that of traditional Islamic scholarship in that its audience is broader and its methods of address-ing that audience are more flexible and varied accord-ing to the sociopolitical context.

fatwa: An opinion offered by an Islamic scholar, rooted in the precepts of Islamic legal reasoning, in response to a specific question. *Fatwas* are nonbinding on the ques-tioner and are intended to serve as a form of guidance. Who is legitimately allowed to give a *fatwa* is a matter of contention, particularly when conflicting opinions are offered for the same or similar questions.

fellah (pl. fellahin): An Egyptian peasant farmer. The term can also refer more broadly to anyone who is associated with a rural sociocultural background, even if not engaged in agriculture or village life. Its usage is ambiguous: city people often use *fellah* derogatorily to refer to ignorance and lack of civilization; however, the *fellah* is also simultaneously romanticized as the bearer of true, authentic Egyptian values.

fiqh: The discipline of Islamic jurisprudence to produce legal rulings designed to regulate all aspects of public, pri-vate, and commercial life, based on interpretation of the scriptural sources.

galabiyya: The long, ankle-length robe that is traditional Egyp-tian dress.

hadith:	A saying of the Prophet Muhammad that carries the weight of being a scriptural source when authenticated. In contemporary Egypt, as elsewhere in the Muslim world, *hadiths* often take the form of aphorisms that have significant spiritual weight when used to comment on social practice.
halal:	That which is permissible under Islamic precepts. As a technical term of Islamic jurisprudence, what is *halal* is simply that which is not forbidden or considered sinful and can include both practices that are discouraged and those that are seen as neutral. However, in everyday parlance, *halal* bears a positive connotation to indicate the spiritual and moral value of a particular practice.
haram:	That which is forbidden or sinful (i.e., those acts that will weigh against the offender on the Day of Judgment), both under Islamic precepts and as a technical term of Islamic jurisprudence. In contemporary speech it also has a broader meaning that indicates something pitiful or upsetting. For example, a person might say: "Oh *haram*—that old man has only one leg!
hurma:	That which is sacrosanct or inviolable, and etiologically related to the word *haram*. *Hurma* is often used in connection to the dead body and its status as an object that must be treated with utmost care.
ifta':	The practice of issuing a *fatwa*.
istifta':	The practice of seeking out a *fatwa*.
maslaha:	The principle that one must consider the public interest in crafting rulings that form the shari'a. The notion of *maslaha* as a tool of jurisprudence has been of intense interest among the Muslim reformers of the twentieth century as a mechanism for how to modernize Islamic law. This has led to considerable debate and tension over whether it can serve as an independent source of law or can be appropriate only in the absence of specific guidance from the Qur'an or the teachings of the Prophet Muhammad *(sunna)*. In more general parlance *maslaha* has come to refer to acts that have greater benefit than harm, particularly on the level of the individual.
maslaha 'ama:	The consideration of social welfare in efforts to determine the value and ethical standing of certain social practices, often focusing on the balance between the benefit to the general public and the potential harm to an individual or small group.

mufti:	A scholar who issues a *fatwa*.
al-sabr:	A value that can be glossed as patience, forbearance, fortitude in the face of struggle, and steadfastness in one's faith.
sadaqa:	Charity and the spiritual rewards associated with it.
sadaqa jariyya	(pronounced as "gariyya" in the Egyptian dialect): The notion of the continual accrual of spiritual rewards, even after death, stemming from an act of charity that has a perpetual nature, such as building a mosque.
salat:	Ritual prayer performed in Arabic, can refer to the obligatory five daily prayers or to superorotory prayers.
shariʿa:	The rules and regulations governing the social lives of Muslims as derived from the sources of the Qurʾan and prophetic sunna, though some understand shariʿa literally as the "path" to follow God's command, which they contrast with *fiqh*. Others claim there can be no shariʿa without fiqh, and still others claim there is little or no distinction between the two.
shaykh:	In Egypt, usually a term of respect given to someone who has attained a level of Islamic scholarship. *Shaykh* is also used as the official title for Islamic scholars who are appointed to positions of leadership in the major state institutions of religious authority.
al-shirk:	Specifically, acts that deny the oneness of God. By extension, in everyday usage *al-shirk* also carries the broader meaning of idolatry, polytheism, and heresy.
al-tawakkul:	Utter reliance on God. While this concept has often been described in English as the concept of fatalism, the connotation in Arabic is far more positive and linked to the fundamental meaning of the word *islam*, namely, submission to the will of God. *Tawakkul* is something that many Muslims strive to cultivate in establishing the closeness of their relationship to the divine.
usul al-fiqh:	The principles guiding the construction of Islamic jurisprudence through the methodological extrapolation of rules from revelation.

References

'Abd al-Hafiz, G., M. 'Arafa, et al. 2007. Drinking Water Crisis Spills Over Provinces. al-Misri al-Yawn.

Abdeldayem, H. 2010. Transparency and Living Donor Liver Transplantation in Egypt. Nile Liver Journal 1(1):7–13.

'Abduh, M. 1966. *The theology of unity.* Trans. Ishaq Musa'ad and Kenneth Cragg, eds. London: George Allen and Unwin Ltd.

Abu-Lughod, L. 2005. *Dramas of nationhood: The politics of television in Egypt.* Chicago: University of Chicago Press.

Afifi, A. 2000. *The Egyptian Renal Registry: 5th annual report of the Egyptian Society of Nephrology for the year 2000,* 1–11.Cairo: Egyptian Society of Nephrology

———. 2001. *The Egyptian Renal Registry: 6th annual report of the Egyptian Society of Nephrology for the year 2001.* Cairo: Egyptian Society of Nephrology.

———. 2003. *The Egyptian Renal Registry: 7th annual report of the Egyptian Society of Nephrology for the year 2003.* Cairo: Egyptian Society of Nephrology.

Afifi, A., and M. Abdel Karim. 1996. *Renal replacement therapy in Egypt: First annual report,* 1–11.Cairo: Egyptian Society of Nephrology.

Agamben, G. 1998. *Homo sacer: Sovereign power and bare life.* Stanford, CA: Stanford University Press.

Agrama, H.A. 2010. Ethics, tradition, authority: Toward an anthropology of the fatwa. *American Ethnologist* 37(1): 2–18.

El-Agroudy, A., M. Sobh, et al. 2004. A prospective, randomized study of coadministration of ketoconazole and cyclosporine A in kidney transplant recipients: Ten-year follow-up. *Transplantation* 77(9): 1371–76.

Al-Ahali. 2007. Al-Qamh al-musartan amam al-na'ib al-'am (The cancerous wheat before the district attorney). May 16.

Al-Ahram. 2009. Al-mufaraqa al-mudhhila! (What a difference!) Letter to the editor. March 24.

Amin, H. 2002. Freedom as a value in Arab media: Perceptions and attitudes among journalists. *Political Communication* 19: 125–35.

Amin, T. 2007a. Documentary unveils brokerage for selling kidneys among the poor living in slums. *Al-Misri al-Yawm*, English edition, July 15. www .almasry-alyoum.com/article2.aspx?ArticleID = 68776 (last accessed 8/22/2011).

Al-ʿArabi. 2007. 6000 tin min al-qamh al-musartan fi al-Daqahliyya (6,000 tons of canerous wheat in Daqahliyya). May 20.

ʿArafa, M. 2007. 5,000 people demonstrate against thirst. *Al-Misri al-Yawm*, English edition, July 14.

Aramesh, K. 2007. Human dignity in Islamic bioethics. *Iranian Journal of Allergy, Asthma and Immunology* 6(suppl. 5): 25–28.

Arendt, H. 1951. *The origins of totalitarianism: Imperialism.* New York: Harcourt.

Armbrust, W. 1996. *Mass culture and modernism in Egypt.* Cambridge: Cambridge University Press.

———. 2000. *Mass mediation: New approaches to popular culture in the Middle East and beyond.* Berkeley: University of California Press.

Asad, T. 1986. *The idea of an anthropology of Islam.* Occasional Papers Series, Center for Contemporary Arab Studies. Washington DC: Georgetown University Press.

———. 1993. *Genealogies of religion: Discipline and reasons of power in Christianity and Islam.* Baltimore: Johns Hopkins University Press.

———. 2003. *Formations of the secular: Christianity, Islam, modernity.* Stanford, CA: Stanford University Press.

El-Aswad, e.-S. 1987. Death rituals in rural Egyptian society: A symbolic study. *Urban Anthropology* 16(2): 205–41.

Atighetchi, D. 2007. *Islamic bioethics: Problems and perspectives.* New York: Springer.

Awad, M. 2008. Organ trafficking reaches new heights in Egypt. *Al Arabiya News,* English edition, November 18. www.alarabiya.net/articles/ 2008/11/18/60359.html (last accessed 8/22/2011).

Bakr, M.A. 2000. Renal Transplantation in Egypt. *Organs and Tissues* (1): 39–44.

Barsoum, R. S. 2002. Overview: End-stage renal disease in the developing world. *Artificial Organs* 26(9): 737–46.

———. 2003. End-stage renal disease in North Africa. *Kidney International* 13 (suppl. 83): S111–S114.

Beauchamp, T. L., and J. F. Childress. 2001. *Principles of biomedical ethics.* Oxford: Oxford University Press.

Beck, U. 1992. *Risk society: Towards a new modernity.* London: Sage.

Biehl, J. 2007. *Will to live: AIDS therapies and the politics of survival.* Princeton: Princeton University Press.

al-Bishri, T. 2001. *Naql al ʿadaaʾ fi duʾ al-shariʿa wal qanun.* Al-Qahira: Nahdat-misr.

al-Bisi, S. 2006. *Al-Ahram,* January 26.

Bouzid, A. 1998. Man, society and knowledge in the Islamist discourse of Sayyid Qutb. PhD dissertation, Science and Technology Studies, Virginia Polytechnic Institute.

Briggs, C. 2003. *Stories in the time of cholera: Racial profiling during a medical nightmare.* Berkeley: University of California Press.

Brooke, J.H. 1991. *Science and religion: Some historical perspectives.* Cambridge: Cambridge University Press.

Budiani, D. 2005. Sheikhs, labs, doctors, and bodies: The Egyptian transplant theater. Paper delivered at the American Anthropological Associations (AAA) 104th annual meeting, Washington DC, December.

———. 2006. Towards a world of ethical solutions for organ and tissue supplies. Washington DC: Council for Organ Failure Solutions.

———. 2007. Facilitating organ transplants in Egypt: An analysis of doctors' discourse. *Body and Society* 13(3): 125–49.

Budiani, D., and O. Shibly. 2006. Islam, organ transplants, and organ trafficking in the Islamic world. Paper delivered at the Islam and Bioethics Conference, Penn State University, March 27–28.

———. 2008. Islam, organ transplants, and organ trafficking in the Muslim world: Paving a path for solutions. In *Muslim medical ethics: From theory to practice,* ed. J. Brockopp, 138–50. Columbia: University of South Carolina Press.

Budiani-Saberi, D.A. 2010. *Organ SOS: A plea from the shadows: 40 minutes.* Documentary film. Council for Organ Failure Solutions.

Budiani-Saberi, D.A., and F.L. Delmonico. 2008. Organ trafficking and transplant tourism: A commentary on the global realities. *American Journal of Transplantation* 8: 925–29.

Burgel, C.I. 1976. Secular and religious features of medieval Arabic medicine. In *Asian medical systems: A comparative study,* ed. C. Leslie, 44–62. Berkeley: University of California Press.

Chu, J. 2010. *Cosmologies of credit: Transnational mobility and the politics of destination in China.* Durham, NC: Duke University Press.

Cohen, L. 1998. *No aging in India.* Berkeley: University of California Press.

———. 1999. Where it hurts: Indian material for an ethics of organ transplantation. *Daedalus* 128(4): 135–65.

———. 2001. The other kidney: Biopolitics beyond recognition. *Body and Society* 7(2–3): 9–29.

———. 2005. Operability, bioavailability, and exception. In *Global assemblages: Technology, politics, and ethics as anthropological problems,* A. Ong and S.J. Collier, eds., 79–90. Malden: Blackwell Publishing.

Comaroff, J.C., and J. Comaroff. 2000. Millennial capitalism: First thoughts on a second coming. *Public Culture* 12(2): 291–343.

Cowan, R. 2008. *Heredity and hope: The case for genetic screening.* Cambridge: Harvard University Press.

Cromer, E.B. 1908. *Modern Egypt.* London: Macmillan.

Crowley-Matoka, M. 2005. Desperately seeking "normal": The promise and perils of living with kidney transplantation. *Social Science and Medicine* 61: 821–31.

Crowley-Matoka, M., and M. Lock. 2006. Organ transplantation in a globalised world. *Mortality* 11(2): 166–81.

Daar, A. S., and B. A. Khitamy. 2001. Bioethics for clinicians: 21. Islamic bioethics. *Canadian Medical Association Journal* 164(1): 60–63.

Dallal, A. 2000. Appropriating the past: Twentieth-century reconstruction of pre-modern Islamic thought. *Islamic Law and Society* 7(1): 325–58.

Daniels, N., B. Kennedy, et al. 1999. Why justice is good for our health: The social determinants of health inequalities. *Daedalus* 128(4): 215–51.

Dar al-Ifta' al-Misriyya. 2007. Al-Mawdu': Naql wa zira'at al-'ada' al-bashariyya. May 20. www.dar-alifta.org (last accessed 8/22/2011).

Das, V. 1999. Public good, ethics, and everyday life: Beyond the boundaries of bioethics. *Daedalus* 128(4): 99–133.

Durrah, A. 2007. The thirsty in Mahalla: "Arrest us—perhaps we will find clean water to drink in prison." *Al-Misri al-Yawm*, English edition, July 11.

Early, E. A. 1993. *Baladi women of Cairo: Playing with an egg and a stone.* Boulder: Lynn Rienner.

Eickelman, D. F. 1992. Mass higher education and the religious imagination in contemporary Arab societies. *American Ethnologist* 19(4): 643–55.

———. 2000. Islam and the languages of modernity. *Daedalus* 129(1): 119.

Eickelman, D. F., and J. W. Anderson, eds. 2003. *New media in the Muslim world: The emerging public sphere.* Bloomington: Indiana University Press.

EIPR (Egyptian Initiative for Personal Rights). 2009. Joint report by a coalition of Egyptian human rights NGOs on the universal periodic review of Egypt. September.

El-Zanaty, F., and A. Way. 2009. *Egypt Demographic and Health Survey* 2008. Cairo, Egypt: Ministry of Health, El-Zanaty and Associates, and Macro International.

Ernst, C. W. 2003. *Following Muhammad: Rethinking Islam in the contemporary world.* Chapel Hill: University of North Carolina Press.

Esmat, G., A. Yosry, et al. 2005. Donor outcomes in right lobe adult living donor liver transplantation: Single-center experience in Egypt. *Transplantation Proceedings* 37: 3147–50.

Essamie, M., A. Soliman, et al. 1995. Serious renal disease in Egypt. *International Journal of Artificial Organs* 18(5): 254–60.

Evans, R., M. Barer, et al., eds. 1994. *Why are some people healthy and others not? The determinants of health of populations.* Hawthorne, NY: Aldine de Gruyter.

Fadiman, A. 1998. *The spirit catches you and you fall down.* New York: Macmillan.

Farmer, P. 1992. *Aids and accusation: Haiti and the geography of blame.* Berkeley: University of California Press.

———. 1997. On suffering and structural violence: A view from below. In *Social Suffering,* V. Das, A. Kleinman, and M. Lock, eds. 261–84. Berkeley: University of California Press.

———. 1999. *Infections and inequalities: The modern plagues.* Berkeley: University of California Press.

———. 2003. *Pathologies of power: Health, human rights, and the new war on the poor.* Berkeley: University of California Press.

Farquhar, J. 1994. *Knowing practice: The clinical encounter in Chinese medicine.* Boulder: Westview Press.

Fassin, D. 2001. Culturalism as ideology. In *Cultural perspectives on reproductive health,* ed. C. M. Obermeyer, 300–318. Oxford: Oxford University Press.

———. 2003. The embodiment of inequality: AIDS as a social condition and the historical experience in South Africa. *EMBO Reports* 4: S1, S4–S9.

———. 2007. *When bodies remember: Experiences and politics of AIDS in South Africa.* Berkeley: University of California Press.

Fischer, M. M. J. 2003. *Emergent forms of life and the anthropological voice.* Durham: Duke University Press.

Fleishman, J., and N. El-Hennawy. 2008. When the body becomes an ATM. *Los Angeles Times,* March 13.

Fouad, S. 2005. Egypt national health accounts 2001–02. In *The Partners for Health Reform Plus Project.* (USAID Report, November). url (last accessed 8/22/2011): www.healthsystems2020.org/content/resource/detail/1810/

Fox, R. C. 1996. Afterthoughts: Continuing reflections on organ transplantation. In *Organ transplantation: Meanings and realities,* S. J. Youngner, R. C. Fox, and L. J. O'Connell. Madison: University of Wisconsin Press.

Fox, R. C., and J. P. Swazey, eds. 1974. *The courage to fail: A social view of organ transplants and dialysis.* Chicago: University of Chicago Press.

———. 1992. *Spare parts: Organ replacement in American Society.* New York: Oxford University Press.

———. 2008. *Observing bioethics.* Oxford: Oxford University Press.

Frank, C., M. Mohamed, et al. 2000. The role of parenteral antischistomal therapy in the spread of hepatitis C virus in Egypt. *The Lancet* 355(9207): 887–891.

Gawande, A. 2003. *Complications: A surgeon's notes on an imperfect science.* New York: Picador.

———. 2007. *Better: A surgeon's notes on performance.* New York: Metropolitan Books.

Gershoni, I., and J. Jankowski, 1995. *Redefining the Egyptian nation 1930– 1945.* Cambridge: Cambridge University Press.

Gerth, H. H., and C. W. Mills. 1965. *From Max Weber: Essays in sociology.* Oxford: Oxford University Press.

El-Ghobashy, M. 2006. *Taming leviathan: Constitutional contention in contemporary Egypt.* Department of Political Science. New York: Columbia University.

Ghods, A.J. 2002. Renal transplantation in Iran. *Nephrology Dialysis Transplantation* 17: 222–28.

Ghoneim, M.A., M.A. Bakr, et al. 2001. Live-donor renal transplantation at the Urology and Nephrology Center of Mansoura: 1976–1998. In *Clinical transplants*, J.M. Cecka and P.I. Terasaki, eds., 167–78. Los Angeles: UCLA Immunogenetics Center.

al-Ghumari, A. 1987. *Taʿrif ahl al-Islam bi-an naql al-ʿaduw haram.* Cairo: Dar Misr lil-Tabaʿa.

Ginsburg, F.D. 1989. *Contested lives: The abortion debate in an American community.* Berkeley: University of California Press.

Gordon, E.J. 2001. "They don't have to suffer for me": Why dialysis patients refuse offers of living donor kidneys. *Medical Anthropology Quarterly* 15(2): 245–67.

Gordon, J. 2002. *Revolutionary melodrama: Popular film and civic identity in Nasser's Egypt.* Chicago: Middle East Documentation Center.

Goyal, M., R.L. Mehta, et al. 2002. Economic and health consequences of selling a kidney in India. *Journal of the American Medical Association* 288(13): 1589–93.

Gran, P. 1979. Medical pluralism in Arab and Egyptian history: An overview of class structures and philosophies of the main phases. *Social Science and Medicine* 13(B): 339–48.

Gregg, J., and S. Saha. 2006. Losing culture on the way to competence: The use and misuse of culture in medical education. *Academic Medicine* 81(6): 542–47.

Guda, S. 2008. The Shaykh's approach. *Al-Misri al-Yawm*, English edition, July 10.

Gusterson, H. 1996. *Nuclear rites: A weapons laboratory at the end of the Cold War.* Berkeley: University of California Press.

Gutmann, M. 2007. *Fixing men: Sex, birth control, and AIDS in Mexico.* Berkeley: University of California Press.

Hacking, I. 1999. *The Social construction of what?* Cambridge, MA: Harvard University Press.

Haeri, N. 2003. *Sacred language, ordinary people: Dilemmas of culture and politics in Egypt.* New York: Palgrave Macmillan.

Hafez, S. 2011 *An Islam of her own: Reconsidering religion and secularism in women's Islamic movements.* New York: New York University Press.

Hafiz, S.E., and E. Rogan. 1995. Press law 93. *Index on Censorship* 25(2): 56–60.

Hallaq, W. 1997. *A history of Islamic legal theories: An introduction to Sunni Usul al-fiqh.* Cambridge: Cambridge University Press.

———. 2001. *Authority, continuity, and change in Islamic law.* Cambridge: Cambridge University Press.

Hamdy, S.F. 1998. God's gift to women: Ideologies of motherhood, womanhood, and fertility in Egypt. MA thesis, Department of Anthropology, Stanford University.

————. 2005. Blinding ignorance: Medical science, diseased eyes, and religious practice in Egypt." *Arab Studies Journal* 7/8(2/1): 26–45.

————. 2008. When the state and your kidneys fail: Political etiologies in an Egyptian dialysis unit. *American Ethnologist* 35: 553–69.

————. 2009. Islam, fatalism, and medical intervention: Lessons from Egypt on the cultivation of forbearance (sabr) and reliance on God (tawakkul). *Anthropological Quarterly* 82(1): 173–96.

Hamdy, S. F., and L. Nasir. 2007. *Culture and medicine in the Arab world.* Oxford: Radcliffe.

Haraway, D. J. 1985. Manifesto for cyborgs: Science, technology, and socialist feminism in the 1980s. *Socialist Review* 80: 65–108.

————. 1988. Situated knowledges: The science question in feminism and the privilege of partial perspective. *Feminist Studies* 14(3): 575–99.

————. 1989. *Primate visions: Gender, race, and nature in the world of modern science.* New York: Routledge.

Harding, S. 2006. *Science and social inequality: Feminist and postcolonial issues.* Urbana: University of Illinois Press.

Hasan, M. 1990. *Muhammad Mutwalli al-Sha'rawi: Min al-qarya ila al-'alamiyya.* Cairo: Maktab al-Turath al-Islami.

Hassan, A. M. 2010. Egypt: Cairo scoffs at new Nile water agreement. http://latimesblogs.latimes.com/babylonbeyond/2010/05/egypt-cairo-scoffs-at-new-nile-water-agreement.html (last accessed 5/16/2010).

Hassan, A.M., H. Sheashaa, et al. 2005. Study of ochratoxin A as an environmental risk that causes renal injury in breast-fed Egyptian infants. *Pediatric Nephrology IPNA* 21: 102–5.

Hassan, N., N. El-Ghorab, et al. 1994. HIV infection in renal dialysis patients in Egypt. *AIDS* 8: 853.

Haykel, B. 2003. *Revival and reform in Islam: The legacy of Muhammad al-Shawkani.* Cambridge: Cambridge University Press.

Helmreich, S. 1998. *Silicon second nature: Culturing artificial life in a digital world.* Berkeley: University of California Press.

Hirschkind, C. 2006. *The ethical soundscape: Cassette sermons and Islamic counterpublics.* New York: Columbia University Press.

Hoffmaster, B., ed. 2001. *Bioethics in social context.* Philadelphia: Temple University Press.

Hogle, L. F. 1996. Transforming "body parts" into therapeutic tools: A report from Germany. *Medical Anthropology Quarterly* 10(4): 675–82.

————. 1999. *Recovering the nation's body: Cultural memory, medicine, and the politics of redemption.* New Brunswick: Rutgers University Press.

Hourani, A. 1962. *Arabic thought in the liberal age, 1798–1939.* Cambridge: Cambridge University Press.

El-Husseini, A., F. El-Basuony, I. Mahmoud, A. Donia, N. Hassan, N. Sayed-Ahmed, and M. Sobh. 2004. Effect of concomitant administration of cyclosporine and ketoconazole in children with focal segmental glomerulosclerosis. *American Journal of Nephrology* 24: 301–6.

El-Husseini, A., F. El-Basuony, I. Mahmoud, H. Sheashaa, A. Sabry, R. Hassan, N. Taha, N. Hassan, N. Sayed-Ahmad, and M. Sobh. 2005. Long-term effects of cyclosporine in children with idiopathic nephrotic syndrome: a single-centre experience. *Nephrology Dialysis Transplantation* 20: 2433–38.

El-Husseini, A., M. Foda, Y. Osman, and M. Sobh. 2006. Characteristics of long-term live-donor pediatric renal transplant survivors: A single-center experience. *Pediatric Transplantation* 10: 1–6.

Ibrahim, A. 2007. Dangers of imported meat! *Al-Ahram*, June 3.

Ibrahim, S. E. 1996. *Egypt, Islam, and democracy.* Cairo: American University in Cairo Press.

'Imad al-Shadhili, A., and N. al-Kashif. 2007. Citizens in Damietta live on jerrycans for twelve years. *Al-Misri al-Yawm*, July 13.

Inhorn, M. 1994. *Quest for conception: Gender, infertility, and Egyptian medical traditions.* Philadelphia: University of Pennsylvania Press.

———. 1996. *Infertility and patriarchy: The cultural politics of gender and family life in Egypt.* Philadelphia: University of Pennsylvania Press.

———. 2003. *Local babies, global science: Gender, religion, and in vitro fertilization in Egypt.* New York: Routledge.

IPEN (International POPs Elimination Project). 2006. *Health status in the impact zone of the El Kafr El-Zayat chemical plant.* Egypt Sons Association for Development and Environmental Protection, Cairo. www.ipen.org/ ipepweb1/library/ipep_pdf_reports/4egy%20health%20status%20el% 20kafr%20el-zayat%20impact%20zone.pdf (last accessed 8/22/2011).

Iqbal, M. 2002. *Islam and science.* Burlington, VT: Ashgate Publishing Co.

IRIN (Integrated Regional Information Networks). 2006. *Egypt: Poverty pushes poor Egyptians to sell their organs.* IRIN report, UN Office of the Coordination of Humanitarian Affairs, May 30. www.irinness.org/Report .aspx?ReportId = 26926 (last accessed 8/22/2011).

———. 2008. *Egypt: Selling a kidney to survive.* IRIN report, UN Office of the Coordination of Humanitarian Affairs, December 16. www.irinnews.org/ Report.aspx?ReportId = 81973 (last accessed 8/22/2011).

al-'Irqsusi, 'A. 1998. *Anqadhuna . . . fishash wa kalawi al-Misriyin lil biy'!* Cairo: Mu'assassat al-ahram.

Jackson, S. A. 1999. The alchemy of domination? Some Ash'arite responses to Mu'tazalite ethics. *International Journal of Middle Eastern Studies* 31: 185–201.

Jacob, M.-A. 2009. The shared history: Unknotting fictive kinship and legal process. *Law and Society Review* 43(1): 95–126.

Jain, S. L. 2010. The mortality effect: Counting the dead in the cancer trial. *Public Culture* 22(1): 89–117.

Jasanoff, S. 2005. *Designs on nature: Science and democracy in Europe and the United States.* Princeton: Princeton University Press.

Johansen, B. 1999. *Contingency in a sacred law: Legal and ethical norms in the Muslim fiqh.* Leiden: E. J. Brill.

Johnston, C. 2009. Egypt orders seizure of Russian wheat. Reuters, May 13.

Johnston, D. 2004. A turn in the epistemology and hermeneutics of twentieth century usul al-fiqh. *Islamic Law and Society* 11(2): 234–82.

Jonsen, A. 1998. *The birth of bioethics.* New York: Oxford University Press.

Joralemon, D. 1995. Organ wars: The battle for body parts. *Medical Anthropology Quarterly,* 9(3): 335–56.

Kamal, M.M. 2004. Fi nas wa fi nas: Class culture and illness practice in Egypt. In *Health and identity in Egypt,* H. Sholkamy Hania and F. Ghannam, eds., 65–90. Cairo: American University in Cairo Press.

Kamali, M.H. 1991. *Principles of Islamic jurisprudence.* Cambridge: Islamic Texts Society.

El-Kataney, E. 2009. Giving life after death. *Egypt Today.* April 8. http://egypt today.com/article.aspx?ArticleID=8461 (last accessed 8/22/2011).

Kaufman, S. 2000. In the shadow of "death with dignity": Medicine and cultural quandaries of the vegetative state. *American Anthropologist,* n.s. 102(1): 69–83.

Kaufman, S., and L. Morgan. 2005. The anthropology of the beginnings and ends of life. *Annual Review of Anthropology* 34: 317–41.

Kaufman, S., A.J. Russ, et al. 2006. Aged bodies and kinship matters: The ethical field of kidney transplant. *American Ethnologist* 33(1): 81–99.

Keller, E.F. 1992. *Secrets of life, secrets of death: Essays on language, gender, and science.* New York: Routledge.

Kerr, M.H. 1966. *Islamic reform: The political and legal theories of Muhammad 'Abduh and Rashid Rida.* Berkeley: University of California Press.

Al-Khader, A.A. 1999. Cadaveric renal transplantation in the Kingdom of Saudi Arabia. *Nephrology Dialysis Transplantation* 14: 846–50.

Khalidi, R. 2004. *Resurrecting empire: Western footprints and America's perilous path in the Middle East.* Boston: Beacon Press.

———. 2009. *Sowing crisis: The cold war and American dominance in the Middle East.* Boston: Beacon Press.

Kienle, E. 2001. *A grand delusion: Democracy and economic reform in Egypt.* New York: I.B. Tauris.

Kierans, C. 2005. Narrating kidney disease: The significance of sensation and time in the emplotment of patient experience. *Journal Culture, Medicine and Psychiatry* 29(3): 341–59.

Kleinman, A. 1995. *Writing at the margin: Discourse between anthropology and medicine.* Berkeley: University of California Press.

———. 1999. Moral experience and ethical reflection: Can ethnography reconcile them? A quandry for "the new bioethics." *Daedalus* 128(4): 69–97.

Kleinman, A., and P. Benson. 2006. Anthropology in the clinic: The problem of cultural competency and how to fix it. *PLoS Medicine* 3(10): 1673–76.

Kleinman, A., V. Das, et al., eds. 1997. *Social suffering.* Berkeley: University of California Press.

Krawietz, B. 1991. *Die Hurma: Schariatrechtlicher Schutz vor Eingriffen in die körperliche Unversehrtheit nach arabischen Fatwas des 20 Jahrhunderts.* Berlin: Duncker and Humblot.

———. 1997. Darura in modern Islamic law: The case of organ transplantation. In *Islamic law: Theory and practice*, R. Gleave and E. Kermeli, eds., 185–93. London: I. B. Tauris.

———. 2003. Brain death and Islamic traditions: Shifting borders of life? In *Islamic ethics of life: Abortion, war, and euthanasia*, ed. J. Brockopp, 194–213. Columbia: University of South Carolina Press.

Kugle, S. 2007. *Sufis and saints' bodies: Mysticism, corporeality, and sacred power in Islam*. Chapel Hill: University of North Carolina Press.

Kuppinger, P. 2000. Death of a midwife. In *Situating globalization: Views from Egypt*, C. Rouse, ed., 255–82. Bielefield: Transcript Verlag.

Kurzman, C. 2002. *Modernist Islam, 1840–1940: A sourcebook*. New York: Oxford University Press.

Lambert-Zazulak, P., P. Rutherford, et al. 2003. The International Ancient Egyptian Mummy Tissue Bank at the Manchester Museum as a resource for the palaeoepidemiological study of schistosomiasis. *World Archaeology* 35(2): 223–40.

Lane, S. D. 1994. Research bioethics in Egypt. In *Principles of health care ethics*, ed. A. L. R. Gillon, 885–94. New York: John Wiley.

Lane, S. D., B. I. Mikhail, A. Reizian, P. Courtright, R. Marx, and C. R. Dawson. 1993. Sociocultural aspects of blindness in an Egyptian delta hamlet: Visual impairment vs. visual disability. *Medical Anthropology Quarterly* 15: 245–60.

Langford, J. 2002. *Fluent bodies: Ayurvedic remedies for postcolonial imbalance*. Durham: Duke University Press.

———. 2009. Gifts intercepted: Biopolitics and spirit debt. *Cultural Anthropology* 24(4): 681–711.

Latour, B. 1987. *Science in action: How to follow scientists and engineers through society*. Cambridge: Harvard University Press.

———. 1988. *The Pasteurization of France*. Cambridge: Harvard University Press.

———. 1993. *We have never been modern*. Cambridge: Harvard University Press.

———. 2005. From realpolitik to dingpolitik: How to make things public. In *Making things public: Atmospheres of democracy*, B. Latour and P. Weibel, eds., 1–31. Cambridge: MIT Press.

Leila, R. 2007. Blood feud: The saga of the defected blood bags continues. *Al-Ahram Weekly* (Cairo), 849, June 14–20. http://weekly.ahram.org.eg/2007/849/eg6.htm (last accessed 8/22/2011).

Leslie, C. 1976. The ambiguities of medical revivalism in modern India. In *Asian medical systems: A comparative study*, ed. C. Leslie, 356–67. Berkeley: University of California Press.

Lock, M. 1993a. Cultivating the body: Anthropology and epistemologies of bodily practice and knowledge. *Annual Review of Anthropology* 22: 133–55.

————. 1993b. *Encounters with aging: Mythologies of menopause in Japan and North America.* Berkeley: University of California Press.

————. 1995. Transcending mortality: Organ transplants and the practice of contradictions. *Medical Anthropology Quarterly* 9(3): 390–93.

————. 2001. Situated ethics, culture, and the brain death "problem" in Japan. In *Bioethics in social context,* ed. B. Hoffmaster, 39–68. Philadelphia: Temple University Press.

————. 2002a. Inventing a new death and making it believable. *Anthropology and Medicine* 9(2): 97–115.

————. 2002b. *Twice dead: Organ transplants and the reinvention of death.* Berkeley: University of California Press.

Lock, M., and V.-K. Nguyen, eds. 2010. *An anthropology of biomedicine.* Malden: Wiley-Blackwell.

Lombardi, C. 2006. *State law as Islamic law in modern Egypt: The incorporation of the shariʿa into Egyptian constitutional law.* Leiden: E.J. Brill.

Machledt, D. E. 2007. Moving risk: Tuberculosis, migration, and the scope of public health at the U.S.-Mexico border. Ph.D. dissertation, Department of Anthropology, University of California, Santa Cruz.

MacIntyre, A. C. 1984. *After virtue: A study in moral theory.* Notre Dame, IN: University of Notre Dame Press.

Mahmood, S. 2005. *Politics of piety: The Islamic revival and the feminist subject.* Princeton: Princeton University Press.

Malinowski, B. 1961. *Argonauts of the western Pacific: An account of native enterprise and adventure in the archipelagoes of Melanisian New Guinea.* New York: E.P. Dutton.

Mamdani, M. 2004. *Good Muslim, bad Muslim: America, the cold war, and the roots of terror.* New York: Pantheon Books.

Martensen, R. 2001. The history of bioethics: An essay review. *Journal of the History of Medicine* 56(2): 168–75.

Mashhur, S. 2007. A British report says Hani Sorour exposed medical solutions to the sun. *Al-Misri al-Yawm,* May 26.

Masud, M.K., B. Messick, et al., eds. 1996. *Islamic legal interpretation: Muftis and their fatwas.* Cambridge, MA: Harvard University Press.

McAlister, M. 2001. *Epic encounters: Culture, media, and U.S. interests in the Middle East, 1945–2000.* Berkeley: University of California Press.

McGrath, C. 2009a. Egypt: Move to end organ trafficking. Inter-Press Service Agency. May 18. http://ipsnews.net/news.asp?idnews=46886 (last accessed 8/22/2011).

————. 2009b. Viral time bomb set to explode. Inter-Press Service Agency. May 5. http://ipsnews.net/news.asp?idnews = 46723.

El-Mehairy, T. 1984. *Medical doctors: A study of role concept and job satisfaction: The Egyptian case.* Leiden: E.J. Brill.

Messick, B. 1993. *The calligraphic state: Textual domination and history in a Muslim society.* Berkeley: University of California Press.

————. 1996. Media muftis: Radio fatwas in Yemen. In *Islamic legal interpretation: Muftis and their fatwas*, M. K. Masud, B. Messick, and D. S. Powers, eds., 310–20. Cambridge: Harvard University Press.

Al-Misri al-Yawm. 2007a. As the match stared, hospitals stopped working. English edition, April 7.

————. 2007b. Shahada ʿam ismaʿil ʿidam al-qamh al-musartan (Uncle Ismail witnessed the destruction of the cancerous wheat). May 19.

————. 2007c. Demonstration with machetes and jerrycans in front of people's assembly. English edition, August 1.

————. 2010a. "ElBaradei to visit Mansoura." English edition, March 31. www .almasryalyoum.com/en/node/23987/ (last accessed 8/22/2011).

————. 2010b. "ElBaradei for president of Egypt 2011." English edition, April 4. www.almasryalyoum.com/en/node/24570 (last accessed 8/22/2011).

Mitchell, R. 1993. *The society of the Muslim Brothers*. New York: Oxford University Press.

Mitchell, T. 2002. *Rule of experts: Egypt, techno-politics, modernity*. Berkeley: University of California Press.

Mittermaier, A. 2011. *Dreams That Matter: An Anthropology of the Imagination in Contemporary Egypt*. Berkeley: University of California Press.

Moazam, F. 2006. *Bioethics and organ transplantation in a Muslim society*. Bloomington: Indiana University Press.

Moazam, F., R. M. Zaman, et al. 2009. Conversations with kidney vendors in Pakistan. *Hastings Center Report* 39(3): 29–44.

Mol, A. 2008. *The logic of care: Health and the problem of patient choice*. New York: Routledge.

Moosa, E. 1998. Transacting the body in the law: Reading fatawa on organ transplantation. *Afrika Zamani* 5 and 6: 291–317.

————. 1999. Languages of change in Islamic law: Redefining death in modernity. *Islamic Studies* 38(2): 305–42.

————. 2005. *Ghazali and the poetics of imagination*. Chapel Hill: University of North Carolina Press.

Morsy, S. 1988. Islamic clinics in Egypt: The cultural elaboration of biomedical hegemony. *Medical Anthropology Quarterly* 2(4): 355–69.

————. 1993. *Gender, sickness, and healing in rural Egypt: Ethnography in historical context*. Boulder, CO: Westview Press.

Al-Mousawi, M. T. H., and H. Al-Matouk. 1997. Views of Muslim scholars |on organ donation and brain death. *Transplantation Proceedings* 29: 3217.

Muntasar, S. 1989. Al-nas al-kamil li-hadith al-Shaʿrawi lil-tilifizyun wa aladhi athara al-dajja wa fataha malaf al-qadiyya (The entire transcript of Shaʿrawi's television appearance that caused a shock and opened the topic up for discussion). *October Weekly Magazine* 642 (February 12), 3–7.

Murad, A.-H. N.d. Islamic spirituality: The forgotten revolution. www.masud .co.uk/ISLAM/ahm/fgtnrevo.htm (last accessed 4/21/2006).

Al-Mutlaq, H., and K. Chaleby. 1995. Group psychotherapy with Arab patients. *Arab Journal of Psychiatry* 6(2): 125–36.

Narayan, K. 1993. How native is a "native" anthropologist? *American Anthropologist* 95(3): 19–32.

Nasr, S. H. 2002. *The heart of Islam: Enduring values for humanity.* New York: HarperCollins.

New York Times. 1981. Egypt-U.S. wheat deal. December 23.

Nguyen, V.-K. 2005. *The embodiment of health inequalities: The case of rapidly expanding access to antiretrovirals in West Africa.* Keynote address delivered at Rethinking Inequalities and Differences in Medicine: An Interdisciplinary Conference, Vanderbilt University, Center for Medicine, Health and Society, Nashville, April 29–May 1.

———. 2010. *The republic of therapy: Triage and sovereignty in West Africa's time of AIDS.* Durham: Duke University Press.

Nguyen, V.-K., and K. Preschard. 2003. Anthropology, inequality and disease: A review. *Annual Review of Anthropology* 32: 447–74.

Nuwayhid, I., M. Khawaja, and S. Jabbour, eds. Forthcoming. *Public health in the Arab world: Towards a multidisciplinary perspective.* Cambridge: Cambridge University Press.

Ong, A., and S. J. Collier. 2005. *Global assemblages: Technology, politics, and ethics as anthropological problems.* Malden: Blackwell Publishing.

Opwis, F. 2005. *Maslaha* in contemporary Islamic legal theory. *Islamic Law and Society* 12(2): 182–223.

Petryna, A. 2002. *Life exposed: Biological citizens after Chernobyl.* Princeton: Princeton University Press.

———. 2009. *When experiments travel: Clinical trials and the global search for human subjects.* Princeton: Princeton University Press.

Pharma and Healthcare Insight. 2010. Organ trafficking crackdown treats symptoms not the disease. October. www.pharmaceuticalsinsight.com/file/93095/organ-trafficking-crackdown-treats-symptoms-not-the-disease.html (last accessed 8/22/2011).

Porter, R. 1998. *The greatest benefit to mankind: A medical history of humanity.* New York: W. W. Norton.

Qureshi, E., and M. Sells. 2003. *The new Crusades: Constructing the Muslim enemy.* New York: Columbia University Press.

Ramadan, K. 2007. Al-Massiri: A harsh lesson. *Al-Misri al-Yawm,* May 27.

Rapp, R. 1997. Real-time fetus: The role of the sonogram in the age of monitored reproduction. In *Cyborgs and citadels: Anthropological interventions in emerging sciences and technologies,* G. L. Downey and J. Dumit, eds., 31–48. Santa Fe: School of American Research Press.

———. 1999. *Testing women, testing the fetus: The social impact of amniocentesis in America.* New York: Routledge.

Rashad, A., F. Phipps, and M. Haith-Cooper. 2004. Obtaining informed consent in an Egyptian research study. *Nursing Ethics* 11(4): 394–99.

Razack, S. 2007. *Casting out: The eviction of Muslims from Western law and politics.* Toronto: University of Toronto Press.

Rosaldo, R. 1993. *Culture and truth: The remaking of social analysis.* Boston: Beacon Press.

Russ, A.J., J.K. Shim, et al. 2005. "Is there life on dialysis?" Time and aging in a clinically sustained existence. *Medical Anthropology* 24(4): 297–324.

Rutherford, B. 2008. *Egypt after Mubarak: Liberalism, Islam, and democracy in the Arab world.* Princeton: Princeton University Press.

Saad, R. 1998. Shame, reputation, and Egypt's lovers: A controversy over the nation's image. *Visual Anthropology* 10: 401–12.

Sabiq, S. 1994. *Fiqh al-sunna.* 3 vols. Cairo: Maktabat al-Qahira.

Sabry, A., A. El-Agoudy, et al. 2005. HCV associated glomerulonpathy in Egyptian patients: Clinicopathological analysis. *Virology* 334: 10–16.

Sachedina, A.A. 1999. Can God inflict unrequited pain on His creatures? Muslim perspectives on health and suffering. In *Religion, health, and suffering,* J.R. Hinnells and R. Porter, eds., 65–84. London: Kegan Paul International.

———. 2009. *Islamic biomedical ethics: Principles and application.* Oxford: Oxford University Press.

Said, E. 1979. *Orientalism.* New York: Vintage.

Salah, Muhammad. 2009. Ighlaq mustashfayy al-marwa wal-sudan (Shutting down of Sudan and Marwa hospitals). *Al Wafd,* March 13. http://alwafd .org/details.aspx?nid = 14927 (last accessed 4/9/2009).

Salvatore, A. 1997. *Islam and the political discourse of modernity.* Reading, UK: Garnet Publishing.

Salvatore, A., and D. Eickelman. 2004. *Public Islam and the common good.* Leiden: E.J. Brill.

El-Sayed, N.M., P.J. Gomatos, et al. 2000. Epidemic transmission of human immunodeficiency virus in renal dialysis centers in Egypt." *Journal of Infectious Diseases* 181: 91–97.

Scheid, V. 2002. *Chinese medicine in contemporary China: Plurality and synthesis.* Durham: Duke University Press.

Scheper-Hughes, N. 1992. *Death without weeping: The violence of everyday life in Brazil.* Berkeley: University of California Press.

———. 1996. Theft of life: The globalization of organ stealing rumours. *Anthropology Today* 12(3): 3–11.

———. 2000. The global traffic in human organs. *Current Anthropology* 41(2): 191–224.

———. 2001. On organ theft narratives. *Current Anthropology* 42(4): 556–58.

———. 2002. The ends of the body: Commodity fetishism and the global traffic in organs. *SAIS Review* 22(1) (Winter–Spring): 61–80.

———. 2003. Rotten trade: Millennial capitalism, human values and global justice in organ trafficking. *Journal of Human Rights* 2(2): 197–226.

———. 2005. The last commodity: Post-human ethics and the global traffic in "fresh" organs. In *Global assemblages: Technology, politics, and ethics as anthropological problems,* ed. A. Ong and S. J. Collier, 145–68. Malden, MA: Blackwell Publishing.

———. 2007. The tyranny of the gift: Sacrificial violence in living donor transplants. *American Journal of Transplantation* 7: 507–11.

Schiebinger, L. 1993. *Nature's body: Gender in the making of modern science.* Boston: Beacon Press.

Schiezer, J. 2010. Kidney transplants generally safe for lupus patients. *Renal and Urology News.* February. www.renalandurologynews.com/kidney-transplants-generally-safe-for-lupus-patients/article/156779/ (last accessed 8/22/2011).

Shaheen, J. 2009. *Reel bad Arabs: How Hollywood vilifies a people.* New York: Olive Branch Press.

al-Sha'rawi, M. M. 1999. *Al-Fatawa: Kul ma yuhim al-muslim fi hayatihi yawmihi wa ghadihi.* Cairo: Maktab al-Tawfiqiyya.

———. 2002. *Al-Fatawa al-Kubra.* 3rd ed. Cairo: Maktab al-Turath al-Islami

Sharp, L. A. 1995. Organ transplantation as a transformative experience: Anthropological insights into the restructuring of the self. *Medical Anthropology Quarterly,* 9(3): 357–89.

———. 2000. The commodification of the body and its parts. *Annual Review of Anthropology* 29: 287–328.

———. 2001. Commodified kin: Death, mourning, and competing claims on the bodies of organ donors in the United States. *American Anthropologist* 103(1): 112–33.

———. 2006. *Strange harvest: Organ tranplants, denatured bodies, and the transformed self.* Berkeley: University of California Press.

———. 2007. *Bodies, commodities, and biotechnologies.* New York: Columbia University Press.

Sholkamy, H. 1999. Why is anthropology so hard in Egypt? In *Between field and text: Emerging voices in Egyptian social science,* S. Shami and L. Herrera, eds., 119–38. Cairo: American University in Cairo Press.

———. 2004. Conclusion: The medical cultures of Egypt. In *Health and identity in Egypt,* H. Sholkamy and F. Ghannam, eds., 111–28. Cairo: American University in Cairo Press.

Sholkamy, H., and F. Ghannam, eds. 2004. *Health and identity in Egypt.* Cairo: American University in Cairo Press.

Shukrallah, A. 2012. Egypt in crisis: Politics, healthcare, and social mobilisation for health rights. In *Public health in the Arab world: Towards a multidisciplinary perspective,* R. Giacaman, I. Nuwayhid, M. Khawaja, and S. Jabbour, eds. Cambridge: Cambridge University Press.

Siminoff, L. A. S., and C. M. Saunders. 2000. African-American reluctance to donate: Beliefs and attitudes about organ donation and implications for policy. *Kennedy Institute of Ethics Journal* 10(1): 59–74.

Singerman, D. 1994. *Avenues of participation: Family, politics, and networks in urban quarters of Cairo.* Princeton: Princeton University Press.

Skovgaard-Petersen, J. 1997. *Defining Islam for the Egyptian state: Muftis and fatwas of the Dar al-Ifta*. Leiden: E.J. Brill.

Smith, D.J. 2001. Romance, parenthood, and gender in a modern African society. *Ethnology* 40(2): 129–51.

Smith, D.J., and B. Mbakwem. 2007. Life projects and therapeutic itineraries: Marriage, fertility, and antiretroviral therapy in Nigeria. *AIDS* 21(suppl. 5): S37–S41.

Smith, J., and Y. Haddad. 2002. *The Islamic understanding of death and resurrection*. Oxford: Oxford University Press.

Smith, N. 2001. Scales of terror and the resort to geography: September 11, October 7. *Society and Space* 19: 631–37.

Solomon, N. 1997. From folk medicine to bioethics in Judaism. In *Religion, health and suffering*, J. Hinnells and R. Porter, eds., 166–86. London: Kegan Paul International.

Sontag, S. 2001. *Illness as metaphor* and *AIDS and its metaphors*. New York: Picador.

Sowers, Jeannie. 2007. Nature reserves and authoritarian rule in Egypt: Embedded autonomy revisited. *Journal of Environment and Development* 16(4, December): 375–97.

Sowers, J., E. Weinthal, and A. Vongosh. 2010. Climate change, water resources, and the politics of adaptation in the Middle East and North Africa. *Climatic Change*, April 23. http://pubpages.unh.edu/~jlu36/Climatic Changepiece.pdf.

Spivak, G. 1988. Can the subaltern speak? In *Marxism and the interpretation of culture*, C. Nelson and L. Grossberg, eds., 271–313. Chicago: University of Illinois Press.

Stevens, M.L.T. 2000. *Bioethics in America: Origins and cultural politics*. Baltimore, MD: Johns Hopkins University Press.

Tabishat, M. 2000. Al-daght: Pressures of modern life in Cairo. In *Situating globalization: Views from Egypt*, ed. C.N.a.S. Rouse, 203–30. Bielefield: Transcript Verlag.

———. 2003. Shaikhs and doctors: The debate on organ transplantation in the Egyptian press. Paper presented at the Egypt, Law, and Society Conference/Symposium, Graduate Center, City University of New York.

Thomas, A. 2010. Continuing the definition of death debate: The report on the president's Council on Bioethics on controversies in the determination of death. *Bioethics* (March).

Trotter, J.F., R. Adam, et al. 2006. Documented deaths of hepatic lobe donors for living donor liver transplantation. *Liver Transplantation* 12: 1485–88.

Tsing, A.L. 2005. *Friction: An ethnography of global connection*. Princeton: Princeton University Press.

Tucker, J. 2000. *In the house of the law: Gender and Islamic law in Ottoman Syria and Palestine*. Berkeley: University of California Press.

Turner, B.S. 1997. The body in Western society: Social theory and its perspectives. In *Religion and the body*, ed. S. Coakley, 15–41. Cambridge: Cambridge University Press.

Turner, V. 1974. *Dramas, fields, and metaphors*. Ithaca, NY: Cornell University Press.

Viorst, M. 1998. *In the shadow of the Prophet: The struggle for the soul of Islam*. New York: Anchor Books.

Warren, K. 2010. The illusiveness of counting "victims" and the concreteness of ranking countries: Trafficking in persons from Colombia to Japan. In *Sex, drugs, and body counts: The politics of numbers in global crime and conflict*, P. Andreas and K. Greenhill, eds., 110–26. Ithaca: Cornell University Press.

Watson, H. 1992. *Women in the city of the dead*. Trenton: Africa World Press.

Weir, A. 2009. Israeli organ harvesting. August 28. www.middle-east-online.com/english/?id = 33961 (last accesseed 8/22/2011).

Whitmarsh, I., A.M. Davis, et al. 2007. A place for genetic uncertainty: Parents valuing an unknown in the meaning of disease. *Social Science and Medicine* 65(6): 1082–93.

WHO. 2007. World Health Organization statistics database: Egypt. www.who.int/whosis/database/core/core_select_process.cfm (last accessed 8/22/2011).

Wickham, C.R. 2002. *Mobilizing Islam: Religion, activism, and political change in Egypt*. New York: Columbia University Press.

Wilkinson, R., and K. Pickett. 2010. *The spirit level: Why greater equality makes societies stronger*. New York: Bloomsbury Press.

Williams, J.H., T.D. Phillips, et al. 2004. Human aflatoxicosis in developing countries: A review of toxicology, exposure, potential health consequences, and interventions. *American Journal of Clinical Nutrition* 80: 1106–22.

Winegar, J. 2006. *Creative reckonings: The politics of art and culture in contemporary Egypt*. Stanford: Stanford University Press.

Winner, L. 1980. Do artifacts have politics? *Daedalus* 109(1): 121–36.

Youngner, S.J. 1996. Some must die. In *Organ transplantation: Meanings and realities*, ed. S. J. Youngner, R.C. Fox, and L.J. O'Connell, 32–55. Madison: University of Wisconsin Press.

Youngner, S.J., R.C. Fox, and L.J. O'Connell, eds. 1996. *Organ transplantation: Meanings and realities*. Madison: University of Wisconsin Press.

Zalat, Ali, and Maha al-Bahnasawi. 2007. "Kidney advertiser: Sale is the only way to pay my debts and maintain my daughters' reputation." *Al-Misri al-Yawm*, August 28. www.almasry-alyoum.com/article.aspx?ArticleID=74077 (last accessed 8/22/2011).

Zhan, M. 2001. Does it take a miracle? Negotiating knowledges, identities and communities of traditional Chinese medicine. *Cultural Anthropology* 16(4): 453–80.

Index

'Abduh, Muhammad, 98, 281n36
absolutism, 3, 233–34, 237, 248
Abu-Lughod, Lila, 91
Abu Rish Children's Hospital,
    272–73n3
Academy of Islamic Jurisprudence
    (Majma' al-Fiqh al-Islami), 268n12
access to health care, 13, 31–32, 59, 96,
    110, 247, 263n25, 272n42, 281n35
accident victims, 49, 87, 94, 105,
    268n12, 46fig.
Afghanistan, U.S. war with, xxii, 76
aflatoxins, 182, 289n17
Agamben, Giorgio, 106, 213
agricultural land: and compensation
    for water buffalo, 85; and environ-
    mental risks, 10, 13, 28–29, 59, 182,
    183fig.
Al-Ahram, 29, 181, 217, 257–58n5
AIDS. See HIV/AIDS
Ain Shams University, 272n1,
    294–95n28; Medical School, 273n5;
    Teaching Hospital, 83, 87, 90, 203,
    272–73nn2,3,5
al-Akhbar, 29
al-Arabiya television station, 232
Alexandria, 10, 216, 253
Algeria, 268n12, 277n2
alternative medicines, 36, 243
altruism, 35, 67, 137, 185,
    267n7, 285n13, 290n26; and

commodification of organs, 210,
    216, 223–24, 234–36
ambivalences, 44, 61, 64, 276n36; and
    ethics of scale, 147, 167, 170
American University in Cairo, 293n16
'Amr, Shaykh (religious scholar),
    39–43, 118–19, 265–66nn38–40
anesthesiology/anesthesiologists, 49,
    51, 58–63, 71
aneurisms, 142–43, 284n4
anthropology/anthropologists, 2. See
    also names of anthropologists;
    and bioethics, 7–8, 259nn20,23;
    and commodification of organs,
    209, 228, 235, 293n15; and crises
    of authority, 27, 43–44, 264n27,
    266n42; and defining death, 51, 66,
    78, 267nn3,6; on environmental
    risks, 185–86; on individual behav-
    iors, 259n20; medical anthropol-
    ogy, 7, 176, 209, 259n20, 264n27,
    273–74n12, 293n15; "native ethnog-
    raphers," 51, 267n3; on patient sup-
    port/group therapy, 176; on social
    relations/resources, 27, 191
antigen matching. See tissue typing
Arab Gulf states, 87, 210, 216, 219,
    222, 270n22, 293–94n19, 294–95n28
Arabic language, 40, 264–65n33;
    Egyptian Arabic, 25, 117, 159, 178,
    262nn12,16

Arabic literature/poetry, 56, 99–101, 241, 275n25
Arab–Israeli War (1967), 76, 99, 283n1
Arab Spring, 253–55, 264n32, 269n17
Armbrust, Walter, 91
army, Egyptian, 159–61, 163–66, 168, 190, 286n19
art/artists, 119, 278n10
Asad, Talal, 260n26, 295–96n3
Ashʿari school, 280n23, 282–83n48
Aswan High Dam, 259n19
ʿAtiyya, Kamal, 274n23
authority, Islamic, 1, 5–6, 244, 247, 249–50, 295–96n3. See also fatwas; muftis; religious scholars; and bioethics, 9, 11, 13–15, 17–19, 260n26; crisis of, 6, 21, 24, 33–44, 265–66n38, 41fig.; on defining death, 54–59, 63–64, 76, 271n35; and gender, 11; and Shaʿrawi, Shaykh, 121, 129, 278n6; and spiritual risks, 188, 290n23; and untrustworthy religious scholars, 5–6
authority, medical, 1–2, 249. See also experts, medical; transplant surgeons; names of physicians; and bioethics, 9, 11, 14, 18–19; and cornea transplants, 90, 111; crisis of, 6, 21–39, 43–45; on defining death, 48, 55–56, 75, 80; and doctors of confidence, 36–39, 47, 55–56, 130, 242–43, 264nn28,29; and gender, 11; and untrustworthy physicians, 5–6, 29, 37–39, 175–79, 184, 217, 257–58n5
autopsies, 55, 108, 253
Ayurvedic medicine, 36, 266n42
al-Azhar University, 39–40, 118, 128, 244, 267n9, 277n1; affiliated schools, 150; Faculty of Medicine, 142; fatwa committee at, 11; Mosque, 40, 41fig.; Rector (Shaykh) of, 57, 72, 102, 160, 269n17

"backwardness": and cornea transplants, 2, 84–85, 92–97, 100, 275n25; and Islam, 5, 44, 68–70, 73, 84, 241,

246, 271n33; and Shaʿrawi, Shaykh, 120–22, 131
Badrawi Hospital, 280n34
"bare life," 106, 213, 292n12
Barnard, Christian, 267n2
Barsum, Rashad, 289n18
Beachamp, Tom, 258n10
Bilharz, Theodor, 261n7
bilharzias, 16–17, 180, 261n7. See also schistosomiasis
Biltagi, Muhammad, 270n26
bioethics, 6–9, 247, 250. See also ethics, medical; scale, ethics of; and commodification of organs, 209–10, 234; and cornea transplants, 34–35; and defining death, 49, 60, 78–80, 272n42; defining scope of problem, 9–15; embodied, 15–19; as moving target, 12–15, 259nn20,23; myopic universalisms of, 8; neo-Kantian philosophy in, 7; rebinding of, 8–9, 19; Shaykh Shaʿrawi's views on, 115, 121, 279n13; in U.S., 6–9, 147, 258n10, 260n24
Bishbiysh (Mahalla), 181
al-Bishri, Tariq, 282n46
al-Bisi, Sanaʾ, 257–58n5
black market in human organs, 244–45; brokers of, 155, 210, 216–17, 228–29, 232, 237; in Cairo, 3–4, 10–12, 24, 30, 37, 209, 231–35, 294n24; Coptic Christians' views on, 259n22; and cornea transplants, 34, 96; and crises of authority, 29–30, 34–35, 37–39, 44; and defining death, 48, 56–57, 69, 79; Egyptian Medical Syndicate's regulation of, 221–26, 294–95n28; and ethics of scale, 155–56; and Hani (kidney-failure patient/organ buyer), 154–55, 157–58, 285n16; and Iman (kidney-failure patient), 227–31; and kidney transplants, 29–30, 35, 79, 155–56, 199, 209–10, 215–17, 220–21, 226, 228–29; and middle-men, 210, 217, 220; and Nagla (kidney-failure patient), 212–14, 292n5;

and Shadya (kidney-failure patient), 149–54, 158, 171, 203, 285n14, 287–88nn9,10; Shaykh Sha'rawi's views on, 131–32

blindness, 11, 16, 30, 33, 84, 90–92, 94, 107–10, 112, 260n27, 263n23, 277n40. *See also* cornea opacity/ transplants; and environmental risks, 181; in *The Lamp of Umm Hashim* (1968 film), 99–100, 275n25; and Light and Hope Foundation (Mu'asasat al-Nur Wal-'Amal), 107, 276n38; and Ragia, 25–26, 262n16; Shaykh Sha'rawi's views on, 124; and World Health Organization, 275–76n28

blood banks, 107, 282n43

blood cupping *(higama/hajim)*, 133, 282n45

blood transfusions, 25–26, 30, 216, 262n15; al-Bishri's views on, 282n46; Mufti Shaf'i's views on, 282n43; risks/benefits of, 175, 177, 287n7; Shaykh Sha'rawi's views on, 121, 123, 133–34, 279n15, 282n43

blood types, 150, 189, 205, 219

body belongs to God. *See* God's ownership of bodies

brain death, 3–4, 17, 47–80, 267nn1,2, 269n15, 270nn22,26,27; and accident victims, 49, 87, 268n12, 46*fig.*; circuits of doubt about, 48; and "clash of civilizations," 61, 76–80, 84, 272n40; as clinical death, 65, 68; and commodification of organs, 220, 232; and cornea transplants, 84–85, 274nn13,16, 276n36; criteria outside of, 78–79; and diagnostic error, 62, 70, 270n22; and kidney transplants, 127, 155, 166, 200, 286n22; and liver transplants, 222, 292n6; Lotfy's views on, 48, 58–66, 69–70, 77, 270n26; Marmush's views on, 15, 68–70, 271nn32,33; proponents of, 68–72; Shaykh Gad al-Haqq's views on, 48, 55–57, 60–63, 66,

268nn11,12, 269n17; Shaykh Guma'a's views on, 48, 72–77, 127, 265–66n38, 268–69n13, 74*fig.*; Shaykh Tantawi's views on, 48, 56–57, 72–73, 75–76, 267n1; "slippery slope" of, 63, 77; and the soul, 52, 56, 60–61, 65–67

Brazil, 273–74n12

breast milk, 289n18

Brooke, John Hedley, 284n8

Brown, Jonathan, 277n1

Budiani, Debra, 219–20, 292n7, 293nn15,16, 294n23

Bulgaria, 95

cadavers/cadaveric procurement, 16, 38, 265n36; and commodification of organs, 210, 232; and cornea transplants, 16, 83, 87–89, 265n36, 273n6; and defining death, 47–48, 56–57, 65, 67, 70–72, 79, 268n12, 269n16; and kidney transplants, 200, 286n22

Caine, Mark, 266n43

Cairo, 10, 41, 239, 241, 243; black market in human organs, 3, 10–11, 24, 30, 37, 209, 215, 231–35, 294n24; commodification of organs in, 209–11, 218–19, 221, 225, 227–28, 292n7; cornea transplants in, 11, 32–33, 83, 85–88, 101–2, 272n1, 275–76n28; "counterpublic" of, 43–44; Duqqi Quarter, 90; kidney transplants/dialysis in, 23–24, 35, 141–46, 148, 150, 152, 154–55, 158, 160, 162–63, 166, 168, 170, 179, 211–12, 261nn7,9, 283–84n2, 292n5; liver transplants in, 271n31; Old Cairo, 40, 41*fig.*; private medical clinics/hospitals in, 10, 24, 154, 158; refugee populations in, 293n16; and tourism, 216; in *Wahid min al-nas* (television news program), 259n18

Cairo University Faculty of Medicine. *See* Kasr el Aini

Camp David Accords, 182

Canada, 79

cancer, 182, 184; "cancerous wheat"
(al-qamh al-musartan), 182,
289n19
capitalism, 4–5, 202, 232–33, 237, 250,
291n32
Cartesian dualism, 66
cassette sermons, 44
cataracts, 263n24
cement factories, 183fig.
Center for Arab Studies Abroad, 241,
258n11
chemical fertilizers, 13, 29
childbearing. See reproduction
Childress, James, 258n10
China, 36, 287n7; Chinese medicine, 36
Christianity, 124, 160. See also Coptic
Christians
Chu, Julie, 106
class disparities, 11–12, 84, 91,
94–96, 111, 244–45, 255, 273n10,
277nn40,42; and black market in
human organs, 215–16, 294–95n28;
and commodification of organs,
210–11, 214, 219, 235; and environmental risks, 182; and ethics of scale,
146, 154; and Shaʿrawi, Shaykh,
117–18
cloning organs. See stem cell research
Cohen, Lawrence, 213, 228–29, 292n12
collagen diseases, 199
colonialism, 73–74, 127, 251, 268–
69n13, 295–96n3
commodification of organs, 2–3, 209–
37, 246, 208fig. See also black market in human organs; and Ahmad
(kidney-failure patient), 214; Badr's
views on, 154–56, 218, 292n7;
(com)modification, 43, 266n43; and
cornea transplants, 84; and crises
of authority, 24, 27, 29, 35, 43,
263n19; and defining death, 48, 55,
57–58, 74, 267n7, 268–69nn12,13;
and documentation/monitoring,
221–27, 232, 234, 236, 293–94n19;
and donor-sellers, 212–15, 218–26,
228–33, 235–37, 292–93nn7,11–16,
293–94n19, 294–95nn28,31;

and Emad (donor-seller), 218,
292nn11,12; and ethics of scale,
146–48, 154–59, 284–85nn11,17;
and gender, 292n4; greater transparency in, 231, 236–37, 294n23;
and honor, 215, 218, 232; and Iman
(kidney-failure patient), 227–31;
and kidney transplants, 24, 27, 126–
27, 146–48, 154–59, 191, 194, 206,
211–13, 219, 221, 227–30, 234–35,
263n19, 284–85nn11,17, 292n5,
294n22; Kotb's views on, 146–47,
211; and liver transplants, 209, 213,
219, 221–22, 292n6; and Nagla
(kidney-failure patient), 212–14,
292n5; and ongoing relationship
with donor, 214, 292n7; precautions that paid donor not escape,
213; price of organs, 213, 218–19,
229, 233, 292n5; risks/benefits of,
191, 194, 202, 206, 233–34, 237; and
shame, 216–19; Shaykh Gumaʿa's
views on, 126–27; Shaykh Tantawi's
views on, 130, 137; statistics on, 209,
215, 291n1, 292nn8,9; transnational
organ sales, 210, 215–18, 220–21,
232–35, 292n2; "underground," 215,
220, 229, 232, 237, 247, 293–94n19,
294–95n28
common people (al-ʿawwam), 117, 136
common sense, 18, 178, 196, 198, 214
consent procurement, 24, 35, 55,
70–71, 191, 267n7, 290n26; and
commodification of organs, 231;
for cornea donation, 34, 83–84,
86–92, 95–96, 108–11, 274n17, 276–
77nn39–41; from families, 4, 66,
71, 83, 95, 108–9, 111, 115, 268n12,
276–77nn39–41; informed consent, 4, 70, 84, 95–96, 231, 274n17;
Shaykh Shaʿrawi's views on, 132
contamination, 10, 13. See also
environmental risks; pollution/
pollutants; of agricultural land, 10,
13, 28–29, 59, 182; of blood transfusions, 25, 177, 262n15, 287n7;
of food, 179–82, 289n17; of water

supplies, 10, 13, 16, 29, 59, 175, 179–81, 259n18, 287n7

Coptic Christians, 14, 92, 160–62, 209, 259n22, 266n42, 279n13, 293–94n19; Coptic Orthodox Church, 92, 160; the Pope, 92, 160

cornea opacity/transplants, 2, 4, 21, 30–35, 83–112, 263n25, xx*fig. See also* blindness; public eye banks/hospitals; and accident victims, 87, 105; and "backwardness," 2, 84–85, 92–97, 100, 275n25; and bioethics, 11, 16, 260n27; and "breaking bones of the dead," 106–8, 276n37; and cadaveric procurement program, 16, 83, 87–89, 265n36, 273n6; and "conditions of dire necessity" *(darura)*, 87, 107–8, 276–77n39; consent for transplants, 34, 83–84, 86–92, 95–96, 108–11, 274n17, 276–77nn39–41; and cornea grafting, 2, 33–34, 83–87, 92, 96, 110, 263n25, 274n18; and cornea tissues, 33–35, 44, 80, 84, 86–87, 91, 111; and crises of authority, 33–34, 43–44, 265n36; earliest in Egypt, 86, 96, 98; elderly patients, 31; and eye globes, 83, 87, 89, 97–98; and eye theft, 4, 29, 83, 85, 263n25, 272–73nn1,3; and fatwas, 93, 107–10, 276–77n39; and ignorance, 16, 44, 84, 86, 90, 93–95, 99–100, 104–5, 111, 274n21, 275n25; imported grafts for, 95–96, 263n25, 274n18; "intentions and actions," 101–6, 108–10; in *The Lamp of Umm Hashim* (1968 film), 99–100; in *The Lamp of Umm Hashim* (Haqqi), 101; national campaign for cornea donation, 92–93, 95–96, 98, 109, 111; and national eye bank program, 107, 110, 273n5; "for overall public benefit" *(maslaha 'ama)*, 87; and perennial charity *(sadaqa jariyya)*, 103–4, 110–11, 277n41; preservation techniques for transplants, 86–87, 274n18; public outreach programs for, 11, 92–93,

95, 31*fig.*; and scandals, 83–84, 90, 110, 221, 257n3; and Shaykh Ma'mun, 107–9, 276–77n39; and Shaykh Sha'rawi, 120, 279n15; and Shaykh Tantawi, 92–93, 101–4, 107, 109–11, 275–76n28; statistics on, 87; in U.S., 87, 93, 101, 274n16, 275n27, 277n42; waiting lists for transplants, 272–73n3; young *(shabab)* patients, 31–33, 263n26

corruption, 2, 5, 12–13, 241, 243, 246, 255. *See also* black market in human organs; organ/eye theft; and blood transfusions, 177, 287n7; and cornea transplants, 90; and crises of authority, 24, 28, 31, 37–39; and environmental risks, 13, 28, 184; of government, 24, 31, 177, 184, 253, 287n7; in medical education, 38; and medical malpractice/mistreatment, 177, 179, 206, 287n7; in Pakistan, 264n31; in public/private medical institutions, 37, 39, 90, 177, 179, 287–88nn7,10; and Sha'rawi, Shaykh, 117

costs of medical treatment, 145, 148–54, 168, 170, 284n9, 285nn12,13

The Courage to Fail (Fox and Swazey), 144–45

CPR, 50, 53, 61–62

cultural difference, 14, 79, 97–98, 272nn40,42, 274n22

Cushing's syndrome, 200

cyborg, 183–84, 250

cyclosporine, 294n22

Daqahliyya Province, 182, 240, 289n19. *See also* Mansoura

Dar al-'Ulum University, 270n26

Dar al-Hilal al-Tibbi, 68

Dar al-Ifta', 11, 71, 93, 107, 129, 187–88, 258nn15,16, 267–68n10, 269n17, 271n37, 278n6

Darura. *See* jurisprudence, Islamic

al-Daruriyyat al-khamsa. *See maqasid*

The Days (al-Ayam) (Hussein), 275n25

death. *See also* brain death: and afterlife, 44, 84, 94, 103–4, 106, 159, 168,
205; and bare afterlife, 106; and bioethics, 6, 15, 115; "breaking bones of
the dead," 106–8; cardiopulmonary,
49, 53, 78, 80, 95, 230–31, 274n13,
291n33; certitude of, 59–62, 80,
106, 200, 270n22; of children, 60,
88; "clinical death" *(al-mawt al-
kliniki)*, 65, 274n13; coming "back
to life," 62, 270n22; and cornea
transplants, 33–34, 83–84, 86–89,
91–98, 100–101, 103–11, 265n36,
273n4, 274nn13,22, 275n27,
276–77n39; and crises of authority,
21–22, 26, 33–35, 43, 45, 265n36;
criteria of "dead donors," 78–79;
dead as sentient, 106; dead bodies,
22, 33–34, 43, 84–89, 91, 94, 97–98,
100–101, 103–12, 240, 265n36,
274n22, 275n27, 276–77n39, 292n2;
and diagnostic error, 62, 70, 270n22;
and dignity *(hurma)* of dead,
107–9; as divine sign, 60–61; and do
not resuscitate (DNR) orders, 78,
291n33; and ethics of scale, 150–53,
158–59, 163, 170, 285n14; irreversibility of, 62–63, 83–84, 91, 274n13;
of kidney-failure patients/donors,
15, 26, 150–52, 170, 174, 177, 193,
200–201, 203, 212, 232, 235–36,
258n14; of liver-failure patients/
donors, 15, 260n25, 271n31; and
material body, 34, 67, 73, 75, 91,
103–4, 111, 122–23, 128; "mercy
killing," 77; "non-heartbeating
donors" (NHBDs), 78; preparation
for, 63; redefining, 6, 21, 47–80, 249,
267n7; respect for the dying/dead,
63, 107–9, 111, 270n23; rights of
dead, 33, 47, 91, 106, 112; rites for
the dead, 104–7, 276n35; sacralizing
the dead, 66–67, 136; of Shadya
(kidney-failure patient), 152–53,
158, 203, 285n14; Shaykh Sha'rawi's
views on, 119, 122–24, 128–29,

145–46, 280n34, 281nn35,39; and
the soul, 52, 56, 60–61, 65–67, 84,
275n27; and terminal illness, 120,
137, 155, 193–94, 203–4, 219, 223,
246, 279n14
democracy, 4, 22
Demographic and Health Survey,
Egyptian (2008), 288n11
depression, 184
diabetes, 25–26, 89, 151, 178, 180, 184,
191, 194, 199, 212, 288n14
dialysis machines/clinics, 10, 22–30,
246, 250–51, 262nn13,14, 284n10,
140*fig.*, 172*fig.*; and 'Abduh, Sayyid,
200–204, 291nn34–36; and Ahmad
(kidney-failure patient), 214;
and 'Ali (kidney-failure patient),
159–68, 228, 286n19; and bioethics, 6, 8–9, 14–15; and blackouts/
brownouts, 26; and commodification
of organs, 212–14, 225, 227, 292n5;
early machines, 263nn20,21; and
environmental risks, 179–81, 183–
86; and "good" solvents, 176–77,
250, 287n7; and Hani (kidney-failure patient/organ buyer), 154–55,
158, 285n16; and Iman (kidney-
failure patient), 227–31; and Khadra
(kidney-failure patient), 186–89;
and Khalid (kidney-failure patient),
190–94, 193*fig.*; and Madame Sabah
(kidney-failure patient), 165–66;
and Mahdi (kidney-failure patient),
179–80; and Mahmud (kidney-
failure patient), 238*fig.*; and medical
malpractice/mistreatment, 174–79,
287–88nn3,6–8,10,12; and Muhammad (kidney-failure patient), 174,
203–5; and Muna (kidney-failure
patient), 27–28; and Nagla (kidney-
failure patient), 212–14, 292n5;
and Ragia (kidney-failure patient),
25–26, 20*fig.*; and Sa'id (kidney-
failure patient), 196; and Shadya
(kidney-failure patient), 149–54,
158, 287–88n10; and social risks,

190–92, 196–200, 203, 190*fig.*; and spiritual risks, 186–89; statistics on, 258n13; and Tamir (kidney-failure patient), 150, 153–54; transplant as "vacation from dialysis," 177; and "washing" *(ghasil)*, 25–26, 178, 194, 262nn13,14

diglossic society, 262n12

dignity, 2, 66, 90, 107–10, 219, 235, 243, 253–55

disability, 63, 90, 184, 187–89

"disappeared" children, 4

divine property *(inna al-jasad milk allah)*, 28. *See also* God's ownership of bodies

divine will. *See* God's will

divorce, 197–98, 207, 293–94n19

doctors of confidence, 130, 242. *See also* experts, medical; transplant surgeons; *names of physicians*; as "close to God" *('arif rabbina)*, 37, 264n29; and crises of authority, 36–39, 264n28; on defining death, 47, 55–56; and ethics of scale, 146, 156

donors. *See* organ/eye donors

Dream satellite channel, 259n18

driver's license checkoffs, 17, 93, 159

droughts, 259n19

drugs: anti-retroviral, 286n1, 290n27; black market in, 155; cost of, 13, 148, 155, 177, 285n12, 294n22; cyclosporine, 294n22; immunosuppressive, 22–24, 34, 59, 200, 228–29, 234, 261n5, 285n12, 286n21, 294n22; and kidney transplants/dialysis, 22–24, 26, 30, 148, 155, 175, 177, 179–80, 203, 261n5, 288nn11,12; and medical malpractice/mistreatment, 175, 177, 179–80, 288nn11,12; side effects of, 13, 26, 148, 180, 200

Duqqi Quarter (Cairo), 90

eclampsia *(tasammum haml)*, 187

economics, 1–2, 4–5, 8–9, 12–15, 29, 45. *See also* financial resources; and

defining death, 68, 71, 73–75, 77; and environmental risks, 182–85; and Sha'rawi, Shaykh, 116–18, 137

education, Egyptian, 32–33; al-Azhar schools, 150; citizen education on mass media, 92–93, 95; and cornea transplants, 92–95; and crises of authority, 28–29, 264–65nn33,34,36,37,38; equal opportunity in, 38, 264–65n33; medical education, 38–39, 99, 264–65nn33,34,36,37; national high school exams, 264–65n33; nepotism in, 38, 265n37; and private lessons, 264–65n33; and religious scholars, 39–40, 265–66nn38,39; tuition for, 264–65nn33,34

efficacy, medical, 12, 14, 17, 22, 111, 116, 170, 203, 244, 246–47, 272n42

Egyptian Medical Syndicate, 5, 24, 221–26, 232, 234, 236, 264n32, 265n37, 293–94n19, 294–95n28; president of, 64, 215, 292n8

Egyptian National Medical Ethics Committee (al-Jama'iyya al-Misriyya li-l Akhlaqiyyat al-Tibbiyya), 58, 270n21

"Egyptian ophthalmia." *See* trachoma

Egyptian Society of Nephrology, 177, 180, 258n13, 284–85n11, 287n8, 291n1

El Baradei, Mohamed, 242

England. *See* Great Britain

English language, 198, 201, 262n12, 264–65n33

Enlightenment, Egyptian *(nahda)*, 69, 84, 91, 275n25

environmental risks, 174–75, 179–86, 206, 288n14, 289–90nn16–19, 183*fig. See also* contamination; pollution/pollutants

Ernst, Carl, 282–83n48

erythropoietin injections, 262n15

ethics, medical, 1, 4, 6–8, 21, 28, 36, 250. *See also* bioethics; scale, ethics of; and commodification of organs, 209–10, 213, 231, 233–37; and cornea transplants, 34, 97; and crises of authority, 22, 34, 36–37, 39, 44; and defining death, 47–54, 58–60, 63, 73, 75–76, 78–79, 267n1, 270n21; and doctors of confidence, 36–38, 264nn28,29; "do no harm," 8; in Japan, 49; and kidney transplants, 142, 144, 146, 148, 151–52, 155, 166–68, 170–71, 196; and Sha'rawi, Shaykh, 116, 282–83n48; and stem cell research, 28; in U.S., 28

ethics, religious, 18, 244, 246–50, 255. *See also* scale, ethics of; and commodification of organs, 209–10, 213, 231, 234–37; and cornea transplants, 103, 108–9, 111; and crises of authority, 22, 24, 37, 39–44; and defining death, 47–48, 51–55, 63, 70–71, 73, 75–76, 79, 271n33; and doctors of confidence, 37; and kidney transplants, 151–52, 166–68, 170–71, 174–75, 188, 191–92, 206; and risks/benefits of treatment, 174–75, 188, 191–92, 195–96, 199, 203, 206–7, 290n23; and Sha'rawi, Shaykh, 126–27, 137, 282–83n48

Europe. *See also names of European countries*: and commodification of organs, 210–11, 216, 221, 223–24, 233–34, 292n6; cornea transplants in, 93, 98–100; defining death in, 51–53, 55, 58–59, 61, 65–67, 75–76, 78, 267nn5,8, 268n12; kidney transplants in, 155, 175, 211, 284n10; in *The Lamp of Umm Hashim* (1968 film), 99–100; liver transplants in, 292n6; media in, 244–45; medical journals in, 37, 58–59, 65; and Sha'rawi, Shaykh, 118, 281n35; "shortage of organs" discourse in, 155

euthanasia, 75

experiential knowledge, 251; and bioethics, 6–8, 12, 15, 17; and cornea transplants, 32–35, 104; and crises of authority, 32–35, 45; and environmental risks, 179, 183, 185; and gender, 12

experts, medical. *See also* authority, medical; doctors of confidence; transplant surgeons; *names of medical experts and physicians*: in bioethics, 6–7, 11–12; and circuits of doubt, 48; and class, 11–12; on commodification of organs, 210–12, 214–15, 295n29; on cornea transplants, 84–85, 92–98, 101–4, 110–11, 274n21, 275–76n28; and crises of authority, 28–29, 35–39, 43, 45; on defining death, 47–49, 51–66, 68–71, 73–77, 79–80, 269n19, 270nn26,27, 271n35; elitism of, 23–24, 64, 68, 85, 97, 100, 108, 211, 215, 220–21, 236; on environmental risks, 180, 185–86; and ethics of scale, 151, 160; and experiential knowledge, 6–7; and gender, 11–12; on kidney transplants/dialysis, 28–29, 134, 151, 160, 180, 185–86, 195–96; on liver transplants, 295n29; and medical malpractice/mistreatment, 178, 287n9; as organ/eye donors, 94–95, 102, 274n16; and Sha'rawi, Shaykh, 115, 120, 129–31, 134; on social risks, 195–96, 203–5

experts, religious. *See* religious scholars

exploitation. *See also* medical malpractice/mistreatment: and black market in human organs, 215–18; and commodification of organs, 210–11, 216–17, 220, 223, 231, 233; and cornea transplants, 84; and crises of authority, 28–29, 34, 37; and defining death, 75, 105; of kidney transplants, 247; of poor, 3–4, 10, 12, 75, 84, 131, 136, 210, 216–17, 220, 231, 239, 245, 259n18; sexual, 233 extremists, 5, 38, 41, 64, 68, 72, 85, 245; ʿAli (kidney-failure patient) as, 167; Shaykh Shaʿrawi as, 131, 136, 167

eye banks. *See* public eye banks/hospitals

eye theft, 4, 29, 83, 85–89, 91, 263n25, 272n1

Facebook, 253

family, 12, 15–17, 240, 244, 246–47, 250, 295–96n3; and commodification of organs, 210–14, 217–31, 233–35, 293–94nn19,20; Coptic Christians' views on, 259n22; and cornea transplants, 30–33, 83–84, 86–91, 93–95, 97–100, 104–6, 108, 111–12, 265n36, 272n1, 276–77n39; and crises of authority, 23, 26–28, 30–33, 35–36, 39, 44, 263n19, 265n36; and defining death, 48–51, 61, 66–68, 70–71, 80, 267n7, 268n12, 270–71nn30,34; in England, 97; and environmental risks, 16, 179–81, 185–86; and ethics of scale, 148–50, 152–53, 157–71, 284–85n11; and kidney transplants/dialysis, 23, 26–28, 30, 32, 35–36, 116, 126, 148–50, 152–53, 157–71, 173–74, 179–81, 185–206, 211–12, 239, 246, 263n19, 269n18, 284–85n11, 291nn33,34; in *The Lamp of Umm Hashim* (1968 film), 99–100; and medical malpractice/mistreatment, 173–76, 179; and rites for the dead, 104–7, 276n35; and Shaʿrawi, Shaykh, 116–17; and social risks, 189–99, 203–6; and spiritual risks, 186–89; and "three brothers" tale, 199–203, 291n34; and "tyranny of the gift," 70, 191, 203–7, 271n34

al-fard al-ʿayn, 276n35

al-fard al-kifaya, 276n35

Farmer, Paul, 14

Farouk, King, 260n27

Fassin, Didier, 295–96n3

fatalism, 28, 30, 167, 169, 286n23

fatwas: and cornea transplants, 93, 107–10, 276–77n39; and kidney transplants, 145–47, 185; of Shaʿrawi, Shaykh, 117, 119–22, 126–31, 136, 278nn6,11, 279n14, 280n29, 114*fig.*

fellahin, 85, 94, 294n20

feminist scholars, 295–96n3

femtosecond, 159, 168

fertility. *See* reproduction

films: on black market in human organs, 4, 216–17, 294n24, 208*fig.*; on class disparities, 91; on cornea transplants, 99–100, 274n23, 275nn24,25

financial resources, 15, 35, 272n42. *See also* economics; and black market in human organs, 216–18, 294–95n28; and commodification of organs, 209–14, 218–26, 228, 230–31, 233–37, 293n17; and cornea transplants, 31, 96, 263n25, 274n18; and defining death, 62, 65, 70–71, 79; and kidney transplants/dialysis, 145, 148–61, 167, 170–71, 174–75, 177–78, 180, 186–89, 194–95, 197–99, 202–4, 206–7, 284n9, 285nn12,13,17, 286–87nn19,2; and medical malpractice/mistreatment, 174–75, 177–78, 180, 286–87n2; and social risks, 194–95, 197–99, 204–7; and spiritual risks, 187–89; and "three brothers" tale, 202–3

fiqh. *See* jurisprudence, Islamic

food security/storage, 16, 179–83, 259n19, 289n17; breast milk, 289n18; "cancerous wheat" *(al-qamh al-musartan)*, 182–83, 289–90nn19,20; genetically modified food, 134, 179, 181

foreign aid/debts, 9, 29, 182–84, 264n32, 289–90n20

Fox, Renée, 144–45, 191, 257n1

France, 52, 271n31

fraud, 177, 287–88n10

Free Officers' Coup (1952), 260n27

fungi. *See* aflatoxins; ochratoxins

futility, medical, 53, 116, 279n14

Gad al-Haqq, Shaykh, 48, 55–57, 60–63, 66, 268nn11,12, 269n17, 277n40

Gawande, Atul, 245

gender, 11, 246, 255, 271n33, 292n4, 295–96n3; and kidney transplants/dialysis, 27, 196–99, 287n3, 291nn30–32, 292n4; and social risks, 196–99, 291nn30–32

genetically modified food, 134, 179, 181

genetics, 13, 32, 199, 247, 250, 291n34

Germany, 52, 77, 267n5

Gharbiyya Province, 26, 292n5. *See also* Tanta

al-Ghazali, 266n41

Ghoneim, Mohamed, 22–24, 36–37, 141, 241–43, 260n2, 261–62nn7,9, 264n30; on commodification of organs, 211, 221, 293n17, 294n22

al-Ghumari, 'Abdallah, Shaykh, 277n1

gift, tyranny of, 70, 191, 203–7, 271n34

glaucoma, 263n24

God, remembrance of *(al-dhikr)*, 124–25

God's benevolence/compassion *(al-rahma)*, 169

God's omnipotence, 98, 104, 124, 132, 251

God's ownership of bodies, 1–2, 244, 247, 238*fig.*; and bioethics, 9, 19, 24; the body as trust *(amana)*, 162, 187, 202; and commodification of organs, 211, 233; Coptic Christians' views on, 259n22; and cornea transplants, 34–35, 102; and crises of authority, 24, 27–28, 34–36, 38, 44; and defining death, 59, 63; and ethics of scale, 159, 167, 169; and kidney transplants, 27–28, 36, 159, 167, 169, 206–7, 246, 290n26; Shaykh al-Ghumari's views on, 277n1; Shaykh

Sha'rawi's views on, 3, 27, 115–16, 120, 122–26, 130–32, 135, 137–38, 159, 163, 251, 279n19, 280n31, 290n26; Shaykh Tantawi's views on, 130, 137

God's trials *(al-ibtila')*, 30, 128, 175, 184, 205

God's will, 22, 30, 43, 68, 250, 271–72n38; and ethics of scale, 150, 153, 162, 166–69, 171, 286n23; and risks/benefits of treatment, 194–95, 202; Shaykh Sha'rawi's views on, 123–25, 136–37, 167

God's work, 37, 264n28, 264n31

Goffman, Erving, 124

goiter operations, 153–54

graft survival, 24, 132, 228, 261–62n9, 285n16, 286n21, 294n22

Great Britain: British Empire, 97, 268–69n13; cornea transplants in, 96–98, 274n22; defining death in, 59, 61–62, 65; English Eye Institute, 96–97; kidney transplants in, 177

Guma'a, 'Ali, Shaykh, 48, 72–77, 97, 126–27, 132, 265–66n38, 268–69n13, 271nn36,37, 277n40, 280nn26,27, 74*fig.*

Gutmann, Matthew, 266n42

Habib, Tariq, 120–22, 279nn12,13

hadith, 64, 103, 106–10, 270n24, 276nn32,34,37, 277n1, 283n52, 286n24; "breaking bones of the dead," 106–10, 276n37

hajj, 156

halal, 41, 69, 71, 107, 161

Haqqi, Yahya, 99–101, 275n25

haram: and commodification of organs, 209, 211, 213; and cornea transplants, 88, 91, 93, 107, 276n30; and crises of authority, 33–35, 37, 41; and defining death, 52, 59, 69, 71; and ethics of scale, 142–46, 150, 160–64, 166–67, 170; and kidney transplants, 142–46, 150, 160–64, 166–67, 170, 187, 191–92, 200, 202–3, 244; Kotb's views on, 142–46;

and risks/benefits of treatment, 187,
191–92, 200, 202–3; Shaykh al-
Ghumari's views on, 277n1; Shaykh
Sha'rawi's views on, 120, 134, 137,
145, 170, 279n19, 281n37

harm, 8, 35, 39, 55, 59, 70–71, 107–9,
246, 250, 266n41. *See also* risks/
benefits; and commodification
of organs, 212, 233; and ethics of
scale, 144, 148, 154, 157, 164, 167,
171; Shaykh Sha'rawi's views on,
130–34, 137; and suicide/"suicide
operations," 144

Harvard Medical School: Ad Hoc
Committee . . . to Examine the Definition of Death, 49

heart disease/transplants, 51–52, 178,
243, 267n2, 268n12; coronary artery
bypass grafts, 142–43, 284n4

hemodialysis treatment, 26, 148–49,
168, 178, 260n3, 261–62n9. *See also*
dialysis machines/clinics

hepatitis C, 16–17, 153, 177, 212, 234,
287n8, 295n29

hijab, 271n33

Hinduism, 67

Hirschkind, Charles, 43–44, 104,
270n23

HIV/AIDS, 59, 177, 273–74n12,
286n1, 290n27, 295–96n3

Hogle, Linda, 267n5

hukm, 127

al-Husayn, the Sayyid, 118

Hussein, Taha, 275n25

el-Husseini, 'Amr, Dr., 290n28

hypertension, 154, 178, 180, 184, 191,
196, 200, 203, 288n11

iatrogenesis (treatment-induced illness), 174, 288n14

Ibrahim, Muhammad (ophthalmolo-
gist/major figure in eye banking),
90, 96–98, 274nn19–21

ignorance, 6, 12, 41, 73, 111, 258n6;
and cornea transplants, 16, 44,
84, 86, 90, 93–95, 99–100, 104–5,
274n21, 275n25; in *The Lamp of*

Umm Hashim (1968 film), 99–100,
275n25; and Sha'rawi, Shaykh,
120–22, 281n35; and social risks,
198

ijma' (consensus). *See* jurisprudence,
Islamic

Ilhaquna! (Save Us!; film), 216–17,
208*fig.*

Imam al Du'a' (Leader of the Preachers; television program), 136

immunosuppressants, 22–24, 34, 59,
200, 228–29, 234, 261n5, 285n12,
286n21, 294n22

imperialism, 4, 76–78, 97

'Imran, Abdul Mu'ti, 127, 280n30

India, 36, 215, 228–29, 266n42

indigenous healing practices, 36,
264n27, 266n42

inequalities, social, 2, 4, 241, 246, 255.
See also class disparities; poor/
poverty; and bioethics, 7–8, 14–15;
and commodification of organs, 214,
237; and cornea transplants, 84; and
defining death, 73, 77, 79; and environmental risks, 184–86; and ethics
of scale, 147, 156, 171; in medical
education, 265n37; and uncertainty
in medicine, 288n13

infitah ("Open Door Policy"), 5,
257n4, 273n11

insurance, health, 29, 262n15; army
insurance, 159–61, 163, 166, 286n19;
in England, 177; universal health
coverage, 29, 177

intellectuals, Egyptian, 77, 118–19,
136, 216, 241, 275n25, 278n5,
290n21

intentions and actions, 101–6, 108–10,
123

International POPs Elimination Project (IPEN), 288n14

internet, 253

Iran, 57, 79, 249, 268n12; Islamic
Revolution (1979), 76; U.S. hostage
crisis (1979–80), 76

Iraq war, 26, 76

al-'Irqsusi, 'Abd al-Hamid, 39, 217

Islam, 1–5, 244–50. *See also* authority, Islamic; ethics, religious; God's
ownership of bodies; jurisprudence,
Islamic; Muslims; and "backwardness," 5, 44, 68–70, 73, 84, 271n33;
and bioethics, 11–15, 18–19, 24,
260n26; and charity, 103–4, 110–11,
277n41; and "clash of civilizations,"
61, 76–80, 84, 272n40; and commodification of organs, 209, 211,
227; and cornea transplants, 86,
93–95, 98, 101–10, 273n4; and crises
of authority, 22, 24, 27–28, 30, 33,
39–44, 265–66nn38–42, 41*fig.*; and
Day of Judgment, 67; and defining death, 47–48, 51, 53–66, 68–72,
75–78, 267nn8,9, 268–69nn11–13,
270n21, 271nn32,33,37; and ethics
of scale, 158, 160–62, 285n18; and
fate *(nasib)*, 154, 285n15; framework *(al-itar al-islami)*, 42; and hajj,
156; humans as God's viceregents
(khalafa), 271–72n38; hyperobjectification of, 161–62, 169, 248–49,
285n18; "intentions and actions,"
101–6, 108–10, 123; "Islam as the
solution" *(al-islam huwwa al-hal)*,
68; Islamic tradition, 104, 117, 119,
124, 127, 135–36, 246, 276n34,
282n45; and kidney transplants/
dialysis, 22, 27–28, 30, 55, 144,
158, 160–62, 167–69, 187–89, 200,
285n18; logic *('ilm al-mantiq)*, 265–
66n38; and modernity, 42, 44, 127,
280n29; *niqab*, 153; permissibility
of organ donation, 3, 107–9, 120–21,
123, 128–30, 132–35, 145, 151,
162, 167–71, 192, 203, 281nn37,40,
290n26; philology *('ilm al-lugha)*,
265–66n38; "pope of Islam," 126;
and prayer, 104, 106, 117, 161–62,
191, 203–5, 242, 276n35, 286n20,
248*fig.*; religious principles *(usul
al-din)*, 265–66n38; and revelation, 122, 134–35, 281n36, 282–
83nn45,48; and risks/benefits of
treatment, 175–76, 187–89, 191–92,

200, 207, 290nn23,26; and saints, 98,
100, 104; *salat al-istikhara* (seeking
the good), 161–62, 286n20; salvation in, 124–25; Shaykh Sha'rawi's
views on, 118–30, 135–38, 145,
167, 170–71, 279nn13–15, 280n29;
al-shirk, 98, 100–101; and slavery,
73–74, 268–69n13; and spiritual
rewards, 3, 33, 67, 70, 94, 101–4,
109–10, 130, 150, 202, 275n27; and
spiritual struggle *(jihad)*, 164; and
suicide/"suicide operations," 122,
130, 144, 279n19; *sunna*, 276n34;
traditional curriculum *(al-manhaj
al-Islami)*, 40, 265–66n38

Islamic jurisprudence *(fiqh)*, 11, 40–42,
55–56, 58, 63, 75–76, 108, 118, 126–
28, 130–33, 247, 265–66nn38,41,
267n8, 268nn11–13, 270n21,
271n37, 276n30, 279n14, 280n26,
281nn36,37,40,41, 282–83nn46,48,
41*fig.*; *darura* (conditions of dire
necessity), 87, 107–8, 130, 132,
135, 276–77n39; *al-fard al-'ayn*,
276n35; *al-fard al-kifaya*, 276n35;
hukm, 127; *ijma'* (consensus),
268–69n13; *madhhab*, 126, 280n26;
maslaha 'amma (public benefit/
social good), 42, 87, 107–10, 131–33,
135–36, 144–46, 266n41, 277n40,
283nn49,51; and modernity, 42, 44,
127, 280n29; *sadaqa jariyya*, 103–4,
110–11, 277n41; *sadd al-dhara'i'*
(blocking the means), 132, 276n30,
281–82n41; transnational legal
coalitions, 13, 57; *usul al-fiqh*
(methodologies of), 11, 265–66n38,
276n30; *wara'* (road of caution),
127, 280n30

Islamic Research Academy (Majma'
'al-Buhuth al-Islamiyya), 57,
268–69n13

Islamic revival *(al-sahwa al-islamiyya)*, 1, 5, 21, 38, 44, 250, 260n1.
See also Muslim Brotherhood; and
cassette sermons, 44; and cornea
transplants, 104; and defining death,

54, 70–71, 267nn8,9; as "Islamic trend" *(al-tiyar al-islami)*, 64, 278n7; and Sha'rawi, Shaykh, 116, 118; and spiritual risks, 188
ISO certificates, 287n7
Israel, 76, 95, 182–83, 292n2; Arab–Israeli War (1967), 76, 99, 283n1
Istabl Antar slum, 294n24

January 25 uprisings (Egypt's Arab Spring), 253–55, 264n32, 269n17
Japan, 49, 78, 271n31, 292n6
Jordan, 79, 268n12
journalists. *See* media
jurisprudence. *See* Islamic jurisprudence. *See also* Majma' al-Fiqh al-Islami; shari'a

Kafr al-Zayat (Gharbiya), 181, 289n16
Kafr al-Zayat Pesticides and Chemicals Company (KZPC), 181, 289n16
Kasr el Aini, 38, 64–65, 83, 87–89, 142, 272–73nn1–3; Department of Nephrology, 288n14; Faculty of Medicine, 58, 272n1
kidney disease/transplants, 1–2, 245–46, 284n10. *See also* dialysis machines/clinics; and 'Abduh, Sayyid, 200–204, 291nn34–36; and Ahmad (kidney-failure patient), 25, 214; and 'Ali (kidney-failure patient), 159–69, 171, 228, 285n18, 286nn19,21; and Amin (kidney-failure patient), 175–76; Badr's views on, 68, 70, 154–58, 171; and bioethics, 9–12, 19, 258n14, 259n18; and black market in human organs, 29–30, 35, 79, 155–56, 216; in Cairo, 23–24, 35, 141–46, 148, 150, 152, 158, 160, 162–63, 166, 168, 170, 212, 261nn7,9, 283–84n2, 292n5; and commodification of organs, 24, 27, 126–27, 146–48, 154–59, 191, 194, 206, 209–21, 223–25, 227–30, 232, 234–35, 263n19, 284–85nn11,17, 292n5, 294n22; cornea transplants compared to, 85, 105, 112; and

creatinine levels, 176, 197, 287n4; and crises of authority, 21–30, 34–37, 43; and defining death, 55–57, 59, 71, 79, 268n12; earliest transplants in Egypt, 3, 4, 21, 23, 36–37, 141–43, 146, 211, 283–84n2; elderly patients, 186, 195, 269n18, 288n14; and environmental risks, 9–10, 16, 23, 25, 28–29, 179–86, 288n14; and ethics of scale, 147–71, 284–85nn9–11,14; in Europe, 155, 175, 284n10; and fatwas, 145–47, 185; and gender, 27, 196–98, 287n3, 291nn30–32; government-sponsored treatment *(nafaq al-dawla)*, 149, 285n13; and Hani (kidney-failure patient/organ buyer), 154–55, 157–58, 285n16; and Iman (kidney-failure patient), 227–31; in Iran, 268n12; and Khadra (kidney-failure patient), 186–89; and Khalid (kidney-failure patient), 190–94, 193*fig.*; Kotb's views on, 135, 141–47, 170, 203, 211, 284n6; and Madame Sabah (kidney-failure patient), 165–66; and Mahdi (kidney-failure patient), 179–80; and Mahmud (kidney-failure patient), 238*fig.*; in Mansoura, 22–25, 36–37, 71, 141, 152–53, 241, 261–62nn7,9,10, 285n14; and *maslaha*, 144–46; and medical malpractice/mistreatment, 174–79, 288nn11,12; and Muhammad (kidney-failure patient), 174, 203–5; and Muna (kidney-failure patient), 27–28; and Nagla (kidney-failure patient), 212–14, 292n5; and one-fourth a kidney, 185, 192; in Pakistan, 264n28; and Raghida (kidney-failure patient), 189; and Ragia (kidney-failure patient), 25–26, 28, 20*fig.*; and rebirth/reproduction, 192–93, 196–98, 203–5, 290n27, 193*fig.*; risks/benefits of treatment, 14–15, 144, 146–49, 151, 156–57, 170–71; and Sa'id (kidney-failure patient), 196; and Samira

kidney disease/transplants (*continued*)
(kidney-failure patient), 197; second kidney as "spare part," 74–75,
186, 212; "shadow market" in, 234,
269n18; and Shadya (kidney-failure
patient), 149–54, 158, 171, 203,
285n14, 287–88nn9,10; Shaykh
Guma'a's views on, 126–27; Shaykh
Sha'rawi's views on, 123, 133–34,
137–38, 145; Shaykh Tantawi's
views on, 133–34, 137; and social
risks, 173, 189–200, 203, 290n29,
291nn30,31, 190*fig.*, 193*fig.*; and
spiritual risks, 186–89; statistics on,
23–24, 148–49, 215, 261n5, 262n10,
284–85n11, 286n22, 290n28,
291n31, 292nn8,9; and stress (*al-
daght*), 180; and Tamir (kidney-
failure patient), 150, 153–54, 171;
in Tanta, 10–11, 25–28, 42, 149–52,
154, 158–68, 179, 186–87, 199,
20*fig.*, 172*fig.*; and third kidney,
201–2, 291n35; and "three brothers" tale, 199–203, 291n34; tissue
typing for, 151–52, 154–55, 161–63,
165–66, 168–69, 191, 205, 219, 224–
25, 228–30, 286n21, 294n21; transplant as "vacation from dialysis,"
177; and urine, 141, 144, 152, 240;
in U.S., 23, 28, 149, 155, 162, 164,
166, 175, 261–62nn5,9, 269n18,
286n22; in *Wahid min al-nas*
(television news program), 259n18;
waiting lists for transplants, 149,
166, 198, 211–12, 284n10, 286n22;
young (*shabab*) patients, 189, 195,
199, 288n14
Kifayya political party, 289n19
kinship. *See* family
Koran. *See* Qur'an
Kotb, Abdel Kader, 135, 141–47, 152,
170, 203, 211, 244, 284nn6,8
Krawietz, Birgit, 135, 283n51
Kulthum, Umm, 129, 280n34
Kuwait, 57, 70, 79, 220, 268n12,
270n22

labor conditions, 175, 179, 198, 234, 237
Laher, Suheil, 277n1
The Lamp of Umm Hashim (1968
film), 99–100, 104, 274n23,
275nn24,25
The Lamp of Umm Hashim (Haqqi),
99–101, 275n25
Lane, Sandra, 263n23, 274n17
Langford, Jean, 106
laws/legislation, 21, 34, 116, 248,
281n37; on commodification of
organs, 215, 220–21, 223, 232; on
defining death, 47–49, 53–54, 58–59,
62, 67–68, 78–79; Law 44 on Family
Status ("Jihan" law), 268n11; for
national eye bank program, 107–8,
110–11, 273n5, 276–77n39; for
national organ transplant program,
3, 47–49, 51, 53, 55, 58, 65, 67, 79,
199, 215, 236
al-Laythi, 'Amr, 259n18, 263n22
Lebanon, 57, 76
leukemia, 290n21
life-support systems, 3–4, 6, 49–53, 55,
58, 61–62, 67, 69, 78, 267n6; Shaykh
Sha'rawi's views on, 128–29,
280n34
Light and Hope Foundation
(Mu'asasat al-Nur Wal-'Amal),
107–8, 276n38
literacy/illiteracy, 21, 86, 93, 122, 159,
224, 274n17, 278n6
liver disease/transplants, 1, 15–17, 245,
259n18, 271n31; and Amin (kidney-
failure patient), 175–76; and bilhar-
zias/schistosomiasis, 16–17, 180,
295n29; and commodification of
organs, 209, 213, 216, 219–22, 234,
292n6, 295n29; and defining death,
56, 59, 68, 271n31; and environmental risks, 16, 29, 180, 182, 184;
and liver lobes, 4, 15–16, 56, 144,
209, 213, 221–22, 260n25, 271n31,
292n6; and medical malpractice/
mistreatment, 175–76; in Saudi Arabia, 268n12; statistics on, 260n25,

295n29; in *Wahid min al-nas* (television news program), 259n18

Liwaʾ al-Islam, 279n18

al-Liwaʾ al-Islami, 122–27, 129, 132, 277n1, 279n18, 280n30

lobbyist groups, 58, 64, 68, 84

Lock, Margaret, 49, 65–66, 235, 267n6, 270n29, 274n16

Lotfy, Safwat, Dr., 48, 58–66, 69–70, 77, 106, 270n26

lupus, 149–51, 178, 285n14, 287n9

Maʿadi Hospital (Cairo), 154, 162–63, 165, 168

Maʿadi suburb, 294n24

Maʾmun, Hasan, Shaykh, 107–9, 276–77n39

madhhab, 126, 280n26

Maghraby, Akef, 273n5, 273n7

El-Maghraby Eye and Ear Hospitals and Centers, 32, 263n25, 273n5, 82*fig.*

Maghraby Eye Hospital (Cairo): Al Noor Society, charitable wing of, xxvi*fig.*, 82*fig.*

Majmaʿ al-Fiqh al-Islami, 132, 281n40

Mansoura, 10, 41; commodification of organs in, 210, 212, 224, 227, 231, 294nn20,22; defining death in, 71, 271n33; kidney transplants/dialysis in, 22–25, 36–37, 141, 148, 152–53, 157, 165–66, 195–99, 211–12, 227–28, 230–31, 239–41, 261–62nn7,9,10, 290n28, 291n31

Mansoura Kidney Center, 23–24, 68, 148, 152, 157, 166, 187, 195–98, 203, 212, 227, 230, 239–41, 243, 261–62nn4,7–9, 290n29, 295n1, 240*fig.*, 242*fig.*, 248*fig.*

Mansoura University Hospital, 23, 261n4

Mansoura Urology and Nephrology Center. *See* Mansoura Kidney Center

maqasid, 266n41

maslaha ʿamma (public benefit/social good), 42, 87, 107–10, 131–33,

135–36, 144–46, 266n41, 277n40, 283nn49,51

al-Massiri, ʿAbd al-Wahhab, 290n21

media, 1, 22, 115, 245, 258n11. *See also* newspapers; television; and bioethics, 7–10, 12, 17; on black market in human organs, 39, 83, 210, 215–17, 231–32, 237, 292n2, 293–94n19; for citizen education, 92; on commodification of organs, 2, 210, 220, 292n2; on cornea transplants, 83–86, 91–93, 98, 103, 110, 272–73nn1,3, 275–76nn27,28; on corruption, 185; and crises of authority, 7, 22, 29–30, 38–39, 43; on defining death, 48–49, 56–57, 59, 64–65, 68–70, 73, 75, 78–79, 270nn21,22, 271n32; on exploitation of poor organ sellers, 3, 10; on eye theft, 83, 272n1; on Ghoneim, 264n30; on "ignorant masses," 6, 12, 258n6; in Japan, 49; on kidney transplants, 3, 21, 39, 141, 162, 188, 271n33; on medical education, 38; on medical malpractice/mistreatment, 29–30, 175, 177; and Nasser, 5; opposition-party press, 12, 13, 29, 38, 54; as "pumpkin-seed journalism," 280n27; and Sadat, 5; on scandals, 21, 30, 39, 110; on Shaʿrawi, Shaykh, 117, 120–27, 131, 136–38, 233, 278n6, 279n18, 280n27, 281n35, 283n52; Shaykh Gumaʿa's views on, 127, 280n27; on social injustice, 76; state-run, 3, 12, 126, 233; in U.S., 17, 78, 244–45, 275n27, 295–96n3

medical malpractice/mistreatment, 24, 29–30, 37–39, 185, 239, 270n23; and black market in human organs, 216–17; and "breaking bones of the dead," 106–10, 276n37; and cornea transplants, 94–96, 98, 102, 105–12, 273n8, 277n40; risks of, 174–80, 287–88nn7–10; Shaykh Shaʿrawi's views on, 115, 131, 136

Medical Syndicate. *See* Egyptian Medical Syndicate

middle classes, 5, 68, 136, 182, 233
migrant workers, 21, 216, 295–96n3
military hospitals, 154, 162–63, 165,
    168, 190, 287n3
Min al-alif ila al-ya' (From A to Z;
    television program), 120, 279n12
Ministry of Education, Egyptian, 38
Ministry of Health, Egyptian, 4–5,
    38, 92–93, 102, 149, 181, 186, 232,
    276n29, 287–88n10, 294nn24,26,27;
    Free Treatment Section, 232
Ministry of Security, Egyptian, 209
Minufiyya, 4, 168
Al-Misri al-Yawm, 121, 184, 218, 241,
    287–88nn7,10
modernity, 42, 44, 78, 98–100, 245,
    250, 275n25; and *maslaha*, 135–36,
    283n49; and Sha'rawi, Shaykh, 117–
    19, 121, 127, 135–36, 280n29
moral lesson (*'ibra*), 203, 291n37
morgues, 4, 29, 83, 85–88, 100, 105,
    110, 272–73nn1,3, 277n41
Morsy, Soheir, 264n27
Al-Mousawi, Dr., 57–58, 64, 66,
    269n19
Mu'tazali theological school,
    282–83n48
Mubarak, Husni, 3, 5, 29, 118, 217,
    253, 255, 264n32, 278n7
muftis, 11, 244, 247, 249. *See also*
    religious scholars; *names of muftis
    and grand muftis*; on commodi-
    fication of organs, 233; on cornea
    transplants, 92–93, 102, 107–10,
    276–77nn39,40; on defining death,
    47–48, 53–58, 62–64, 69, 72–76,
    267–68nn9–12, 269nn17,19,
    271n35, 271n37; grand muftis, 11,
    48, 53–57, 72–75, 92, 107–9, 126,
    129, 137, 265–66n38, 267–68nn10–
    12, 269n17, 271n37, 281n36,
    74*fig.*; on kidney transplants, 188,
    284n5; as *qadi* (judge), 281n37; and
    Sha'rawi, Shaykh, 115, 117, 119,
    126–27, 131, 136–38, 281n36; on
    spiritual risks, 188; as state officials,
    47–48, 54–57, 63–64, 75, 115, 117,

119, 126, 129, 131–32, 135–37,
    267–68nn9,10,13, 269n17, 281n37,
    282–83n48, 284n5
Muhammad, the Prophet, 41, 99, 101,
    117, 120, 127, 146, 271n33, 280n23;
    and blood cupping *(higama/hajim)*,
    133, 282n45; granddaughter Zaynab,
    99–101; grandson Husayn, 118;
    hadith, 64, 103–4, 106–8, 137, 169,
    270n24, 276nn32,34,37, 277n1,
    283n53, 286n24; *sunna*, 276n34
Muslim Brotherhood, 4–5, 24, 54,
    70–71, 118, 240, 264n32, 267n8,
    279n18, 289n19
Muslims, 245–46, 248, 251. *See also*
    Islam; *names of Muslims*; biomedi-
    cine as "universal science," 36; and
    commodification of organs, 293–
    94n19; and cornea transplants, 98,
    103–6, 108; and crises of authority,
    36–37, 39–44, 265–66nn38–41; and
    defining death, 48, 55, 57–64, 67,
    75–79; and ethics of scale, 143, 156,
    159, 162, 170, 285n18, 286n20; and
    "Islamic bioethics," 13–15, 18–19;
    and kidney transplants, 143, 156,
    159, 162, 170, 285n18, 286n20; and
    perennial charity *(sadaqa jariyya)*,
    103–4, 110–11, 277n41; and prayer,
    104, 106, 117, 161–62, 191, 203–5,
    242, 276n35, 286n20, 248*fig.*; and
    rites for the dead, 104–7, 276n35;
    and Sha'rawi, Shaykh, 119, 121–33,
    135–36, 145, 279nn13,19, 280n23,
    282–83nn45,48,49; and Sufi dis-
    cipline/practice, 40, 42, 121, 124,
    266n40, 277n1, 280n23; Sunni Mus-
    lims, 126, 269n17, 282–83n48

Nasser, Gamal Abdel, 4–5, 38, 92, 116,
    273n11, 275n24
Nasser Institute (Cairo), 203
national eye bank program, 107, 110,
    273n5
nationalism, 4, 12, 38, 40, 78, 121,
    156, 159, 245, 250; in China/India,
    36; and commodification of organs,

215–16, 232, 293–94n19; and crises
of authority, 36, 38, 40, 44, 264n28
national organ transplant program, 2,
3, 55, 67, 79–80, 149, 199, 221, 236,
257–58n5; and commodification of
organs, 210, 215, 220; and defining
death, 47–49, 51, 53, 56–57, 65
national public health campaign for
cornea donation, 92–93, 95–96, 98,
109, 111
natural environment, 18–19
neoliberalism, 22, 234, 237, 286–87n2
nephrology/nephrologists, 10, 35, 51,
68, 70, 260n3, 261n7, 267n4, 140fig.
See also names of nephrologists;
on commodification of organs, 220,
227; on environmental risks, 181,
289n18; on medical malpractice/
mistreatment, 177, 288n12; on
social risks, 195–99, 290nn28,29
Netherlands, 23
newspapers, 1, 5, 12–13, 241, 260n25.
See also media; *names of newspapers*; on black market in human
organs, 24, 215–17, 226; on blood
transfusions, 287n7; on commodification of organs, 218–20; on cornea
transplants, 85, 92–93, 107, 110,
272n1; on defining death, 57–58,
63; on environmental risks, 13,
179, 181–82, 184, 289n19; fatwas
published in, 110, 267–68n10; on
kidney transplants, 21, 24, 162; on
living donors, 115; opposition-party
press, 12, 13, 24, 29, 54, 83, 85,
115, 181–82, 184, 226, 287n7; on
Sha'rawi, Shaykh, 117, 120–27, 129,
279n18; state-owned, 5–6, 12–13,
24, 29, 92, 115, 120, 122, 181–82,
217, 226, 279n18; on untrustworthy
physicians, 5–6, 29, 257–58n5; on
"water wars" *(fitnat al-miyah)*, 181
NGO projects, 288n14
Nguyen, Vinh-Kim, 286n1
Nigeria, 290n27
Nile Delta, 22–23, 26, 41, 182, 289n19,
292n5. *See also* Mansoura; Tanta

niqab, 153
niyya/niyyat. See intentions and
actions
Nobel Prize, 159, 242
al-Noor Society (charitable wing of
Maghraby), xxvifig., 82fig.
North America. *See* Canada; United
States
nouveaux riches, 91, 273n11

Oaxaca (Mexico), 266n42
ochratoxins, 182, 289n18
October 1973 War, 141–42, 283n1,
284n3
Oman, 57
ophthalmology/ophthalmologists,
11. *See also names of ophthalmologists*; and cornea transplants,
84–85, 87–92, 94–98, 112, 221, 272–
73nn1,3,5–7, 274nn13,16,19–21;
and crises of authority, 29, 33–34,
93, 263n25, 265n36; and defining
death, 51–53; as organ/eye donors,
94–95, 274n16; triage mindset of,
90–91, 273–74n12
Opwis, Felicitas, 133, 281–82nn36,41,
282–83nn48,49
organ/eye donors, 4, 6, 9, 115. *See
also* black market in human organs;
commodification of organs; checking box on driver's licenses, 17, 93,
159; Coptic Christians' views on,
259n22; and cornea transplants,
33–34, 86–89, 91–98, 103–9, 111–12,
274nn16,21, 277n42; cousins as,
223–24, 294n20; and crises of
authority, 23–24, 26–28, 30, 33–37;
criteria of "dead donors," 78–79;
and defining death, 15, 47, 51–53,
55–67, 69–75, 78–80, 258n14,
260n25, 267nn2,7, 268–69nn12,13,
270–71nn26,30, 276n36; "donation after cardiac death" (DCD),
78; donor-sellers, 212–15, 218–21,
292–93nn7,11–16; and ethics of
scale, 141, 143, 146–52, 154–66, 169,
171, 283–84n2, 286n22; executed

organ/eye donors (*continued*)
prisoners as, 58, 88, 291n33; family
as, 126, 137–38, 148–50, 154, 157,
160–65, 167, 169, 173–75, 185–203,
205–6, 211–12, 214, 221–25,
227–30, 234–35, 239, 283n54, 284–
85nn11,17, 290nn25,28, 291n30,
293–94nn19,20; and "fast cash," 30,
35, 147, 152, 155; and gender, 12;
and kidney transplants, 4, 23–24,
26–28, 30, 36, 48, 141, 143, 146–52,
154–66, 169, 171, 173–75, 185–92,
283–84n2, 285n17, 286n22, 291n31;
and liver transplants, 4, 15, 144,
260n25; living donors, 4, 9, 12,
15, 24, 47, 55–56, 70, 79, 115–16,
143–44, 146, 148–49, 171, 174, 185,
200, 209–15, 218–21, 224, 227, 235,
284n6, 286n22, 292–93nn6,7,11–16;
national campaign for cornea
donation, 92–93, 95–96, 98, 109,
111; "non-heartbeating donors"
(NHBDs), 78; parents as, 23, 126,
137–38, 149–50, 165, 167, 173,
189–98, 205–6, 211, 229, 236, 246,
290nn25,28, 291n30, 190*fig.*; and
perennial charity *(sadaqa jariyya)*,
103–4, 110–11, 277n41; Shaykh
Sha'rawi's views on, 118, 122–34,
137–38, 281n39, 283n54; and social
risks, 189–91, 290n25; sociological studies on, 157, 191, 285n17,
291n31; and spiritual risks, 187–89;
spouses as, 187, 190, 198–99, 211–
12, 227–31, 284–85n11, 293–94n19;
and "tyranny of the gift," 70, 191,
203–7, 271n34; "unrelated living
donors," 36, 146, 148, 202, 220,
223–26, 284–85n11; in U.S., 78,
274n16
organ/eye theft, 216–17, 220, 231,
234, 245–46, 293n16; Coptic Christians' views on, 259n22; and crises
of authority, 24, 29, 34, 39, 263n25;
eye theft, 4, 29, 83, 85–89, 91,
105, 109–10, 115, 263n25, 272n1,
277n41; kidney theft, 4, 24, 83, 216–
17, 208*fig.*; liver lobe theft, 222
organ failure. *See* kidney disease/
transplants; liver disease/transplants
organ trade. *See* black market in
human organs; commodification of
organs
orphanages, 4, 103
overcrowding, 2, 180, 234, 241

paid donors. *See* black market in
human organs; commodification of
organs
Pakistan, 258n10, 264nn28,31, 268n12,
282n43
Palestine, 76, 182, 292n2
parasites, 16, 23–24, 180–81, 261n7,
288n14
Parliament, 3, 257n3, 281n37. *See also*
laws/legislation; on blood transfusions, 177; on criminalizing recognition of brain death, 65, 270n28; on
defining death, 57, 59, 63–65, 68,
270n28; and environmental risks,
184, 289n19
partial vision, 30–31, 263n23
patients' autonomy/rights, 24, 34, 70,
95, 110–11, 137
pesticides, 9, 13, 16, 28, 179–82, 185,
289n16
Petryna, Adriana, 237
pharmaceutical companies, 155, 275–
76n28. *See also* drugs
physicians. *See* experts, medical; transplant surgeons; *names of physicians*
piety, 118, 125–26, 129, 152, 240,
278n7
pilgrimage. *See* hajj
politics, 2, 8–9, 11–15; and commodification of organs, 209, 237; Coptic
Christians' views on, 259n22; and
cornea transplants, 31, 34; and crises
of authority, 22, 28, 31, 34, 38, 43,
264n32; of defining death, 58–59,
69–70, 73, 272n42; and environmental risks, 180–84, 289n19; and

equal opportunity in education, 38; and ethics of scale, 159, 285n18; political dissent, 2, 181, 253–55, 289n19; political etiologies, 13, 179, 186, 245, 259n22; in Saudi Arabia, 70; and Sha'rawi, Shaykh, 116–18, 137, 278n7; and state of emergency, 210, 264n32; in U.S., 28

pollution/pollutants, 2, 59, 234, 241, 244. *See also* contamination; environmental risks; Coptic Christians' views on, 259n22; and kidney transplants/dialysis, 9–10, 16, 25, 28–29, 158, 175, 180, 185, 206; and liver transplants, 16, 29

poor/poverty, 7–8, 15, 239–41, 243, 245; and black market in human organs, 216–17, 232; and commodification of organs, 210–11, 213–14, 218–20, 231, 233–35, 237, 292n5, 293n16; and cornea transplants, 30, 32–34, 84–87, 90–91, 94–96, 98–100, 110–11, 263n25, 274nn17,21, 275n25; and crises of authority, 22–24, 26–27, 29–34, 37–39, 92, 261n7, 263nn19,25; as downtrodden *(il-ghalaba)*, 176, 287n5; and environmental risks, 179–86, 288n14; equal opportunity in education, 38, 264–65n33; and ethics of scale, 146–48, 154–56, 158, 168; exploitation of, 3–4, 10, 12, 75, 84, 131, 136, 210, 216–17, 220, 231, 239, 245, 247, 259n18; and kidney transplants/dialysis, 23–24, 26–27, 37, 146–48, 154–56, 158, 168, 176, 178–86, 206, 261n7, 263n19, 288nn11,12, 291n32; in *The Lamp of Umm Hashim* (1968 film), 99–100, 275n25; and medical malpractice/mistreatment, 5, 38–39, 175–79, 288nn11,12; rural poverty, 16, 23–24, 27, 30–31, 37, 44, 85–86, 94, 154–55, 179–81, 218, 234–35, 239–40, 288n14; Shaykh Sha'rawi's views on, 120–22, 281n35; in *Wahid*

min al-nas (television news program), 259n18; and "water wars" *(fitnat al-miyah)*, 181

postcolonialism, 27, 36, 73, 77, 97, 267n8

power relations, 9, 37, 90–91, 117, 202, 250, 277n40, 291n32

power supply, 26, 176, 250

pragmatism, 223, 226, 233

prayer, 104, 106, 117, 161–62, 191, 203–5, 242, 276n35, 286n20, 248fig.

pregnancy, 27, 69, 119, 187, 196–98, 227–28, 240, 247, 291n37

press. *See* media

preventative health care, 59, 137, 178

Principles of Biomedical Ethics (Beachamp and Childress), 258n10

prisoners, executed, 58, 88

private medical clinics/hospitals, 7, 239. *See also names of private medical clinics/hospitals*; and black market in human organs, 4, 12, 215, 217, 226, 232, 294–95n28; in Cairo, 10, 24, 32, 90, 294–95n28; and commodification of organs, 218–20, 222, 232, 293–94n19; and cornea transplants, 32, 34, 87, 90, 94–96, 111, 263n25, 273n5; and crises of authority, 22, 24, 28–29, 32, 37–39, 261–62n9, 264–65nn33,37; and ethics of scale, 141, 148, 154, 156–57; and government compensation, 186; and kidney transplants/dialysis, 141, 148, 154, 156–57, 178, 181, 186, 199; and medical education, 38–39, 264–65nn33,37; nepotism in, 38, 265n37; risks/benefits of treatment in, 178, 181, 186, 199

privatization: of health care, 1, 5, 24, 29, 43, 84; of major industries in Egypt, 13, 289n16; of medical education, 38, 264–65n33

progressives, 70, 116, 120, 136, 245, 281n35

the Prophet. *See* Muhammad, the Prophet

prosecutors, 83, 85–87, 90, 287–88n10

public eye banks/hospitals, 2, 33, 83–87, 90, 92–97, 102, 105, 107, 109–11, 263n25, 273nn5,9, 277n41. *See also* cornea opacity/transplants; *names of eye banks/hospitals*; in Cairo, 32–33, 83, 85–87, 95, 263n25, 272–73nn1–3; closing of, 83–84, 86–87, 90, 92, 96, 109, 272–73nn1–3, 275–76n28; donations for, 86, 90, 93, 273n5; earliest in Egypt, 107; in England, 97–98; international nonprofit eye banks, 96, 274n18; National Eye Bank, 92–93; outreach programs of, 11, 44, 92–93, 31*fig.*; and scandals, 83, 109–10, 221, 257n3; in Tanta, 11, 30, 87, 93, 272–73n3

public health, 5, 13, 59, 92, 182; national campaign for cornea donation, 92–93, 95–96, 98, 109, 111

public hospitals, 239. *See also* public eye banks/hospitals; *names of public hospitals*; and commodification of organs, 211–13, 219–20, 225, 228, 236, 293–94n19; and crises of authority, 27, 29, 32–33, 37–39, 263n25, 264n32; defining death in, 49–50, 64–65; and ethics of scale, 148, 154–55, 286n21; risks/benefits of treatment in, 178–79, 186, 189, 199–204, 287n3; teaching hospitals, 7, 10, 29, 38–39, 64–65, 83, 86, 156, 173, 178, 189, 199–204, 211–13, 219–20, 228, 272n1, 293–94n19

qadi (judge), 281n37

Qasr al-ʿAyni. *See* Kasr el Aini

Qurʾan, 41, 271–72n38, 273n4, 276nn34,35; "The Fig" chapter, 143, 284n5; God's creation of humans from "water," 191, 290n24; and recitation for the ill, 230; and kidney transplants, 143–44, 152, 158, 163–64, 169, 284n5; prohibition of wine/intoxicants, 134, 282n47; Shaykh Shaʿrawi's views on, 116–19, 122;

television programs on, 3, 26, 116; "*Ya Sin*" chapter, 158

racial minorities, 261–62n9, 272n40, 277n42

Ramadan, 117, 136, 203

Rapp, Rayna, 247

rationalist objectivism, 134, 138, 282–83n48

al-Rawahi (Cairo), 259n18

refugee populations, 293n16

religious scholars, 1, 3, 246–47, 250. *See also* muftis; *names of religious scholars*; Azhari Islamic scholars, 133; and bioethics, 11–14, 18–19; on commodification of organs, 213–14, 231, 233; on cornea transplants, 34, 84–85, 92–93, 101–4, 107–9, 111, 275–76n28; and crises of authority, 6, 22, 28, 34–35, 39–44, 265–66n38, 41*fig.*; on defining death, 47–48, 54–59, 61–67, 69, 71–72, 76–77, 79–80, 267nn1,9, 269n17, 271n35; elitism of, 40, 54, 57–58, 64; and ethics of scale, 147, 150–51, 161–64, 168, 170; on kidney transplants/dialysis, 147, 150–51, 161–64, 168, 170, 188, 191–92, 290nn23,26; in *The Lamp of Umm Hashim* (Haqqi), 101; questionnaire sent to, 57–58; and Shaʿrawi, Shaykh, 119, 126–27, 133–37; *shaykh fattah*, 40; on social risks, 191–92, 290n26; on spiritual risks, 188, 290n23; untrustworthiness of, 5–6, 64

reproduction, 192–93, 196–98, 203–5, 228, 290n27, 193*fig.*

risks/benefits, 4, 173–207, 245–46, 249; and commodification of organs, 191, 194, 202, 206, 233–34, 237; of cornea transplants, 31, 87, 91–92, 96, 107–10, 112, 277n40; and crises of authority, 28, 31, 35, 39; and defining death, 55, 80; environmental risks, 174–75, 179–86, 206, 288n14, 289n16, 183*fig.*; and ethics of scale, 144, 146–49, 151,

156–57, 170–71; iatrogenic risks, 174, 288n14; individual risk reduction, 259n20; of kidney transplants, 14–15, 28, 144, 146–49, 151, 156–57, 170–71, 173–79, 288nn11,12; and *maslaha*, 42, 87, 107–10, 131, 266n41, 277n40; from medical malpractice/mistreatment, 175–79, 185, 287–88nn7–10; and rebirth/reproduction, 192–93, 196–98, 203–5, 290n27, 193*fig.*; and Sha'rawi, Shaykh, 116, 131–37, 282n47; social risks, 173–74, 180, 189–99, 202–6, 286–87n2, 290n29, 190*fig.*, 193*fig.*; spiritual risks, 174, 186–89, 290n23; and "three brothers" tale, 199–203, 291n34

Royal Nile Hilton (Cairo), 101–3, 275–76n28

rural to urban migration, 21, 99

Saad, Reem, 279n12

Sabah al Khayr ya Misr (Good Morning, Egypt; television program), 143

Sabiq, Sayyid, 286n24

sadaqa jariyya, 103–4, 110–11, 277n41

Sadat, Anwar, 4–5, 23, 54–55; assassination of, 264n32; and Camp David Accords, 182; *infitah* ("opening"), 5, 116, 257n4, 273n11; and Sha'rawi, Shaykh, 116, 118, 278n7

sadd al-dhara'i' (blocking the means), 132, 276n30, 281–82n41

Sahih al-Muslim, 103, 276n32

saints (*awliya'* Allah), 98, 100, 104

salat al-istikhara (seeking the good). *See* prayer

Salvatore, Armando, 285n18

Saudi Arabia, 57, 69–70, 79, 90, 199, 249, 268n12, 270n22, 271n32, 273n7, 277n2; and transnational organ sales, 220, 223, 294–95n28

al-Sayyid, Hamdi, 64, 215, 292n8. *See also* Egyptian Medical Syndicate

scale, ethics of, 15–17, 141–71; and 'Ali (kidney-failure patient), 159–69, 171, 285n18, 286nn19,21; and Badr, 154–58, 171, 285n17; and changes of heart, 162–69; and commodification of organs, 146–48, 154–58, 284–85n11,17; costs of transplants, 145, 148–54, 168, 170, 284n9, 285nn12,13; in decision-making process, 147–49, 152–53, 284–85nn9–11; and defining death, 79–80; and Hani (kidney-failure patient/organ buyer), 154–55, 157–58, 285n16; and Kotb, 141–47, 152, 170, 284nn6,8; seeking the good, 158–62; and Shadya (kidney-failure patient), 149–54, 158, 171, 285n14; and social relations/resources, 147–52, 166–71; and Tamir (kidney-failure patient), 150, 153–54, 171

scandals, 10, 21, 30, 39; and cornea transplants, 83–84, 90, 109–10, 115, 221, 257n3

Scheper-Hughes, Nancy, 202, 235, 237, 291n32, 292n2

schistosomiasis, 16–17, 23, 180–81, 261n7, 288n14, 295n29

science/technology, 17–19, 244–45, 247, 250–51. *See also* life-support systems; and Arabic language, 264–65n33; biomedicine as "universal science," 36–37; and commodification of organs, 228–29; and cornea transplants, 93, 97–100, 108, 111, 274n22; and crises of authority, 27–28, 36–37, 39, 44–45, 264–65n33; and defining death, 48, 50, 66–70, 73; and environmental risks, 183, 289n17; and ethics of scale, 147, 159–60, 170, 284n8; and kidney transplants/dialysis, 27–28, 142, 159–60, 170, 180, 183, 284n8; in *The Lamp of Umm Hashim* (1968 film), 99–100; "science has no homeland," 97; and Sha'rawi, Shaykh, 119; and "truth" of human bodies, 6; ultrasound technology, 119

secularism, 4, 40, 44, 54, 116, 251, 295–96n3; and commodification of organs, 209, 233; and cornea transplants, 104; and defining death, 54, 61, 66–67, 72, 75, 267n8; and Sha'rawi, Shaykh, 116, 119, 278n7
September 11, 2001, 76
sewage systems, 13, 29, 181
sex-change surgery, 75, 267n1
sexual violence, 295–96n3
Sha'rawi, Muhammad Mutwalli, Shaykh, 3, 27, 59, 115–38, 239, 245–47, 251, 277nn1,2, 278nn4–6,8,11, 279nn13–15, 280nn23,29,33, 114fig.; birthday of, 280n23; on blood transfusions, 121, 123, 133, 279n15; cataract operation of, 120; critics of, 117–22, 127–28, 136–38, 167, 279nn13,15, 280n33, 283n54; as da'iya, 126, 129, 131, 138; death of, 117, 136, 280n33, 283n52; defenders of, 127–29, 137; exile of, 116–17; fatwas of, 117, 119–22, 126–31, 136, 278nn6,11, 279n14, 280n29, 114fig.; on God's owner- ship of bodies, 3, 27, 115–16, 120, 122–26, 130–32, 135, 138, 159, 163, 279n19, 280n31, 290n26; Kotb's views on, 145–46; madhhab of, 126, 280n26; and maslaha, 131–33, 135–36, 283nn49,51; as minister of awqaf (religious endowments), 116; on permissibility of organ dona- tion, 120–21, 123, 128–30, 132–35, 145, 167, 170–71, 281nn37,40, 290n26; respect for, 117–19, 136, 138, 278n6; Shaykh Guma'a's views on, 126–27, 280nn26,27; Shaykh Tantawi's response to, 129–32, 137, 281n37; television programs of, 3, 27, 115–18, 120–22, 129, 136, 278n4; on terminal illness, 120, 137, 279n14; theistic subjectivism of, 282–83n48; views on death, 119, 122–24, 128–29, 145, 280n34, 281nn35,39; weighing risks/ben- efits, 116, 131–36

Shafi'i, Muhammad, 268n12, 282n43
sham al-nasim, 242, 295n2
shari'a, 54, 69, 72, 75, 104, 108, 130, 227, 267n8, 270n26, 282n46
al-Sharif, Nur, 216
Sharp, Lesley, 66–67, 78, 232, 234–35, 269n18, 270–71
Shbin al-Qum (Minufiyya, Egypt), 15, 68, 271n31
Shenouda (Pope), 92, 160
Sholkamy, Hania, 286n23
Singapore, Islamic Religious Council of, 268n12
Skovgaard-Petersen, Jakob, 54, 117, 133, 267nn8,9, 278n6, 281n37
slavery, 73–74, 233, 268–69n13
Smith, Daniel J., 290n27
Sobh, Mohamed, 261n7
socialism, 5, 116, 156, 273n11
social justice, 8, 22, 243, 250–51
social relations/resources, 2–3, 245–47, 249. See also class disparities; inequalities, social; and bioethics, 9–10, 17–19; and commodification of organs, 211–12, 214, 218–19, 224–25, 229–31, 235; and defining death, 75–76; and ethics of scale, 147–52, 166–71; and risks/benefits of treatment, 173–74, 180, 189–99, 202–6, 286–87n2, 290n29, 190fig., 193fig.; and Sha'rawi, Shaykh, 133, 137
Somali refugee community, 293n16
Sorour, Hani, 177, 287n7
the soul, 52, 56, 60–61, 65–67, 84, 275n27
Soviet Union, 116
Spain, 96
spiritual risks, 174, 186–89, 290n23
state welfare, 2, 4, 21–22, 32–33, 76
stem cell research, 27–28
sterilization, 16–17
Sudan, 268–69n13; Sudanese refugee community, 293n16, 294–95n28
Suez Canal, 283n1
Sufi discipline/practice, 40, 42, 121, 124, 266n40, 277n1, 280n23

suicide/"suicide operations," 122, 130,
144, 279n19
al-Sukari, ʿAbd al-Salam, 132
sunna, 276n34
Swazey, Judith, 144–45, 191
Syria, 277n1

Tahrir Square (Cairo), 253–55
Tanta, 10–11, 41; cornea transplants
in, 11, 30, 87–88; defining death
in, 49–51; environmental risks in,
179–81; kidney transplants/dialy-
sis in, 10–11, 25–28, 42, 149–52,
154, 158–68, 179–81, 186–87, 199,
292n7, 20*fig.*, 172*fig.*; no functioning transplant program in, 10–11,
258n14
Tanta University: Department of
Medicine, 199; Faculty of Medicine,
258n14
Tanta University Hospital, 30, 87,
93, 105, 180–81, 190, 200, 203–4,
272–73n3
Tantawi, Muhammad Sayyid, Shaykh,
245; on cornea transplants, 92–93,
101–4, 107, 109–11, 275–76n28;
on defining death, 48, 56–57,
72–73, 75–76, 267n1; on kidney
transplants, 160, 284n5; as organ/
eye donor, 92–94, 102; response to
Shaykh Shaʿrawi, 129–32, 134, 137,
281n37; Royal Nile Hilton speech
of, 101–3, 275–76n28
television programs, 5, 12–13, 17,
259n18. *See also* media; *names
of television programs*; on black
market in human organs, 217, 232;
on class disparities, 91, 95, 273n10;
on cornea transplants, 92–93, 95,
100, 105, 275–76nn24,25,28; on
environmental risks, 13, 29, 175,
179, 259n18, 263n22; of Habib,
Tariq, 120–22, 279n12; on kidney
transplants, 4, 21, 142–43, 146–47,
160, 162–64, 168, 188; *The Lamp of
Umm Hashim* (1968 film), 100; on
medical malpractice/mistreatment,

29; Qurʾanic programs, 3, 26, 116;
satellite television, 12–13, 259n18;
of Shaʿrawi, Shaykh, 3, 27, 115–18,
120–22, 129, 136, 278n4; soccer
matches, 203, 230, 287–88n10; state-
owned television, 1, 5–6, 12, 92–93,
95, 116, 162, 275–76n28; and Tantawi, Shaykh, 92, 101–3, 275–76n28;
on untrustworthy physicians, 5–6,
217; in U.S., 17, 146–47
tertiary care centers, 23, 243, 261n7
theft of organs/eyes. *See* organ/eye
theft
theistic subjectivism, 282–83n48
Tissue Banks International (Baltimore,
Md.), 273n5
tissue typing, 151–52, 154–55, 161–63,
165–66, 168–69, 191, 205, 219, 224–
25, 228–30, 286n21, 294n21
tourists, 182, 216
toxicity, 9–10, 237, 244; aflatoxins,
182, 289n17; as environmental risk,
9–10, 13, 16, 25, 28–29, 175, 179,
181–82, 185, 206, 234, 289nn17–20;
and kidney transplants/dialysis, 25,
144, 177, 206, 229, 262n14; ochratoxins, 182, 289n18
trachoma, 16, 93, 100, 260n27, 273n6,
275n25
trafficking of human organs, 210,
215, 217, 220, 231–32, 234, 247,
293nn15,17, 294n24. *See also* black
market in human organs
transnational organ sales, 210, 215–18,
220–21, 232–35, 292n2
transplant surgeons, 1, 3, 10–11,
14–15, 21, 44, 239–40, 260n25. *See
also names of transplant surgeons*;
and commodification of organs,
210–11, 215, 220–23, 226–29,
231–37, 293n16; and defining death,
51, 68; and kidney transplants, 112,
141–46, 152, 162–65, 168, 170; and
Shaʿrawi, Shaykh, 129, 135, 138
trust *(amana)*, 162, 187, 202
Turkey, 95
Turner, Bryan, 124

ʿulamaʾ, 54, 267n9. *See also* religious scholars
Umm Hashim shrine, 99–101
uncertainty, 180, 206, 288n13
unemployment, 2, 265n37
UNESCO, 13
United Nations, 232
United States, 244, 247; African Americans in, 277n42; bioethics in, 6–9, 258n10, 260n24; bumper stickers in, 275n27; and Camp David Accords, 182; and commodification of organs, 210–11, 216, 221, 223–24, 233–34, 292n6; cornea transplants in, 87, 93, 274n16, 275n27, 277n42; defining death in, 49, 51–53, 55, 58, 61, 65–67, 75–80, 267n6, 270–71n30, 272n40, 272n41, 274n16, 276n36; driver's license checkoffs, 17, 93, 159; and environmental risks, 182–83, 289–90nn17,20; Food and Drug Administration (FDA), 289n17; and foreign aid, 182–84, 264n32, 289–90n20; Iranian hostage crisis (1979–80), 76; kidney transplants in, 23, 28, 149, 155, 162, 164, 166, 175, 211, 261–62nn5,9, 269n18, 284n10, 286n22, 291n33; liver transplants in, 292n6; media in, 17, 78, 244–45, 275n27, 295–96n3; medical journals in, 37, 58, 65; militarization in Middle East, 76, 182, 250; Muslim students from, 265–66n38; President's Council on Bioethics, 79, 272n41; rhetoric of "gift of life," 15, 17, 28, 67, 78, 80, 144–45, 210, 224, 260n24, 270–71n30; and Sadat, 116; and Shaʿrawi, Shaykh, 118, 281n35; "shortage of organs" discourse in, 155; stem cell research in, 28; and terrorism, 76, 159; USAID, 182–83; views on uncertainty in medicine, 288n13
universal health coverage, 29, 177
universalisms, 7–8, 19, 22, 108, 135, 234, 260n26; biomedicine as

"universal science," 36; and defining death, 63, 66, 272n42
urology/urologists, 10, 22–23, 37, 51, 190, 235, 260n3, 267n4. *See also names of urologists*

ventilators, 49–50, 61–62, 67, 78. *See also* life-support systems
Viorst, Milton, 244–45
visual disability, 30–31, 263n23

Wahid min al-nas (television news program), 259n18, 263n22
waraʿ (road of caution), 127, 280n30
"washing" *(ghasil)*, 25–26, 178, 194, 262nn13,14
Wasil, Nasir Farid, Shaykh, 277n40
water: contamination of, 10, 13, 16, 29, 59, 175, 179–81, 259n18, 287n7; and perpetual charity *(sadaqa jariyya)*, 103
water buffalo, 85
We are all Khalid Saʿid (Facebook group), 253
Weber, Max, 264n28
welfare state, 273n11
West, 4–5, 22, 37, 44, 220, 244–45, 285n18. *See also* Europe; United States; and Cartesian dualism, 66; and "clash of civilizations," 61, 76–80, 84, 272n40; defining death in, 48, 55, 61, 66–68, 70; and Shaʿrawi, Shaykh, 124
West Africa, 286n1
wheelchairs, 238*fig.*
Wickham, Carrie, 64, 118, 278nn7,10
Winegar, Jessica, 278n10
World Health Organization, 3, 215, 231, 275–76n28, 292n9

Yacoub, Magdi, 243

Zamalek (Cairo), 23, 230, 261n6
Zaynab, the Sayyida, 99–101
Zewail, Ahmed, 159
Zithromax, 275–76n28

Designer: Lia Tjandra
Text: 10/13 Aldus
Display: Aldus
Compositor: BookComp, Inc.
Printer and Binder: IBT-Global

CPSIA information can be obtained
at www.ICGtesting.com
Printed in the USA
JSHW021506241219
3188JS00002B/23